Allergic Diseases and the Environment

Nestlé Nutrition Workshop Series
Pediatric Program, Vol. 53

Allergic Diseases and the Environment

Editors

Erika Isolauri, Turku, Finland

W. Allan Walker, Boston, Mass., USA

19 figures and 31 tables, 2004

KARGER

Nestlé NUTRITION

Nestec Ltd., 55 Avenue Nestlé, CH–1800 Vevey (Switzerland)
S. Karger AG, P.O. Box, CH–4009 Basel (Switzerland) www.karger.com

Printed in Switzerland on acid-free paper by Reinhardt Druck, Basel
ISBN 3–8055–7649–8
ISSN 0742–2806

Library of Congress Cataloging-in-Publication Data
(CIP-Code is available from the Library of Congress on request.)

Contents

Preface

A major pediatric health problem in developed countries is the increasing incidence of allergic diseases during infancy and childhood. Over the last two decades the incidence of atopic dermatitis and asthma has increased several fold and represents a major cause of medical expense, hospitalization, and loss of school/work days for children and their parents. Paradoxically, the incidence of allergic disease has not risen in developing countries over the same time period. This observation has led to careful scrutiny of the environmental differences that exist between the two settings and may account for this discrepancy. As a result of this scrutiny, a hypothesis, the 'hygiene hypothesis', has evolved which suggests that infants born in the 'sterile' environment of modern hospitals in the developed world may not be subjected to the same microbial burden on entering the extrauterine environment as their counterparts in a contaminated setting in the developing world. Therefore, these infants in a 'sterile' environment with a lack of microbial stimulus may not adjust to a balanced mucosal immune response which includes expansion of T-helper (Th) cell subsets that can mediate immune responses (e.g., cellular immune, humoral immune, and oral tolerance). Accordingly, this Workshop was convened to consider in depth the environmental factors that influence the changing pattern of worldwide childhood allergy. Experts in basic research, epidemiology, and clinical investigation from around the world have been asked to provide their perspectives on this dilemma.

The conference began with a clinical overview of the changing patterns in the clinical aspects of pediatric allergic disease. What emerged was the notion of 'the allergic march'. This suggests that once the infant is sensitized there is a progression of sensitization. This concept also suggests that 'allergy-prone' infants will develop clinical symptoms largely based on the nature and route of allergen exposure throughout infancy and childhood. For example, food allergy from the ingestion of foreign proteins in breast milk or formula initially results in gastrointestinal and/or skin manifestations of allergy. As the infant gets older, inhalant allergens become important and result in pulmonary symptoms, with the end result being chronic asthma. The concept further suggests that once sensitized the infant/child may have a progression of allergy leading to a chronic condition. This suggestion, however, has not been proven by clinical studies. A new definition of hypersensitivity was considered and the notion that symptoms ascribed to allergy are not always immunologically mediated and must be carefully evaluated before labeling of an 'atopic' child is made. Clarification between the term 'atopy' and allergy (hypersensitivity) was made. A strong suggestion for a better understanding of the mechanisms in order to distinguish between the terms is needed. Finally a careful appraisal of clinical manifestations of food allergy was considered in the context of an accurate diagnosis and possible strategy for prevention.

In a session on environmental factors contributing to the increased incidence of allergy in infants and children in developed countries, a refinement of the 'hygiene hypothesis' was presented. Careful clinical studies in IgE-mediated allergic infants and children, beginning at birth and prospectively followed, suggest that allergic children take longer to balance their 'T'-helper cell subset response and therefore appear to be more prone to a Th2 (e.g., IgE-mediated) immune response to antigens (allergens). An appropriate initial colonization of the gut may help to prevent this developmental process. Strong evidence that allergy in infants and children was due to an imbalance in Th2 responsiveness was provided, making 'allergy' a Th2-predominant disease. However, by way of considering other mechanisms, clinical studies in African children infested with parasites, an IgE/Th2-mediated response, also appear to be protective against clinical allergic symptoms. These studies suggested that anti-inflammatory cytokines induced by parasite infestation may prevent allergic symptoms.

An important component of the immune response to luminal antigens is the 'muted' systemic response to innocuous antigens such as food proteins and commensal flora, a process called oral tolerance. The current understanding of how this response occurs was discussed and the importance of commensal intestinal flora and innate immune responses underscored. The importance of breast-feeding in modulating an appropriate initial colonization of the neonatal gut was stressed with regard to oral tolerance and gut maturation. In the absence of an appropriate initial colonization, the infant may lack tolerance and inappropriately respond to innocuous antigens in the gut. To further emphasize the importance of the initial colonization process, the role of colonizing bacteria in the maturation of intestinal defenses and their effect in age-related neonatal intestinal infections were considered. 'Cross-talk' between colonizing bacteria in the developing epithelium response to bacterial components was discussed. In addition, new techniques for more precisely defining the myriad of colonizing gut bacteria and the need to examine microbial intestinal contents with feeding was reviewed. Of interest was the observation that partial hydrolysates fed to infants at risk of developing allergy produced a gut flora that was more similar to breast-fed infants' flora than infants fed standard infant formulas.

Finally, we considered whether breast-feeding or protective nutrients fed to infants at risk of developing allergy could prevent or modulate the severity of allergic symptoms. Careful meta-analyses showed that exclusive breast-feeding did not appear to prevent allergy but was protective during nursing. There was also some suggestion of a delay in expression of allergic symptoms in infants on breast milk. Standard protective nutrients such as glutamine, arginine, nucleotides, etc., did not appear to protect infants at risk of allergy. However, a warning was given that using too restrictive a diet in treating infants at risk of developing allergy could lead to severe malnutrition and other complications. Evidence suggested that probiotics, but not prebiotics, may be effective in preventing allergy. This was followed by strong evidence, provided by a carefully considered clinical trial in infants at risk of developing allergy, that probiotics given to the mother in late pregnancy and continued while nursing infants in conjunction with the infants receiving the same probiotic could effectively prevent allergic dermatitis. Other attempts to prevent chronic asthma by early intervention suggested that more prospective multicenter trials are needed. An excellent prospective multicenter trial in Germany, the GINI study, suggests that partial hydrolysates can delay and possibly prevent long-term manifestations of allergy. However, this study needs to be carried out over a longer time period before definitive conclusions can be made.

In general, the comprehensive approach to the environment and clinical allergy was very helpful in answering questions and clarifying concepts for the attendees. However, probing observations from the attendees with extensive clinical experience suggest that additional long-term, multicenter trials are necessary before an approach to reversing this increasing trend in pediatric allergic disease can be made.

Erika Isolauri and W. Allan Walker

Foreword

For this 53rd Nestlé Pediatric Nutrition Workshop, the topic 'Allergic Diseases and the Environment' was chosen as a follow-up to two previous workshops with similar topics, held in 1987 in Munich, Germany ('Food Allergy') and in 1993 in Versailles, France ('Intestinal Immunology and Food Allergy'). However, since then, the evolution and incidence of allergic diseases have changed and there have been many successful advances in the prevention and therapy of allergic diseases. Therefore, it seemed necessary to point out the state-of-the-art of environmental influences upon allergic diseases. With this Workshop, we wanted to determine whether the hygiene hypothesis really would explain some mechanisms in the development of allergic diseases. In addition, how promising are the attempts to enhance oral tolerance and how effective are antioxidants, polyunsaturated fatty acids, pre- and probiotics in the prevention and treatment of allergic diseases? In order to answer these and other questions we sought the knowledge of various experts in different fields to clarify the pathogenesis of and the preventive as well as therapeutic implications for the various manifestations of the atopic syndrome.

I would like to thank the two chairmen, Prof. *Erika Isolauri* and Prof. *Allan Walker*, who are well-known experts in this field, for putting the program together and inviting as speakers the opinion leaders in the field of allergic diseases. Pediatricians invited from 21 countries contributed to the discussions that are published in this book.

We wish to thank Dr. *Philippe Steenhout* from the Nutrition Strategic Business Division (NSBD), Lausanne, Switzerland, who was responsible for the scientific coordination of the Workshop. Our special thanks to the administrative team of the NSBD and the Nestlé Research Center (NRC) for the successful relocation and organization of the Workshop, which should originally have been held in Kuala Lumpar, Malaysia. The last-minute relocation to the NRC in Vers-Chez-les-Blancs, Lausanne, was deemed necessary due to the fear of potential terrorist attacks arising from the war in Iraq.

Prof. Wolf Endres, MD

Vice-President
Nestec Ltd., Vevey, Switzerland

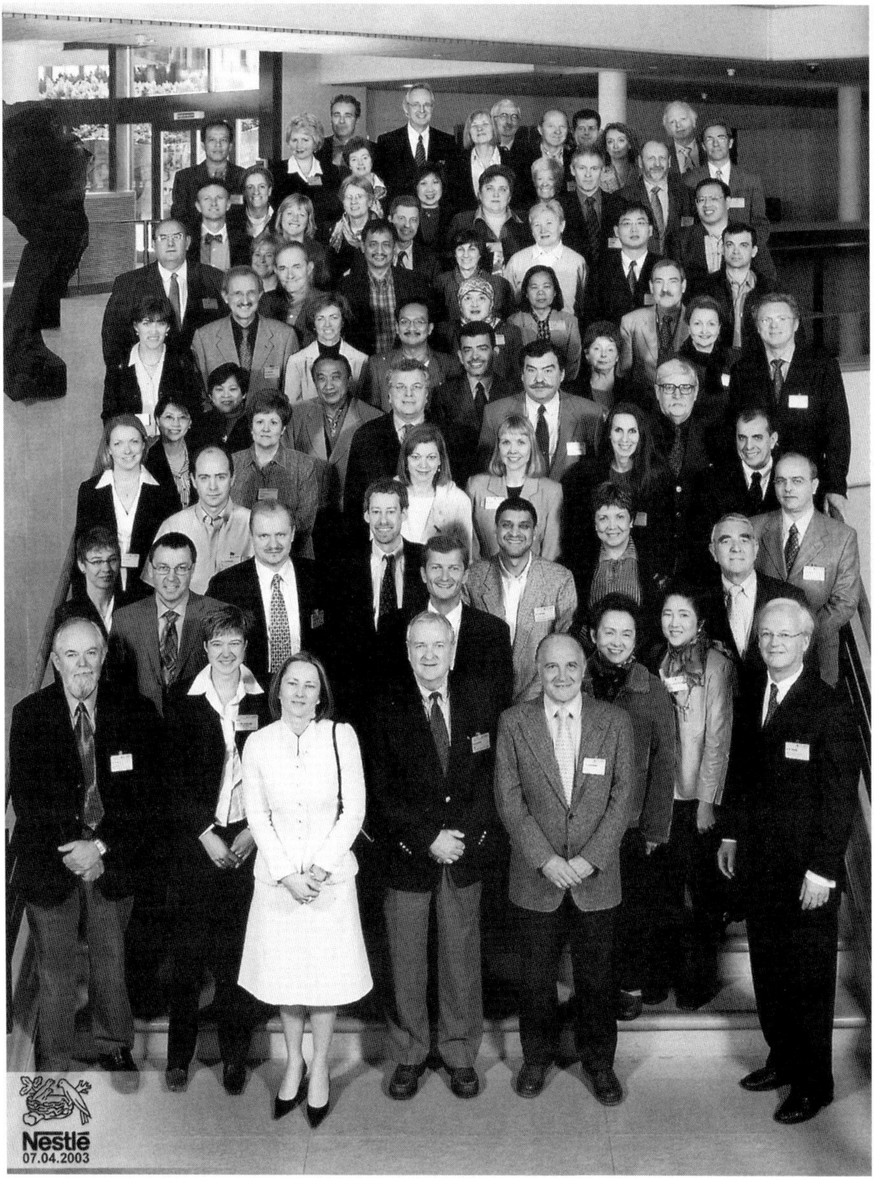

53rd Nestlé Nutrition Workshop
Pediatric Program
Lausanne, April 6–10, 2003

Contributors

Chairpersons, Speakers

Prof. Peter Van Bladeren
Nestlé Research Center
Management
PO Box 44
CH–1000 Lausanne 26
Tel. +41 21 785 88 01
Fax +41 21 785 85 55
E-Mail peter.van-bladeren@rdls.nestle.com

Prof. Renate L. Bergmann
Klinik für Geburtsmedizin
Charité Virchow Hospitals
Humboldt University
Augustenburger Platz 1
DE–13353 Berlin
Germany
Tel. +49 30 450 564 101
Fax +49 30 450 564 908
E-Mail renate.bergmann@charite.de

Prof. Carsten Bindslev-Jensen
Odense University Hospital
Allergy Center
DK–5000 Odense C
Denmark
Tel. +45 6 541 36 24
Fax +45 6 312 15 07
E-Mail carsten.bindslev-jensen@allergi.sdu.dk

Dr. Christopher Duggan
Children's Hospital
Division of GI/Nutrition
300 Longwood Avenue
Boston, MA 02115
USA
Tel. +1 617 355 7612
Fax +1 617 730 0496
E-Mail christopher.duggan@tch.harvard.edu

Dr. David Hill
Department of Allergy
Royal Children's Hospital
Flemington Road
Parkville, Victoria 3052
Australia
Tel. +61 3 9345 5701
Fax +61 9345 4848
E-Mail allergy.clinic@rch.org.au

Prof. Patrick Holt
Division of Cell Biology
Telethon Institute for Child Health Research
PO Box 855
West Perth WA 6872
Australia
Tel. +61 8 9489 7838
Fax +61 8 9489 7707
E-Mail patrick@ichr.uwa.edu.au

Prof. Erika Isolauri
Turku University Central Hospital
University of Turku
Department of Paediatrics
FI–20520 Turku
Finland
Tel. +358 2 313 1460
Fax +358 2 313 2433
E-Mail erika.isolauri@utu.fi

Dr. Simon Murch
Royal Free and University College Medical School
Centre for Paediatric Gastroenterology
Royal Free Campus
Rowland Hill Street
London NW3 2PF
UK
Tel. +44 207 830 2780/830 2779
Fax +44 207 830 2146
E-Mail s.murch@rfc.ucl.ac.uk

Prof. Sergio Romagnani
Università degli Studi di Firenze
Dipartimento di Medicina Interna
Viale Morgagni, 85
IT–50134 Florence
Italy
Tel. +39 55 413663/4296402
Fax +39 55 412867
E-Mail s.romagnani@dmi.unifi.it

Prof. Seppo Salminen
University of Turku
Degree Programme on Healthbiosciences
(Functional Foods Forum)
FI–20014 Turku
Finland
Tel. +358 400 601394
Fax +358 2 3336884
E-Mail seppo.salminen@utu.fi

Dr. Anita van den Biggelaar
Leiden University Medical Center
Department of Parasitology-4
Albinusdreef 2
PO Box 9600
NL–2300 RC Leiden
The Netherlands
Tel. +31 71 526 5062/513 5814
Fax +31 71 526 6907
E-Mail biggelaar@lumc.nl

Prof. Yvan Vandenplas
Free University of Brussels
Academic Hospital
Department of Pediatrics
Laarbeeklaan 101
BE–1090 Brussels
Belgium
Tel. +32 2 477 5780
Fax +32 2 477 5783
E-Mail yvan.vandenplas@az.vub.ac.be

Dr. Andrea von Berg
Marien-Hospital GmbH
Forschungsinstitut zur Prävention von Allergien und Atemwegserkrankungen
Kindes- und Jugendalter der Klinik für Kinder- und Jugendmedizin
Pastor-Janssen-Strasse 8–38
DE–46483 Wesel
Germany
Tel. +49 281 104 1664/1659
Fax +49 281 3191659
E-Mail vonBerg@marien-hospital-wesel.de

Prof. W. Allan Walker
Harvard Medical School
Massachusetts General Hospital – East
Developmental Gastroenterology Laboratory
Charlestown, MA 02129
USA
Tel. +1 617 726 7988
Fax +1 617 726 4172
E-Mail allan_walker@hms.harvard.edu

Moderators

Dr. Rodolphe Fritsche

Nestlé Research Center
Food Immunology
P.O. Box 44
1000 Lausanne 26
Switzerland
Phone: ++41 21 785 86 83
Fax: ++41 21 785 85 44
E-mail:
rodolphe.fritsche@rdls.nestle.com

Dr. Pierre Guesry

Nestlé Research Center
Scientific and General Services
P.O. Box 44
1000 Lausanne 26
Switzerland
Phone: ++41 21 785 80 90
Fax: ++41 21 785 83 08
E-mail:
pierre.guesry@rdls.nestle.com

Dr. José Saavedra

Nestlé Glendale
800 N. Brand Blvd.
91203 Glendale
USA
Phone: +1 (818) 549-6774
Fax: +1 (818) 549-5704
E-mail: jose.saavedra@us.nestle.com

Dr. Eduardo Schiffrin

Nestlé Research Center
NSBD Medical Services
P.O. Box 44
1000 Lausanne 26
Switzerland
Phone: ++41 21 785 86 71
Fax: ++41 21 785 85 65
E-mail:
eduardo.schiffrin@rdls.nestle.com

Dr. Philippe Steenhout

Nestlé Research Center
NSBD Medical Services
P.O. Box 44
1000 Lausanne 26
Switzerland
Phone: ++41 21 785 95 47
Fax: ++41 21 785 85 65
E-mail:
philippe.steenhout@rdls.neste.com

Dr. Thierry von der Weid

Nestlé Research Center
Food Immunology
P.O. Box 44
1000 Lausanne 26
Switzerland
Phone: ++41 21 924 30 07
E-mail:
Thierry.VonDerWeid@nestle.com

Invited attendees

Prof. Magda Carneiro-Sampaio / Brazil
Prof. Emanuel Sarinho / Brazil
Prof. Dirceu Sole / Brazil
Dr. John Dean / Canada
Dr. Antony Ham Pong / Canada
Dr. Peter Nieman / Canada
Mrs. Lesley Scharf / Canada
Prof. Carl-Peter Bauer / Germany
Dr. Chen Chun-Yi / Great China Region (Taiwan)
Dr. Ni Yen-Hsuan / Great China Region (Taiwan)
Dr. Shyur Shyh-Dar / Great China Region (Taiwan)
Prof. Evangelia Mantzourani / Greece
Prof. Santa Nousia Arvanitaki / Greece
Dr. Photini Saxoni-Papageorgiou / Greece
Dr. Konstantinos Siafakas / Greece
Dr. Eva Micskey / Hungary
Dr. Anky Tri Rini Kusumaning Edhy / Indonesia
Dr. Anang Endaryanto / Indonesia
Dr. Yusmala Helmy / Indonesia
Dr. Zakiudin Munasir / Indonesia
Dr. Budi Setiabudiawan / Indonesia
Dr. Dadi Suyoko / Indonesia
Prof. Antonio Marini / Italy

Dr. Rinaldo Zanini / Italy
Prof. Salim Al-Malik /Kingdom of Saudi Arabia
Mrs. Yolanda Meijer / The Netherlands
Mr. Herman Neijens / The Netherlands
Mrs. Johanna Rijntjes / The Netherlands
Dr. Pilar Agnes Andaya / Philippines
Dr. M.A. Stella Paspe / Philippines
Prof. Mieczyslawa Czerwionka-Szaflarska / Poland
Dr. Hanna Szajewska / Poland
Prof. Coriolan Ulmeanu / Romania
Prof. Vera Revyakina / Russia
Dr. Ahmed Ismail Manjra / South Africa
Prof. Luis Ros Mar / Spain
Prof. Juan Carlos Vitoria Cormenzana / Spain
Dr. Christina West / Sweden
Prof. Chalerat Direwattanachai / Thailand
Prof. Jarunghchit Ngamphaiboon / Thailand
Dr. Jonathan Hourihane / UK
Dr. Gideon Lack / UK
Prof. Lesia Besh / Ukraine
Prof. Olga Lasytsya / Ukraine
Prof. Ricardo Sorensen / USA

Nestlé participants

Mrs. Lesley Scharf / Canada
Prof. Mike Possner / Germany
Mr. Elias Papadopoulos / Greece
Dr. Gabriella Metzger / Italy
Mrs. Marjan Skotnicki-Hoogland / The Netherlands
Dr. Olga Netrebenko / Russia
Prof. Wolf Endres / Switzerland
Dr. Bianca-Maria Exl-Preysch / Switzerland
Mr. Rodolphe Fritsche / Switzerland
Dr. Pierre Guesry / Switzerland
Ms. Petra Klassen / Switzerland
Mrs. Florence Rochat / Switzerland
Dr. Eduardo Schiffrin / Switzerland
Ms. Marie-Christine Secretin / Switzerland
Dr. Philippe Steenhout / Switzerland
Dr. Thierry von der Weid / Switzerland
Dr. Janet Aylott / UK
Mrs. Cynthia Brown / USA
Mrs. Linda Hsieh / USA
Prof. Pepe Saavedra / USA

Isolauri E, Walker WA (eds): Allergic Diseases and the Environment.
Nestlé Nutrition Workshop Series Pediatric Program, Vol. 53, pp. 1–25,
Nestec Ltd.; Vevey/S. Karger AG, Basel, © 2004.

Clinical Overview: The Changing Pattern of Clinical Aspects of Allergic Diseases

Yvan Vandenplas

Department of Pediatrics, Academisch Ziekenhuis, Vrije Universiteit Brussel, Brussels, Belgium

Introduction

Allergy is a hypersensitivity reaction initiated by immunological mechanisms. Although wide individual variations may be observed, atopic diseases tend to be related to the first decades of life, and obviously require a juvenile immune system. The incidence of allergic disease can be estimated at about 30% of the population. However, the variation throughout the world in the prevalence of asthma, allergic rhinoconjunctivitis and atopic eczema is striking [1]. A dramatic increase in allergic disease during the last decennia has been noticed, mainly centered in socioeconomically highly developed communities around the world.

Treatment and especially prevention of allergic disease has become a public health priority topic. At least three breeding grounds are needed to develop allergic disease: a genetic background; contact with the causal allergen and adjuvant, and additional environmental factors. Contact with an offending allergen is needed to develop tolerance.

Prevalence

The increase during the last decennia in symptoms compatible with allergic disease (atopic dermatitis, asthma, rhinitis) is beyond doubt, although its etiology has not been clarified. An increase in any reported disease has many contributing factors: there may be an increase in risk factors provoking the disease, but there may as well be a higher professional and public awareness. According to the data from Burr et al. [2], Aberg et al. [3] and Ninan and

Russell [4], there is a twofold increase in allergic diseases during the last decades. An increase of about 5–10% over a period of 10 years (1985–1995) was reported in Norwegian children [5]. Recent data suggest that the incidence of atopic disease in children, exclusively breast-fed during 3 months and born in families with one atopic family member, has reached almost 50% by the age of 2 years [6]. According to the literature, atopic dermatitis has a prevalence varying from 8 to 24%, and a cumulative incidence between 13 and 44%. These data suggest that the prevalence of some phenotypes in defined age groups is truly increasing, and is not simply explicable by an increase in awareness, a change in diagnostic methods, a better knowledge of symptoms, over-reporting of mild symptoms or changes in indoor risk factors.

In a period of 8 years (1990 and 1998), a highly significant increase in all wheezing disorders was reported in 1- to 5-year-old children in Leicestershire, UK [7]. The fact that all preschool wheezing disorders increased, including viral wheeze, makes it probable that factors unrelated to atopy are implicated in the changing epidemiology of wheeze in childhood [7]. This survey suggests an increase in the host response to common viral infections [7]. More than anything else, the increase in wheezing over an almost 10-year period suggests a fundamental change in pulmonary responsiveness to environmental triggers. Among those triggers, there was a significant decrease in parental smoking, increase in nursery and day care attendance, and increase in single households [7]. The increase in wheezing occurred not only in atopic children, wheezing because of multiple triggers, but also in those wheezing only during colds. The fact that many authors suggested that (respiratory) infections acquired early in life may reduce the risk for the development of later atopy (see section 'Infection'), is not in contradiction to the fact that wheezing may occur in the context of infectious and/or allergic disease.

The Allergic March

The allergic march refers to the natural history of atopic diseases, and is characterized by a typical sequence of sensitization and manifestation of symptoms which appear during a certain age period, persist over years or even decades, but then often show a tendency for spontaneous remission with age [8]. Although an 11-week-old fetus can produce IgE, no specific sensitization to food or inhalant allergens has been detected with standard methods. Interleukin (IL)-4 and interferon-γ (IFN-γ) are produced from 22 weeks onwards.

The atopic march starts during the first months of life, and the first IgE responses to food proteins develop, especially to cow's milk and hen's egg [9]. First, sensitization to hen's egg and cow's milk occurs, followed by wheat and soy [9]. Ten years ago Hill et al. [10] showed that in a cohort of 42 children with IgE-mediated cow's milk allergy (CMA), the prevalence of eczema was 57%, asthma 69%, allergy 67%, peanut allergy 55%, and 83% of infants demonstrated positive skin-prick tests to 3 or more allergens [10]. Although many studies report a remission rate of CMA of 90% by the age of 1 year, the remission rate of the IgE-mediated CMA in the population of Hill et al. [10] was only 31% at 2 years. Children with persistent cow's milk protein allergy (CMPA) had a significantly higher incidence and level of skin sensitivity to inhalant and other dietary allergens [10].

Early sensitization to hen's egg proteins may be a predictor of subsequent sensitization to aeroallergens and the development of allergic airway symptoms [11]. At the age of 4 years, the incidence of allergic disorders (asthma, rhinitis and eczema) in a birth cohort of 1,218 children was 28.1% [12]; 19.6% had a positive reaction to more than 1 allergen. Still at 4 years, sensitization to inhalant allergens was relatively common (19.2%) as compared with food allergens (3.5%) [12]. House dust mite (11.9%), grass pollen (7.8%) and cat (5.8%) are the most common positive reactions. Overall, 68.4% of the children sensitized to house dust mite had asthma, eczema and/or rhinitis [12]. Sensitization to environmental allergens from indoor and outdoor sources such as house dust mite and cat allergens requires more time, and is generally observed between 1 and 10 years [9]. Sensitization to dog does not start before the age of 5 years, and is seldom [12]. Sensitization to pollen, birch and grass mostly occurs after the 2nd year of life [9]. Transient sensitization in early childhood in a country with a low allergy prevalence is followed by a downregulation of skin reactivity [13]. There is a dose-response relation between early exposure to cat and mite allergens and the risk of sensitization during the first years of life [8].

Allergic disease starts in young infants with a high incidence of CMPA, which is at its maximum a couple of months after the introduction of cow's milk, thus between 6 and 12 months. Health care costs during the first year of life are substantially higher in cow's milk formula-fed than in breast-fed infants [14]. Therefore, in infants, interest has been focused on the prevention of symptoms of allergic disease related to cow's milk. Although CMPA persists in some infants, and allergy to other food proteins develops, the prevalence of food allergy in older children, adolescents and adults is only a couple of percent. Atopic sensitization can be transitory, and disappear in the 2nd or 3rd year of life. Sometimes manifestations of atopic disease are limited to food allergy and atopic eczema not leading to inhalant allergy or asthma at school age. But if sensitization to food occurs at a young age and sensitization to inhalant allergens also occurs, this is a strong predictive factor for the later development of asthma. Almost simultaneously with food allergy, atopic eczema or dermatitis develops with a peak prevalence around the age of 3 years, and decreases in older children. Eczema frequently starts from the age of 3 months on. Typical hay fever symptoms do not occur before the age of 2, suggesting that at least 2 pollen seasons are necessary to develop the symptoms.

The natural history of wheezing is more complex. Epidemiological data from Europe and the USA suggest that between one third and half of the children have at least one episode of wheezing between the age of 0 and 6 years [9, 15]. However, this wheezing is transient in most of the children. But in some children, especially boys with 1 atopic parent and those who had eczema as baby, the wheezing does not disappear and asthma will develop. When present in wheezing infants, specific IgE >0.35 kU/l to wheat, egg white or inhalant allergens are predictive of later childhood asthma [16]. At the age of 7–10 years, allergic rhinoconjunctivitis develops, reaching a peak incidence at almost 20 years. Asthma starts to develop a few years after rhinoconjunctivitis, and is characterized by a sharper increase, reaching a peak incidence at about the age of 15 years.

Relevant factors for the 'allergic march' are the genetic background, contact with allergens and environmental factors such as air pollution and tobacco smoke, contact with microorganisms.

Genetic Factors

Genetic studies provided evidence for a linkage between certain chromosome regions and manifestations of atopy. Since the study by Kjellman and Croner [17] in the 1970s, the role of family history and thus genetic background is a well-known risk factor. Asthma and other allergic diseases are genetically heterogeneous disorders. Each of the atopic phenotypes is probably the result of a polygenic inheritance and a complex interaction between genes and environmental factors. However, the trend how allergic manifestations develop and present is similar or comparable within members of one family, suggesting a degree of phenotype-specificity. At the phenotype level, there is a closer association between asthma or atopic dermatitis in the child and the same manifestations in its parents and siblings than with other manifestations of atopy [18]. Different studies have provided evidence of remarkable differences in the prevalence of certain atopic phenotypes between continents and countries and even within countries [1]. Genes may increase the susceptibility, but not necessarily lead to full disease expression.

If the chromosomal 'risk' zones for atopic disease become well identified, screening for their presence may be used for prevention, or eventually (genetic) treatment. Various genes predisposing to atopy have been identified. A linkage of atopy to the chromosomal region 11q13 was first reported in 1989 [19]. A linkage between total IgE and several markers in the IgE region, containing genes coding for IL-3, IL-4, IL-5, IL-9, IL-12B and IL-13 was reported [20]. Also a linkage between asthma and total serum IgE was found on chromosome 12q [21]. In the future better knowledge of the genes involved may offer a possibility for a breakthrough in the approach to allergic patients [22]. However, today we do not have this knowledge.

Maternal atopy is the major triggering factor [6, 23]. Male preponderance was observed with most allergens, but is significant only for house dust [12]. The degree to which genetic and environmental factors influence susceptibility to autoimmune and allergic diseases is still not well defined. The best hint derives from concordance rates of such diseases in monozygotic twins [18]. The rate is 75% in case of asthma [24]. Nevertheless, in absolute numbers, atopic manifestations occur more frequently in nonatopic than in atopic families, because the latter regards a relatively small part of the population. Therefore, the majority of prospectively affected children will not be identified at birth by family history.

When East joined West Germany, a lower prevalence of atopic disease was reported in East Germany, despite the absence of genetic difference [25]. The impact of environmental factors may be more important but also more transient than that of genetic background.

Immunologic Markers

In the absence of good genetic markers, immunologic markers may be capable of detecting (a group of) individuals at risk before sensitization occurs. The production of IgE is genetically controlled. Therefore, IgE determination on cord blood was initially thought to be a good screening tool [25, 26]. However, the sensitivity, specificity and predictive value of IgE do not sufficiently discriminate between those who will and will not develop atopic disease. Eosinophils or eosinophilic cationic protein may be a better risk factor for wheezing and asthma.

Fetal T cells have the capacity to respond to contact with an allergen and the response of these cells differs in infants who will and will not later develop atopic disease [27]. In children who will develop atopic disease, a continuation of fetal allergen-specific Th2 response during infancy, and a decreased capacity for production of Th1 cytokine IFN-γ was demonstrated [28]. Up to now, immunologic markers enabling in daily routine a selection of 'at-risk' infants at birth have not been described.

The impressive rise in prevalence emphasizes the potent action of environmental factors in molding this immune disorder which is characterized by inadequate restrained Th2 immune mechanisms (or an imbalance between Th1 and Th2) and IgE production. Atopic disease is a two-stage process, involving a discrete phase for induction which is regulated via interactions between Th1 and Th2 cytokines, followed by a second and more complex effector phase involving the expression in target tissues of sensitized individuals of highly variable levels of Th2 mediated inflammation [29]. Several studies suggest that those children who will go on to have more severe and persistent asthma symptoms already have immune responses skewed toward Th2 at the time of the very first episodes of airway obstruction in infancy [30].

Symptoms

A reason why the prevalence of allergic disease has increased during the past decennia may be related to a better knowledge of symptoms of allergic disease. One allergen can cause different symptoms: wheat allergy may be at the origin of atopic dermatitis, urticaria, baker's asthma, celiac disease, etc. Symptoms of allergic disease are aspecific and can be caused by different pathophysiologic mechanisms. Gastroesophageal reflux can be the consequence of a motility disorder, but is as well an accepted symptom of allergy [31]. Eosinophilic esophagitis is a relatively new entity that is now quite prevalent on the east coast of the USA, but (very) rare in Europe [32].

The hypothesis that exposure induces allergic disease such as asthma with airway inflammation via sensitization has recently been seriously challenged. In a number of countries, the prevalence of asthma has increased independent of allergen exposure [33, 34]. The factor that is common to all situations leading to early sensitization and induces asthma is not clear, but maturation of the immune system of atopic children seems to develop different than in nonatopic children, and is characterized by a predominance of Th2 instead of Th1 cells.

More than 15 years ago Hill et al. [35] identified at least 3 different groups of children with CMA. About one third of CMA children have predominantly urticarial and angioedematous eruptions, developing within 1 h after ingestion, with a high IgE and positive skin-prick tests [35]. A second group is composed by half of the allergic children. These children present with pallor and gastrointestinal symptoms such as vomiting and diarrhea occurring between 1 and 24 h after ingestion, and are relatively IgA-deficient [35]. Finally, about one fourth of patients have eczema, bronchitic or diarrhea symptoms that present more than 24 h after ingestion [35]. Only those with eczema have a positive skin test and high IgE [35]. (The fact that 1 of the 3 patient groups is discretely IgA-deficient, may explain why probiotic bacteria are partially successful in reducing symptoms of allergic disease, since some of the probiotic strains enhance IgA secretion.)

Allergy has been advocated as a cause of symptoms in every known organ system, although many of these symptoms are far from being generally accepted (table 1) [36].

General Life Style

A Western life style may be one of the most relevant determinant factors provoking allergy. Populations with a high socioeconomic status are at the highest risk of developing atopic sensitization. But which factor has the most determinant role is unclear. A change in environmental factors (day care, feeding, living conditions and life style, etc.) is very likely, at least in part,

Table 1. Extra-gastrointestinal symptoms that have been attributed to allergic disease

General	Anaphylaxis
Dermatological	Angioedema, lip swelling,urticaria, (acute/chronic/delayed pressure), atopic eczema, itching
Respiratory	Wheezing, asthma, stridor, (recurrent) cough, chronic otitis, nasal stuffiness, sneezing, Heiner syndrome
Neurologic, psychiatric, behavioral	Migraine, myasthenia gravis, epilepsy, spinal cord syndrome, 'excessive crying', colic, disturbed sleep, vertigo, asthenia, irritability, hyperactivity, hyperkinetic syndrome, affective disorders, schizophrenia, muscular pain
Urinary	Nephrotic syndrome, eosinophilic cystitis, orthostatic albuminuria
Vasculitis	Henoch-Schönlein
Arthropathy	Rheumatoid arthritis

to contribute to the increase in allergic disease. Atopic dermatitis occurs more frequently in urban than rural areas. Some of these environmental factors may have an increasing effect while others may have a decreasing effect. Migrant studies show that the prevalence of atopic dermatitis in immigrants matches that of natives in the adopted country, and not that of the home country [37]. The most important environmental trigger factors that cause allergic disease are food allergens and aeroallergens, irritants, emotional factors, climatic and seasonal factors, pollution and microbial agents such as *Staphylococcus aureus*. Environmental factors can act as an allergen, but are also capable of upregulating existing IgE responses or leading to either disease manifestation or an aggravation of symptoms. Active smoking is consistently related to an increased risk of lower airway diseases such as bronchitis, recurrent wheezing and pneumonia. Whether the same is valid for passive smoking is still matter of debate. But, the influence of smoking is only demonstrable during infancy, when infants spent most of their time in the direct neighborhood of their smoking mother. Children of mothers who smoke have wheezing before 3 years but not at the age of 6; children of atopic mothers have persistent wheezing [15].

Relevant candidate environmental factors include changes in diet, chemical air pollution and (lack of) microbial exposure in developed countries [38]. Much research has focused on the causal role of contact with allergens and the development of asthma. Most epidemiological studies report a correlation between (the type of and the moment of) allergic sensitization and asthma [39]. If sensitization to inhalation allergens occurs at a young age, it would be a risk factor for asthma. If it occurs after the age of 8 years, it would be a risk factor for allergic rhinitis. But, children growing up in an environment with or without house dust mites have a comparable incidence of asthma [40].

The contact organ may also cause confusion. Regarding food allergens, the gastrointestinal tract is the most predominant and logic contact organ. But food allergens may also cause symptoms via skin contact or inhalation. The recent demonstration that sensitization to peanut protein may occur in children through the application of peanut oil to inflamed skin [41], suggests that sensitization may occur via many different ways that may be hard, if not impossible, to discover by taking the history of the individual patient.

Breast-Feeding

The protective role of breast-feeding on infectious and allergic disease is still a matter of debate. There is no convincing evidence that breast-feeding protects from later atopic disease. Breast-fed infants have a lower incidence of infectious diseases such as gastroenteritis and otitis than formula-fed infants. Potentially protective factors for infectious disease are present in higher amounts in feces from breast-fed infant than in those from formula-fed infants, but only during the 1st month of life [42]. A very weak trend towards a slightly increased prevalence of atopic disease in the prolonged breast-fed group could be observed [42]. Recently, this trend was highlighted by Sears et al. [43] in a 26-year follow-up study demonstrating that breast-feeding (for 1 month or more) did not protect from atopy and asthma, and may even increase the risk. Asthma, allergy to cat, house dust mites and grass pollen were even slightly more frequent in the breast-fed group, between 9 and 26 years for asthma [43]. According to a 17-year follow-up study, exclusive breast-feeding for a prolonged period of more than 6 months protects from eczema, respiratory and food allergy at the age of 1 and 3 years [44]. But, at 17 years of age, the prevalence of substantial atopy was lowest in the group that had intermediate breast-feeding during 1–6 months (36%), followed by the group that had prolonged breast-feeding (42%), and the group that had no breast-feeding or less than 1 month (65%) [44]. However, the group consisted of only 238 infants at inclusion and the data of not more than 150 17-year-old adolescents were available for long-term analysis [44]. (Since some studies suggest an even higher incidence of wheezing in formerly breast-fed infants, it could be considered that in some situations the protective role of the mother's milk from infectious diseases has a negative impact on the development of allergic disease.)

It is well known that the breast-fed infants have a different gastrointestinal flora than formula-fed babies [45]. Also pharyngeal colonization differs according to whether the baby is breast- or formula-fed: *Haemophilus influenzae* and *Moraxella catarrhalis* colonize formula-fed infants but not breast-fed infants [46].

Formula Feeding and Other Feeding-Related Variables

Breast-fed children and those fed cow's milk have a different gastrointestinal flora. The composition of the gastrointestinal tract flora differs between newborns in whom allergy develops at a later age and those in whom allergy does not develop [47, 48]. The type, timing and amount of bacteria colonizing the intestine of newborns may determine the immunomodulation of the naive immune system [49].

Obesity is characterized by a similar dramatic increase as allergic disease. Obesity was suggested to increase the incidence of asthma in girls [50]. The role of obesity in asthma is not clear: whether obesity causes wheezing or whether asthma causes obesity is far from being clear.

Nucleotides stimulate the immune function, and may therefore decrease allergic disease [51]. Micronutrients such as iron and zinc also stimulate the immune response [52]. α-Linoleic acid is frequently decreased or low in infants with atopic eczema. Administration of *Lactobacillus rhamnosus* GG did not change the α-linoleic content of phospholipids, whereas bifidobacteria B12 caused a significant increase [53]. But not only bifidobacteria and lactobacilli may decrease allergic disease. Other food ingredients may as well influence the development of allergic disease. Protein hydrolysates, both partial and extensive, have been demonstrated to decrease the incidence of CMA in infants born in families with allergic disease [54]. An allergen-reduced feeding of the mother and infant does not result in a reduced incidence of asthma and allergy at the age of 7 years [55]. In some countries (partial) hydrolysates have a market share of 20% or more, and thus will influence epidemiologic data. Moreover, many formulae for infant feeding nowadays contain hydrolyzed proteins, although only a minority of them have indications in the prevention and treatment of allergic disease. The Zug-Frauenfeld study [56, 57] indicates that systematic use of partial hydrolysates together with other environmental preventive recommendations results in a significant reduction in illness.

Monoglycerides with chain lengths of 8–12 carbons have been shown at least partially to inactivate pathogens such as respiratory syncitial virus, herpes simplex virus type 1, *H. influenzae*, group-B streptococcus [58]. Calcium phosphate was shown to reduce intestinal surfactant concentration, strongly protect against salmonella infection, and stimulate growth of lactobacilli [59]. The addition of n-3 fatty acids to the diet of infants has been suggested to decrease the incidence of wheezing during the first 18 months of life [60]. Vitamin D prevents or decreases autoimmune diseases such as diabetes [61].

Indoor Allergens

Indoor allergen exposure is the environmental factor with by far the strongest impact on the manifestation of asthma. Carpets and cats are more frequently present in the houses of children who were sensitized at least once during the first 3 years [62]. An increased exposure to house dust mite increases the risk for sensitization [63]. Respiratory symptoms during the first year of life are less frequent in infants growing up in an environment with a limited presence of house dust mites and without pets [64]. Whether this is a temporary or persistent effect was not clear [64]. Elimination of dust mites reduces the further development of allergic disease in children born to atopic parents with dermatitis and sensitization to food [65]. Moreover, there seems to be a direct relation between the amount of exposure to carpet and cat allergens and the development of symptoms [62], although also the contrary has been demonstrated. There is evidence suggesting that children growing up with cats and dogs less frequently have asthma than children growing up without regular contact with these pets [66, 67]. Among children whose mothers have no history of asthma, exposure to a cat at the age of 2–3 months is associated with a reduced risk of wheezing between the ages of 1 and 5 years [68]. About 15% of mothers and children exposed to high concentrations of cat, but not mite allergens have serum IgG antibodies without IgE antibodies [69]. This IgG antibody is freely transferred to the infant and might influence IgG antibody production in the child [69]. But then again, exposure to a cat in the home increases the risk of developing IgE sensitization to cats [70], although the higher the exposition to cats, the more the sensitization is reduced [71].

This effect could not be shown for dogs [70]. Dog exposure in early life might prevent the development of asthma-like symptoms, at least in low-risk children with no family history of asthma [71]. Cat allergen exposure was lower on parental mattresses in families with allergic mothers, but dog allergen exposure was not different [24]. However, the impact of a different antigenic load on parental mattresses for infants and children is unclear.

Also mite allergen exposure is lower on mattresses in families with allergic mothers [24]. A close association exists between allergen exposure (especially indoor allergens) and sensitization [11, 72]. There is an inverse relation between endotoxin levels (endotoxins are a product of gram-negative bacteria) in the bedding and the incidence of atopy in children living in rural areas [73]. Avoidance of dietary allergens (milk, egg, fish, nuts, soy, wheat, orange) and house dust mite in genetically ‘at-risk’ infants results in a significant reduction in allergic disease [74].

The avoidance of contact with some environmental allergens may result in a reduced incidence of allergic disease, while for other allergens this could not be proven or may even be the opposite.

Outdoor Allergens

The climate and a number of culturally based differences in behavior may also be important. The role of air pollution is not clear. Children who grow up close to a highway and thus are in contact with gasoline particles eliminated by heavy traffic are sensitized more frequently [75]. An association has been suggested between heavy traffic and allergic rhinitis caused by cedar pollen allergy [76]. However, sociodemographic confounders frequently confuse the outcome of similar studies. On the other hand, data suggest that pollution does not seem to influence the incidence or prevalence of asthma. The difference in allergic disease between cities and rural areas is not related to air pollution, but to living on a farm [77]. Recent studies of Swiss, Bavarian and Austrian children have shown that the prevalence of symptoms of allergic rhinitis and of allergen-specific IgE antibodies is much lower among the offspring of farmers than among other children in these areas [77]. Allergies are less frequent when children are exposed early and for a prolonged period to farm animals and cow's milk [78]. Exposure to large quantities of endotoxin present on a farm could contribute to the explanation as to why the incidence of allergic disease is reduced by living on a farm.

The Role of Microorganisms

It was suggested 25 years ago that 'atopic disease is the price paid by some members of the white community for their relative freedom from diseases due to viruses, bacteria and helminths' [79]. Infections are known to have long-lasting, nonspecific systemic effects on the nature of the immune response to antigens and allergens [80]. Indeed, Gerrard et al. [79] observed that native Indians have higher IgE levels than the white community, although the incidence of asthma, eczema and urticaria was less common. A decline in certain childhood infections or a lack of exposure to infectious agents during the 1st year of life, a factor which is associated with smaller families in the middle-class environment of industrialized countries, could have caused the recent epidemic of atopic disease and asthma. Lower respiratory tract infections in 3-month-old infants are associated with the number of persons in the household and history of atopy [81]. At the age of 6 months, lower respiratory tract infections remain associated with the number of persons in the household, but also with day care center attendance [81]. Young children with older siblings at home and those who attend a day care center during the first 6 months of life have a lower incidence of asthma [82]. Children in small families tend to have a decreased incidence of atopy when they attend a day care center in early childhood [83]. The clear inverse relation between the number of siblings and atopy observed in several studies may be related to a protective role of infections, although specific information is inconclusive [84].

Children living in rural areas have more lactobacilli and less clostridia in their intestinal flora than children living in cities, and these differences in flora could be related to a risk of developing sensitization [85]. Allergic infants have an adult type of bifidobacterium flora with high levels of *Bifidobacterium adolescentis*, and healthy infants have high levels of *Bifidobacterium bifidum* [86]. The adhesion to human intestinal mucus of *B. bifidum* is much better than that of *B. adolescentis* [86]. Not all lactobacilli adhere equally well to the intestinal mucosa [87]. If adhesion is 'good', the contact between intestinal cells and food allergens is reduced. The better the adhesion, the better the immune response, and the more IgA secretion. Systematic administration of lactobacillus GG ATCC 53103 during 7 months to children attending day care centers did not result in significant health benefits [88]. The administration of lactobacilli to pregnant women and their babies significantly decreased the incidence of atopic dermatitis [89]. Lactobacilli decreased atopic dermatitis [90].

Recent evidence suggests that contact early in life with many viral pathogens may result in a reduction in allergic disease [91]. Children who grew up in a large family, on a farm or in a day care center have a reduced risk for allergic disease. Children with repeated episodes of a runny nose before the age of 1 year are less likely to develop asthma by the age of 7 years [92]. This effect may even be life long. The lifestyle of children attending Steiner schools differs in many aspects from daily life of children attending classical schools, resulting in a reduced use of antibiotics (52 versus 90%), extremely reduced vaccination rate for measles, mumps and rubella (18 versus 93%) and increased consumption of fermented food (63 versus 4.5%) [93]. Children from Steiner schools have a lower prevalence of atopy than controls [93]. The relation between the number of characteristic features of an anthroposophic lifestyle and risk of atopy is significant and inverse [93].

Antibiotic use during the 1st year of life has been linked to an increased risk of developing asthma and allergy in children with a genetic predisposition for atopy, but the contrary has also been found [84, 94]. Antibiotics not only attack pathogens, but also alter the composition of the normal gastrointestinal flora. However, the impact of antibiotics on the flora is likely to be transient. Therefore, the knowledge that the flora in infants who will develop atopy and those who will not is different, cannot be extrapolated to antibiotic use and its temporary effect.

Vaccines have turned many childhood diseases into distant memories in industrialized countries. The evidence is limited to nonexisting regarding a direct role of vaccinations for development of conditions such as autism and multiple sclerosis. No substantial evidence links measles-mumps-rubella vaccine to autism, or hepatitis B vaccine to multiple sclerosis [95].

Epidemiologic investigations indicate that viral infections may either promote (respiratory syncytial virus) or inhibit (hepatitis A, measles) atopy, although data are scarce [96, 97]. Recovery of natural measles infection reduces the incidence of atopy, asthma and allergic responses to house dust mites to half that seen in vaccinated children [79, 98]. Some infections induce a systemic and nonspecific switch to Th1 activities, and thus decrease the Th2 response that could be responsible for an inhibition of the development of atopy during childhood [19, 94]. A positive serology for hepatitis A or toxoplasmosis has an inverse relation with the incidence of hay fever, allergic rhinitis and asthma [99]. Positive tuberculin responses predict a lower incidence of asthma, lower serum IgE levels and cytokine profile bias towards Th1 type [100, 101]. But according to recent evidence, Calmette-Guérin bacillus vaccination administered to infants is not associated with reduced risk of development of atopy [102]. And the intestinal flora is likely to enhance Th1-type response [103]. The observation that this occurs both with living and heat-killed lactobacilli [103, 104] suggests that the immune-stimulating effect may be related to membrane proteins. Thus, perinatal (both prenatal as neonatal) bacterial infections are potential modulators for the allergic march. Preterm delivery is often the consequence of bacterial infection during pregnancy. The observation that prematures have a lower prevalence of atopic eczema is consistent with this concept [105].

Infants with milk allergy and atopic dermatitis have milder symptoms and fewer markers of intestinal inflammation if the formula is fortified with lactobacilli. However, more intervention studies are needed before efficacy is demonstrated. Secondly, a comparison between the efficacy of hydrolyzed proteins and/or probiotics should be evaluated. It could be that they act independently, synergetically or antagonistically. Similar, the effect of prebiotics on the development (and treatment) of allergic diseases should be studied. Despite several promising findings, the exact role of normal gut microbiota in the development of allergy remains to be elucidated [106]. For successful interventions, more data concerning a communication between host and specific microbial species are needed [106].

The low prevalence of atopic disease in Estonia may, at least in part, be related to the high endotoxin levels in this country. The findings support that high levels of endotoxin, or other bacterial products with Th1-stimulating properties, might protect children from developing atopic disease [107].

Infestation with helminth parasites, which are potent stimuli for allergen-associated Th2 immunity, is associated with a reduced susceptibility to atopy [108]. The parasite-induced stimulation towards a Th2-mediated sensitization to environmental allergens additionally triggers powerful anti-inflammatory mechanisms that limit the magnitude of ensuing in vivo responses to these allergens [108]. Helminth eradication in children in Venezuela was associated with an increased incidence of immediate hypersensitivity to environmental allergens [109]. Rural children in Kenya have much higher antibodies to ascaris than children living in cities (67 vs. 26%); yet, the incidence of positive skin-prick tests was lower in the rural areas [110]. In the city area in Kenya, an association between atopy and asthma could be demonstrated, but not in the rural area [111]. According to these findings, IL-10 plays an important part in determining the severity of allergic disease in individuals [108].

Drug Therapy

Recent data suggest that early medical treatment with cetirizine in young infants with atopic eczema, a positive family history for atopic disease and an early sensitization to grass pollen and house dust mite, significantly reduces the incidence of asthma [111, 112]. The effect of immunotherapy was recently evaluated: immunotherapy with pollen reduced the risk for asthma [113]. Anti-IgE therapy may be capable of increasing the threshold of sensitivity (to peanut) [114].

Conclusion

The list of lifestyle-related factors which might be associated with the imminent epidemic of the 21st century and might have relevance to the atopic march in children is long. Higher education of the mother, higher household income, living in a single-family home in a less densely populated area with fewer people per room, and being a white household were associated with elevated dust mite, cat, and dog allergens and low cockroach allergen [115]. In contrast, low income, living in a multifamily home in a high population density area with a higher occupancy rate per room, and being a Hispanic or black household were associated with elevated cockroach allergens and low concentrations of dust mite, cat, and dog allergens. Although the presence of an individual allergen is more likely associated with one or more socioeconomic or ethnic factors, most homes typically have multiple allergen burdens in excess of concentrations thought to be associated with sensitization and exacerbation of asthma. Mite and cockroach allergens have distinct and opposite associations with socioeconomic factors and population density [115]. Early use of antibiotics is only one risk factor on the list.

As long as there is no marker that is capable with certainty to predict the development of allergic disease or asthma, it will be difficult to stop the allergic march. It is beyond any doubt that the prevalence of symptoms of allergic diseases is increasing in the industrialized world. The predictive role of cells and cytokines has been disappointing. The best predictive factor remains family history. Genetic markers may offer more promising possibilities in the future. Most epidemiological studies focused on selected at-risk populations. Improved knowledge of symptoms and better reports are insufficient to explain the increase. Since the etiology of allergic diseases is multifactorial, genetic background can also not explain this increase. Changing environmental factors such as hygienic and dietary habits are likely to be among the major contributing factors. Primary prevention measures that are suitable for everybody are breast-feeding and introduction of solid food after the 4th month of life, and the avoidance of passive smoking exposure. Breast-feeding and hydrolysates reduce the incidence of CMA [116], but whether this

Table 2. The allergic march: contributing factors

	Evidence
Increasing the allergic march	
• Genetic background (especially mother)	+++
• Early and persisting sensitization	+++
• High contact with allergens (many allergens, high amounts)	+++
• Low contact with some infectious microorganisms	+++
• 'Environmental factors' (as a group, the individual role of most is still debated)	+++
• Passive smoking (during first months of life)	++
Decreasing the allergic march	
• Breast-feeding, hydrolysate feeding during first months of life	+++
• Feeding solids after 4 months	+
• House dust elimination first months of life	++
• Strict elimination after the first months of life	+
• Probiotics	++
• Prebiotics (theoretical concept, not validated)	?
• Addition n-3 fatty acids	+?
• Other dietary changes (zinc, iron, nucleotides, etc.)	?
• Immunotherapy	+
• Medical therapy (antihistamines)	+

results in a reduced incidence of allergic disease during adulthood is far from being clear. Although there are many valid reasons for encouraging breast-feeding during the first 4–6 months of life, based on the current evidence the prevention of asthma and allergies in not one of them [117]. Introduction of solids after the age of 4 months reduces the risk for eczema. Food and environmental allergen avoidance decreases the development of allergic disorders in infancy [73]. In fact, most of the evidence suggests that early preventive measurements do not decrease the incidence of asthma (although some data indicate the opposite). Difficulties in compliance with allergen avoidance may be a detrimental to explain the contradictory findings. A 'medical indoor environment counselor' may improve this compliance and thus lead to a more clear-cut evaluation of the impact of control of environmental risk factors [118].

Parasitic, viral and bacterial infections at an early age may stimulate an anti-inflammatory response that is capable of reducing sensitization. Since a return to the diseases does not offer a solution, early intervention by inducing the right stimuli with controlled introduction of microorganisms in early life may at least in part reduce allergic diseases.

Evidence for factors that induce and promote the allergic march exist for the genetic background (especially of the mother), early and persisting sensitization, high contact with allergens and reduced contact with microorganisms (tables 2, 3). Factors that possibly temper the allergic march are: strict

Table 3. Recommendations to decrease the allergic march applicable to all children

- Breast-feeding, up to 4–6 months
- If supplements are needed: hydrolysate with proven efficacy
- No solids before 4 months of age
- No contact with tobacco smoke

avoidance of environmental allergens; probiotics; n-3 fatty acids in feeding; immunotherapy, and medical treatment (antihistaminics).

References

1 International Study of Asthma and Allergies in Childhood (ISAAC) Steering Committee: Worldwide variation in prevalence of symptoms of asthma, allergic rhinoconjunctivitis, and atopic eczema. Lancet 1998;351:1225–1232.
2 Burr ML, Butland BK, King S, Vaughan-Williams E: Changes in asthma prevalence: Two surveys 15 years apart. Arch Dis Child 1989;64:1452–1456.
3 Aberg N, Hasselmar B, Aberg B, Eriksson B: Increase of asthma, allergic rhinitis and eczema in Swedish schoolchildren between 1979 and 1991. Clin Exp Allergy 1995;25:815–819.
4 Ninan TK, Russell G: Respiratory symptoms and atopy in Aberdeen schoolchildren: Evidence from two surveys 25 years apart. BMJ 1992;304:873–875.
5 Nystad W, Magnus P, Gulsvik A: Increasing risk of asthma without other atopic diseases in school children: A repeated cross-sectional study after 13 years. Eur J Epidemiol 1998;14: 247–252.
6 Rautava S: Probiotics during pregnancy and breast-feeding might confer immunomodulatory protection against atopic disease in the infant. J Allergy Clin Immunol 2002;109:119–121.
7 Kuehni CE, Davis A, Brooke AM, Silverman M: Are all wheezing disorders in very young (preschool) children increasing in prevalence? Lancet 2001;357:1821–1825.
8 Wahn U: What drives the allergic march? Allergy 2000;55:591–599.
9 Kulig M, Bergmann R, Klettke U, et al: Natural course of sensitization to food and inhalant allergens during the first 6 years of life. J Allergy Clin Immunol 1999;103:1173–1179.
10 Hill DJ, Bannister DG, Hosking CS, Kemp AS: Cow milk allergy within the spectrum of atopic disorders. Clin Exp Allergy 1994;24:1137–1143.
11 Nickel R, Kulig M, Forster J, et al: Sensitization to hen's egg at the age of 12 months is predictive for allergic sensitization to common indoor and outdoor allergens at the age of three years. J Allergy Clin Immunol 1997;99:613–617.
12 Arshad SH, Tariq SM, Matthews S, Hakim E: Sensitization to common allergens and its association with allergic disorders at age 4 years: A whole population birth cohort study. Pediatrics 2001;108:E33.
13 Julge K, Vasar M, Bjorksten B: Development of allergy and IgE antibodies during the first five years of life in Estonian children. Clin Exp Allergy 2001;31:1854–1861.
14 Ball TM: Health care cost of formula-feeding in the first year of life. Pediatrics 1999;103: 870–876.
15 Martinez FD, Wright AL, Taussig LM, et al: Asthma and wheezing in the first six years of life. The Group Health Medical Associates. N Engl J Med 1995;332:133–138.
16 Kotaniemi-Syrjanen A, Reijonen TM, Romppanen J, et al: Allergen-specific immunoglobulin E antibodies in wheezing infants: The risk for asthma in later childhood. Pediatrics 2003;111:E355–E361.
17 Kjellman NIM, Croner S: Cord blood IgE determination for allergy prediction: A follow-up to seven years of age in 1651 children. Ann Allergy 1984;53:571–578.

18 Schultz Larsen F: Atopic dermatitis: A genetic-epidemiologic study in a population-based twin sample. J Acad Dermatol 1993;28:719–723.
19 Cookson WOCM, Sharp PA, Faux JA, Hopkin JM: Linkage between immunoglobulin responses underlying asthma and rhinitis and chromosome 11q. Lancet 1989;i:1292–1295.
20 Marsh DG, Neely JD, Breazeale DR, et al: Linkage analysis of IL4 and other chromsome 5q31.1 markers and total serum immunoglobulin E concentrations. Science 1994;264: 1152–1156.
21 Barnes KC, Neely JD, Duffy DL: Linkage of asthma and total serum IgE concentration to markers on chromosome 12q: Evidence from Afro-Caribbean and Caucasian populations. Genomics 1997;46:159–162.
22 Cookson WOC: Asthma genetics. Chest 2002;121(suppl):7–13.
23 van Strien RT, Koopma LP, Kerkhof M, et al: Mite and pet allergen levels in homes of children born to allergic and nonallergic parents. The PIAMA study. Environ Health Perspect 2002;110: A693–A698.
24 Skadhauge LR, Christensen K, Kyvik KO, Sijsgaard T: Genetic and environmental influence on asthma: A population-based study of 11,588 Danish twin pairs. Eur Respir J 1999;13:8–14.
25 Heinrich J, Hoelscher B, Frye C, et al: Trends in prevalence of atopic diseases and allergic sensitisation in children in eastern Germany. Eur Respir J 2002;19:1040–1046.
26 Vandenplas Y, Sacre L: Influences of neonatal serum IgE concentration, family history and diet on the incidence of cow's milk allergy. Eur J Pediatr 1986;145:493–495.
27 Jung T, Moessner R, Drekhoff K: Mechanisms of deficient interferon-gamma production by CD4-effector T-cells generated from naïve precursors is restored by priming in the presence of either high dose Il-2 or IL-12. Clin Exp Allergy 1999;29:912–919.
28 Prescott SL, Macaubas C, Smallacombe T, et al: Development of allergen-specific T-cell memory in atopic and normal children. Lancet 1999;353:196–200.
29 Holt PG, Macaubas C, Stumbles PA, Sly PD: The role of allergy in the development of asthma. Nature 1999;402:12–17.
30 Martinez FD: Links between pediatric and adult asthma. J Allergy Clin Immunol 2001; 107(suppl 5):S449–S455.
31 Salvatore S, Vandenplas Y: Gastroesophageal reflux and cow milk allergy: Is there a link? Pediatrics 2002;110:972–984.
32 Furuta GT: Eosinophilic esophagitis: An emerging clinicopathologic entity. Curr Allergy Asthma Rep 2002;2:67–72.
33 Charpin D, Birnbaum J, Haddi E, et al: Altitude and allergy to house-dust mites: A paradigm of the influence of environmental exposure on allergic sensitization. Am Rev Respir Dis 1991; 143:983–986.
34 Ingram JM, Sporik R, Rose G, et al: Quantitative assessment of exposure to dog (Can f 1) and cat (Fel d 1) allergens: Relation to sensitization and asthma among children living in Los Alomos, New Mexico. J Allergy Clin Immunol 1995;96:449–456.
35 Hill DJ, Firer MA, Shelton MJ, Hosking CS: Manifestations of milk allergy in infancy: Clinical and immunologic findings. J Pediatr 1986;109:270–276.
36 Vandenplas Y, Loeb H: Extra-digestive manifestations of food allergy. Arch Pediatr 1994; 1:57–60.
37 Staines A, Hanif S, Ahmed S, et al: Incidence of insulin dependent diabetes mellitus in Karachi, Pakistan. Arch Dis Child 1997;76:121–123.
38 Hopkin JM: The use of atopy and links to infection. Allergy 2002;57(suppl 72):5–9.
39 Peat JK, Li J: Reversing the trend: Reducing the prevalence of asthma. J Allergy Clin Immunol 1999;103:1–10.
40 Sporik R, Ingram JM, Price W, et al: Association of asthma with serum IgE and skin test reactivity to allergens among children living at high altitude. Tickling the dragon's breath. Am J Respir Crit Care Med 1995;151:1388–1392.
41 Lack G, Fox D, Northstone K, Golding J: Factors associated with the development of peanut allergy in childhood. N Engl J Med 2003;348:977–985.
42 Kohler H: Antibacterial characteristics of the feces of breastfed and formula-fed infants during the first year of life. J Pediatr Gastroenterol Nutr 2002;34:188–193.
43 Sears MR, Greene JM, Willan AR, et al: Long-term relation between breastfeeding and development of atopy and asthma in children and young adults: A longitudinal study. Lancet 2002;360:901–907.

44 Saarinen UM, Kajosaari M: Breastfeeding as prophylaxis against atopic disease: Prospective follow-up study until 17 years old. Lancet 1995;346:1065–1069.
45 Harmsen HJ, Wildeboer-Veloo AC, Raangs GC, et al: Analysis of intestinal flora development in breast-fed and formula-fed infants by using molecular identification and detection methods. J Pediatr Gastroenterol Nutr 2000;30:61–67.
46 Hokama T: Isolation of respiratory bacterial pathogens from the throats of healthy infants fed by different methods. J Trop Pediatr 1999;45:173–176.
47 Bjorksten B, Sepp E, Julge K, et al: Allergy development and the intestinal microflora during the first year of life. J Allergy Clin Immunol 2001;108:516–520.
48 Kalliomaki M, Kirjavainen P, Eerola E, et al: Distinct patterns of neonatal gut microflora in infants in whom atopy was and was not developing. J Allergy Clin Immunol 2001;107:129–134.
49 Gronlund MM, Arvilommi H, Kero P, et al: Importance of intestinal colonisation in the maturation of humoral immunity in early infancy: A prospective follow-up study of healthy infants aged 0–6 months. Arch Dis Child Fetal Neonatal Ed 2000;83:F186–F192.
50 Castro-Rodriguez JA, Holberg CJ, Morgan WJ, et al: Increased incidence of asthma-like symptoms in girls who become overweight or obese during the school years. Am J Respir Crit Care Med 2001;163:1344–1349.
51 Carver JD: Dietary nucleotides: Effects on the immune and gastrointestinal systems. Acta Paediatr Suppl 1999;88:83–88.
52 Dijkhuizen MA: J Effects of iron and zinc supplementation in Indonesian infants on micronutrient status and growth. A positive double-blind placebo-controlled challenge. J Nutr 2001;131:2860–2865.
53 Kankaanpaa PE: Influence of probiotic supplemented infant formula on composition of plasma lipids in atopic infants. J Nutr Biochem 2002;13:364–369.
54 Vandenplas Y, Heymans H: Primary and secondary prevention of atopic diseases in children. Curr Probl Dermatol 1999;28:173–193.
55 Zeiger RS, Heller S: The development and prediction of atopy in high-risk children: Follow-up at age seven years in a prospective randomised study of combined maternal and infant food allergen avoidance. J Allergy Clin Immunol 1995;95:1179–1190.
56 Exl BM, Deland U, Secretin MC, et al: Improved general health status in an unselected infant population following an allergen-reduced dietary intervention programme: The ZUFF study programme. Part II: Infant growth and health status to age 6 months. Eur J Nutr 2000;39:145–156.
57 Exl BM, Deland U, Secretin MC, et al: Improved general health status in an unselected infant population following an allergen-reduced dietary intervention programme: The ZUFF study programme. Part IV: Infant growth and health status to age 2 years. Eur J Nutr 2003; in press.
58 Isaacs CE: Antimicrobial activity of lipids added to human milk, infant formula, and bovine milk. J Nutr Biochem 1995;6:362–366.
59 Bovee-Oudenhoven IM: Dietary calcium phosphate stimulates intestinal lactobacilli and decreases the severity of a salmonella infection in rats. J Nutr 1999;129:607–612.
60 Mihrshahi S, Peat JK, Marks GB, et al: Eighteen-month outcomes of house dust mite avoidance and dietary fatty acid modification in the Childhood Asthma Prevention Study (CAPS). J Allergy Clin Immunol 2003;111:162–168.
61 Mathieu C, Adorini L: The coming of age of 1,25-dihydroxyvitamin D(3) analogs as immunomodulatory agents. Trends Mol Med 2002;8:174–179.
62 Wahn U, Lau S, Bergmann R, et al: Indoor allergen exposure is a risk factor for sensitization during the first three years of life. J Allergy Clin Immunol 1997;99:763–769.
63 Remes ST, Castro-Rogriguez JA, Holberg CJ, et al: Dog exposure in infancy decreases subsequent risk of frequent wheeze but not of atopy. J Allergy Clin Immunol 2001;108:509–514.
64 Custovic A, Simpson BM, Simpson A, et al: Effect of environmental manipulation in pregnancy and early life on respiratory symptoms and atopy during first year of life: A randomised trial. Lancet 2001;358:188–193.
65 Ehnert B, Lau-Schadendorf S, Weber A, et al: Reducing domestic exposure to dust mite allergen reduces bronchial hyperreactivity in sensitive children with asthma. J Allergy Clin Immunol 1992;90:135–138.
66 Heselmar B, Aberg N, Aberg B, et al: Does early exposure to cat or dog protect against later allergy development? Clin Exp Allergy 1999;29:611–671.

67 Perzanowski MS, Ronmark E, Platts-Mills TA, Lundback B: Effect of cat and dog ownership on sensitization and development of asthma among preteenage children. Am J Respir Crit care Med 2002;166:696–702.
68 Celedon JC, Litonjua AA, Ryan L, et al: Exposure to cat allergen, maternal history of asthma, and wheezing in first 5 years of life. Lancet 2002;360:781–782.
69 Platts-Mills TA, Erwin EA, Allison AB, et al: The relevance of maternal immune responses to inhalant allergens to maternal symptoms, passive transfer to the infant, and development of antibodies in the first 2 years of life. J Allergy Clin Immunol 2003;111:123–130.
70 Linneberg A, Nielsen NH, Madsen F, et al: Pets in the home and the development of pet allergy in adulthood. The Copenhagen Allergy Study. Allergy 2003;58:21–26.
71 Platts-Mills T, Vaughan J, Squillace S, et al: Sensitisation, asthma, and a modified Th2 response in children exposed to cat allergen: A population-based cross sectional study. Lancet 2001;357:752–756.
72 Noertjojo K, Dimich-Ward H, Obata H, et al: Exposure and sensitization to cat dander: Asthma and asthma-like symptoms among adults. J Allergy Clin Immunol 1999;103:60–65.
73 Braun-Fahrländer C, Rieder J, Herz U: Environmental exposure to endotoxin and its relation to asthma in school-age children. N Engl J Med 2002;347:869–877.
74 Arshad SH, Matthews S, Cant C, Hide DW: Effect of allergen avoidance on development of allergic disorders in infancy. Lancet 1992;339:1493–1497.
75 Wyler C, Braun-Fahrlander C, Kunzli N, et al: Exposure to motor vehicle traffic and allergic sensitization. The Swiss Study on Air Pollution and Lung Diseases in Adults (SAPADIA) Team. Epidemiology 2000;11:450–456.
76 Chunling W, Tamura K, Matusumoto Y, et al: Effects of quantity of Japanese cedar pollen, air pollution and urbanization on allergic rhinitis morbidity in Ibaraki prefecture. Nippon Koshu Eisei Zasshi 2002;49:631–642.
77 Braun-Fahrländer C, Gassner M, Grize L: Prevalence of hay fever and allergic sensitisation in farmer's children and their peers living in the same rural community. Clin Exp Allergy 1999;29:28–34.
78 Riedler J, Braun-Fahrlander C, Eder W, et al: Exposure to farming in early life and development of asthma and allergy: A cross-sectional survey. The ALEX Study Team. Lancet 2001;358:1129–1133.
79 Gerrard JW, Geddes CA, Reggin Pl, et al: Serum IgE levels in white and Metis communities in Saskatchewan. Ann Allergy 1976;37:91–100.
80 Farooqi IS, Hopkin JM: Early childhood infection and atopic disorder. Thorax 1998;53:927–932.
81 Bunuel Alvarez JC, Vila Pablos C, Puig Congost M, et al: Influence of type of infant feeding and other factors on the incidence of respiratory tract infections in infants followed at a primary care center. Aten Primaria 2002;29:268–277.
82 Ball TM, Castro-Rodriguez JA, Griffith KA, et al: Siblings, day-care attendance, and the risk of asthma and wheezing during early childhood. N Engl J Med 2000;343:538–543.
83 Kramer U, Heinrich J, Wjst M, Wichmann HE: Age of entry to day nursery and allergy in later childhood. Lancet 1999;353:450–454.
84 Droste JHJ, Wieringa MH, Weyler JJ, et al: Does the use of antibiotics in early childhood increase the risk of asthma and allergic disease? Clin Exp Allergy 2000;30:1547–1553.
85 Bjorksten B, Naaber P, Sepp E, Mikelsaar M: The intestinal microflora in allergic Estonian and Swedish 2-year-old children. Clin Exp Allergy 1999;29:342–346.
86 He F, Ouwehand AC, Isolauri E, et al: Comparison of mucosal adhesion and species identification of bifidobacteria isolated from healthy and allergic infants. FEMS Immunol Med Microbiol 2001;30:43–47.
87 Juntunen M, Kirjavainen, PV, Ouwehand AC, et al: Adherence of probiotic bacteria to human intestinal mucus in healthy infants and during rotavirus infection. Clin Diagn Lab Immunol 2001;8:293–296.
88 Hatakka K, Savilahti E, Ponka A, et al: Effect of long term consumption of probiotic milk on infections in children attending day care centers: Double blind, randomised trial. BMJ 2001;322:1327–1332.
89 Kalliomäki M, Salminen S, Arvilommmi H, et al: Probiotics in primary prevention of atopic disease: A randomised placebo-controlled trial. Lancet 2001;357:1076–1079.
90 Isolauri E, Arvola T, Sutas Y, et al: Probiotics in the management of atopic eczema. Clin Exp Allergy 2000;30:1604–1610.

91 Matricardi PM, Rochetti R: Are infections protecting from atopy? Curr Opin Allergy Clin Immunol 2001;1:413–419.
92 Lau S, Nickel R, Niggemann B, et al: The development of childhood asthma: Lessons from the German Multicentre Allergy Study (MAS). Paediatr Respir Rev 2002;3:265–672.
93 Alm JS, Swartz J, Lilja G, et al: Atopy in children of families with an anthroposophic lifestyle. Lancet 1999;353:1485–1488.
94 Celedón JC, Litonjua AA, Ryan L, et al: Lack of association between antibiotic use in the first year of life and asthma, allergic rhinitis, or eczema at 5 years. Am J Respir Crit Care Med 2002;166:72–75.
95 Kimmel SR: Vaccine adverse events: Separating myth from reality. Am Fam Physician 2002;66:2113–2130.
96 Matricardi PM, Rosmini F, Ferrigno L, et al: Cross sectional retrospective study prevalence of atopy among Italian military students with antibodies against hepatitis A virus. BMJ 1997; 314:999–1003.
97 Pershagen G: Can immunization affect the development of allergy? Pediatr Allergy Immunol 2000;11(suppl 13):26–28.
98 Kondo N, Fukutomi O, Ozawa T: Improvement of food-sensitive atopic dermatitis accompanied by reduced lymphocyte responses to food antigen following natural measles virus infection. Clin Exp Allergy 1993;23:44–50.
99 Matricardi PM, Rosmini F, Panetta V, et al: Hay fever and asthma in relation to markers of infection in the United States. J Allergy Clin Immunol 2002;110:381–387.
100 Herz U, Gerhold K, Grüber C: BCG infection suppresses allergic sensitization and development of increased airway reactivity in an animal model. J Allergy Clin Immunol 1998;102: 867–874.
101 Shirakawa T, Enomoto T, Shimazu S, Hopkin JM: The inverse association between tuberculin responses and atopic disorder. Science 1997;275:77–79.
102 Krause TG, Hviid A, Koch A, et al: BCG vaccination and risk of atopy. JAMA 2003;289: 1012–1015.
103 Shida K, Makino K, Mrishita A: *Lactobacillus casei* inhibits antigen-induced IgE secretion through regulation of cytokine production in murine splenocyte cultures. Int Arch Allergy Immunol 1998;115:278–287.
104 Murosaki S, Yamamoto Y, Ito K: Heat-killed *Lactobacillus plantarum* L-137 suppresses naturally fed antigen-specific IgE production by stimulation of IL-12 production. J Allergy Clin Immunol 1998;102:57–64.
105 Bührer C, Grimmer I, Niggemann B, Obladen M: Low 1-year prevalence of atopic eczema in very low birth weight infants. Lancet 1999;353:1674.
106 Kalliomaki P, Isolauri E: Role of intestinal flora in the development of allergy. Curr Opin Allergy 2003;3:15–20.
107 Bottcher MF, Bjorksten B, Gustafson S, et al: Endotoxin levels in Estonian and Swedish house dust and atopy in infancy. Clin Exp Allergy 2003;33:295–300.
108 van den Biggelaar AHJ, van Ree R, Rodrigues LC: Role of parasite-induced interleukin-10 in children infected by *Schistosoma haematobium*. Lancet 2000;356:1699–1700.
109 Lynch NR, Hagel I, Perez M, et al: Effect of antihelminthic treatment on the allergic reactivity of children in a tropical slum. J Allergy Clin Immunol 1993;92:404–411.
110 Perzanowski MS, Ng'ang'a LW, Carter MC, et al: Atopy, asthma, and antibodies to ascaris among rural and urban children in Kenya. J Pediatr 2002;140:582–588.
111 Diepgen TL, Early Treatment of the Atopic Child Study Group: Long-term treatment with cetirizine of infants with atopic dermatitis: A multi-country, double-blind, randomized, placebo-controlled trial (the ETAC trials) over 18 months. Pediatr Allergy Immunol 2002;13: 278–286.
112 Warner JO, ETAC Study Group: A double-blind, randomized, placebo-controlled trial of cetirizine in preventing the onset of asthma in children with atopic dermatitis: 18 months' treatment and 18 months' posttreatment follow-up. J Allergy Clin Immunol 2001;108:929–937.
113 Möller C, Dreborg S, Ferdousi HA, et al: Pollen immunotherapy reduces the development of asthma in children with seasonal rhinoconjunctivitis (the PAT-study). J Allergy Clin Immunol 2002;109:251–256.
114 Leung DYM, Sampson HA, Yunginger JW, et al: Effect of anti-IgE therapy in patients with peanut allergy. N Engl J Med 2003;348:986–993.

115 Lederer BP, Belanger K, Triche E, et al: Dust mite, cockroach, cat, and dog allergen concentrations in homes of asthmatic children in the northeastern United States: Impact of socio-economic factors and population density. Environ Health Perspect 2002;110:419–425.
116 Terraccino L, Isoardi P, Arrigoni S, et al: Use of hydrolysates in the treatment of cow's milk allergy. Ann Allergy Asthma Immunol 2002;89(suppl 1):86–90.
117 Sly P, Holt P: Breast is best for preventing asthma and allergies – Or is it? Lancet 2002;360: 887–888.
118 de Blay F, Fourgaut G, Hedelin G, et al., and the Scientific Committee of the MIEC Study: Medical Indoor Environment Counselor (MIEC): Role in compliance with a device on mite allergen avoidance and on mite exposure. Allergy 2003:58:27–33.

Discussion

Dr. Isolauri: We had the opportunity recently to measure IgE antibodies in different age groups. The first set of columns shown are the important ones that we need to look at now. These are the total IgE levels for the age groups 7, 27, 47, and 67 years, which were measured some 10 years ago. Therefore these 67-year-old subjects were born before the Second World War. These are unpublished data and I want briefly to share them with you. As can be seen total IgE levels are comparable, while specific IgE against aeroallergies has definitely increased: in the older group it is much higher than in the 7-year-olds. As Dr. Vandenplas mentioned, he was surprised to find that 47% of the at-risk population in Finland have atopic eczema. We have an objective measurement showing that 50% of 7-year-olds have antigen-specific antibodies. Similar results have been obtained for children and young adults [1, 2]. The data also nicely correspond with the results of Bergmann et al. [3] showing that the incidence of atopic diseases in the at-risk population was something like 40%. So we truly do not need to be surprised at seeing these percentages in scientific papers as such high levels of IgE positivity can definitely be found nowadays in our population.

Dr. Vandenplas: I agree with your comment, but to add to that, when we did our non-HA intervention study in the late 1980s, the subjects were followed for 5 years, so that brought us to 1992. We also had an atopic disease incidence of 50–60% in the control group. But at that time it was very hard to convince people that this really was the incidence of atopic disease. What is happening now is that as this high figure is being reported more and more often, it is also becoming accepted as really true. Your slides also show very nicely how difficult it is to get a real image of the change in clinical patterns because some of those changes are probably due to changes in our lifestyle from 50 years ago that only have an impact later on. At this time there is such a difference in lifestyle worldwide that you cannot have anything other than very conflicting results.

Dr. Romagnani: I have a short comment on the slide shown by Dr. Isolauri. In my view, it is not surprising that the levels of total IgE were the same in the 7- and 67-year-old subjects because polyclonal IgE production is mainly a consequence of helminthic infections, which probably disappeared from Finland and other Western countries already before the Second World War. By contrast, the production of IgE specific for aeroallergens has increased in developed countries in the last decades and this certainly accounts for the difference in the levels of IgE against common environmental allergens found between the 7- and 67-year-old subjects.

Dr. van den Biggelaar: There might be a rise in allergen-specific IgE and therefore atopy in the Western world. However, many studies in African countries have shown that the prevalence of atopy, defined as children producing allergen-specific IgE, is very high: despite their sensitization these children don't develop allergy.

Dr. Vandenplas: There is of course a world of difference between sensitization and development of symptoms.

Dr. Walker: I was fascinated by your term 'the allergic march' and I want to ask a clarifying question, if I could. When you talk about early food allergy symptoms, are you talking specifically about IgE-mediated food allergy symptoms or are you talking about the type of condition that we frequently see in infancy, e.g., in the first couple months of life, as proteins are introduced into the newborn's diet?

Dr. Vandenplas: Not specifically IgE.

Dr. Walker: This notion goes against conventional wisdom. What most people think is that the food allergic symptoms that occur early on in life have to do with transient developmental immaturities of the immune system. Therefore this is a situation in which symptoms develop and later disappear, whereas in your notion of the 'allergic march' these non-IgE-mediated and non-IgA developmentally associated symptoms seem to lead to a march of IgE-mediated symptoms for the rest of childhood. Is that what you are saying?

Dr. Vandenplas: That was suggested by the studies that I mentioned. What I tried to stress, especially in very young infants, is that it is very difficult to speak about allergy if you don't have proof of an allergic mechanism being involved. I again use the example of changing the formula for an infant. So many things change when a regular formula is substituted by hydrolysates and the symptoms disappear. But as soon as you challenge by changing back to the regular formula, the symptoms reappear, and that is now the definition of proof of allergic disease. I think this is true for a lot of infants with gastrointestinal symptoms related to cow's milk. It just shows that cow's milk is involved, it does not at all show that there is an immunological mechanism involved in these children. Up to now in most studies, they have all been put together, and that is certainly one of the important weaknesses of these studies. During a certain period there was some relaxation in the definition that if you had a positive challenge it was proof of allergic disease, but I don't think that is true.

Dr. K. Bergmann: We are presently performing a large nationally representative study on the health of children and adolescents in Germany, and I would like to share some results from our pretest with you. We are looking at atopy from 4 facets: one is a written questionnaire; another is a personal computer-assisted interview; the third is examination of the child, and the fourth is looking at specific sensitization. In the pretest we examined 1,630 children, and sensitization was analyzed according to a specific panel of 20 different allergens. At the age of 0–2 years we have about 4% sensitized and this increases in 14- to 17-year-old children to a level of about 40%. I wonder if we had a panel of 100 allergens instead of 20 whether there would be 100% sensitization in this population. The other aspect was attention: what kind of impact does the attention of the persons interviewed have? To look into this we analyzed the influence of the education level. There were 4 levels of education: those who had not completed school were in the lowest level, and the highest level was college education. From no completed education to college education the prevalence of atopic diseases increases by a factor of nearly 3. This is a very large difference if I use the region questionnaire. In this life-time prevalence study, when I examine the children, I still have the influence of education but the difference is only from nearly 3% dermatitis or atopic eczema to 4.5%, the difference is only about an additional 50%. So education apparently has an influence on prevalence but what we see in terms of questionnaires is that attention is stronger on measured prevalence. If we only look at history we probably get a wrong impression, we have to examine the persons.

Dr. Vandenplas: I suppose that education also means that according to different forms of education there are different lifestyles, and according to education there are different income levels. Apparently you find that education itself seems also to be a factor as to how parents look after their children. Your impact for education seems to be bigger than the impact if you look at the children. But for the rest, I think it also confirms other data from the literature showing that higher income is related with a higher incidence of atopic disease and that environmental changes play a role.

Dr. K. Bergmann: My message is if it is done on the basis of history the factor is 3, and if you examine the child it is only 50% more. So education apparently does have an influence, but it is much smaller than the influence of attention.

Dr. Vandenplas: Could it mean that parents overreport?

Dr. K. Bergmann: Or underreport.

Dr. Vandenplas: Because I know some studies on the incidence of gastroesophageal reflux in which both the parents and the children were questioned. It was found that parents consistently underreport their children's symptoms. We recently did a study in the psychological area on the reporting of chronic abdominal pain and headaches, and the parents are the ones who underreported the incidence of manifestations.

Dr. Bindslev-Jensen: I think it is very important to stick to the point between sensitization and clinical disease, especially the data you show from the Wahn group on wheat and soy sensitization. It is not reflected in the clinical situation in most of the patients. Another point in the same direction is that we have to define very clearly, when we are comparing data, what we are talking about. Are we talking about allergic asthma for instance or are we just talking about asthma. Because if we look at the allergic march, which was not coined by Sampson, although he has done many good things, it was first drawn by Wahn and then stolen by all of us, then it is a matter of finding out whether this is sensitization, clinical disease or an allergic disease, and again we have to stick to the difference between a correlation. One of the latest studies was about the increase in asthma correlated to the consumption of paracetamol in the UK. If you think that paracetamol causes asthma then you are probably wrong. You have to find out what the correlation is, what is the causal relationship, and then I would urge everybody to stick to the difference between disease and sensitization, because otherwise it is going to be very difficult to find out what is going on.

Dr. Vandenplas: I fully agree with that. Definitions will be one of the next topics. A lot of those statistics are a mixture of everything, which causes confusion.

Dr. Isolauri: I fully agree with both of you, but I think the new changes in atopy definitions are a personal tendency first to produce antigen-specific IgE antibodies, and second to develop symptoms under familial hereditary risk. So the new definition includes not only sensitization but also some morbidity, and therefore we are becoming partly confused: do we discuss allergic disease, atopic disease, or do we simply stick to specific IgE production per se. Therefore my suggestion is that we talk about prevention or the incidence of atopic disease, and prevention and the incidence of specific IgE production.

Dr. Marini: I would like to call attention to the very low birth weight infant population. In this population there are factors that may promote atopic dermatitis, increased gut permeability, bad flora, but in our neonatology experience, very low birth weight infants have a very low incidence of atopic dermatitis [4]. Actually, extremely low birth weight infants never have atopic dermatitis. I ask why? I don't know why, perhaps different tissue reactivities? This is an interesting point.

Dr. Guesry: But the lack of allergy manifestation, is it during the short period in which the immune system has not yet developed, or do you have a long-term follow-up?

Dr. Marini: Up to 6 years of age.

Dr. Endres: I would like to ask a question that is often asked nowadays concerning pets. How many pets? A cat and a dog, 2, 3, none? Must a high-risk family abandon their pet when a child is born?

Dr. Vandenplas: You saw a picture of my daughter with a cat, so that answer is clear from my point of view. I don't think we really have an answer to that question because of the conflicting data. When it was very popular to say that you need to avoid cats and pets in the home, I always showed slides illustrating that domestic animals stimulate the psychomotor development of children. Just do not kill all the pets. I think there is also more than just atopic disease, there is also chow-chow life and psychomotor development for children. I also like cats, but there is no answer.

Dr. Suyoko: I am interested in your statement about breast-feeding not protecting from atopic diseases. In my country we still promote breast-feeding as the best formula for infancy. Can you differentiate a mother who avoids food allergens and a mother who does not avoid food allergens with the incidence of atopic diseases in children? Because I have read that if the mothers avoid food allergens it will protect the infants from allergic diseases. My second question is whether decreasing infectious diseases could increase immunologic or allergic diseases? In my opinion that does not include viral infections because if allergic patients suffer from viral infection the incidence will be increased, not decreased. The last question is about using probiotics before and after delivery, especially for mothers to prevent atopic disease in their children.

Dr. Vandenplas: First, breast-feeding is of course the best way to feed infants. I only wanted to show a recent provoking study which did not find that mother's milk had any protective effect in the long-term. There are a lot of weaknesses in that study and there are studies which show the opposite. I think there is no way to not promote breast-feeding of course. I think the mother should not follow a restricted diet unless she has to do that for herself. If the mother is allergic of course she needs to follow a diet, but not to prevent the development of allergic disease in her child. There has never been proof that this develops in a population and there is a huge risk of malnutrition for the mother. There are studies from the Netherlands showing that there is much more cow's milk protein present in house dust than you have in the milk of the mother. So if you want a strict elimination of cow's milk, I am convinced that you need to do much more than just change the diet of the mother. I will not answer your last question because I think it is one of the topics that will be discussed during an oncoming session.

Dr. Guesry: I agree with you that breast-feeding remains the best nourishment for a baby. However, I also agree with you that the study by Sears et al. [5] from New Zealand is flawed by many aspects, and the data are increasing. The data from Finland [6] seem to show that breast-feeding is not as protective for babies at risk of developing allergy as it was in studies reported 10–20 years ago [7, 8]. So I think we have to ask this question in scientific terms: why has this effect, which was proven so well 20 years ago, seemed to fade away?

References

1 Nakagomi T, Itaya H, Tominaga T, et al: Is atopy increasing? Lancet 1994;343:121–122.
2 Broadfield A, McKeever TM, Scrivener S, et al: Increase in the prevalence of allergen skin sensitization in successive birth cohorts. J Allergy Clin Immunol 2002;109:969–974.
3 Bermann RL, Bergmann KE, Lau-Schadensdorf S, et al: Atopic diseases in infancy. The German Multicenter Atopy Study (MAS-90). Pediatr Allergy Immunol 1994;5(suppl 6):19–25.
4 Agosti M, Vegni C, Gangi S, et al: Allergic manifestation in very low birth weight infants: A 6-year follow-up. Acta Paediatr 2003;(suppl 441):44–47.
5 Sears MR, Greene JM, Willan AR, et al: Long-term relation between breastfeeding and development of atopy and asthma in children and young adults: A longitudinal study. Lancet 2002;360:901–907.

6 Isolauri E, Tahvanainen A, Peltola T, Arvola T: Breast-feeding of allergic infants. J Pediatr 1999;134:27–32.
7 Chandra RK: Five-year follow-up of high-risk infants with family history of allergy who were exclusively breast-fed or fed partial whey hydrolysate, soy, and conventional cow's milk formulas. J Pediatr Gastroenterol Nutr 1997;24:380–388.
8 Marini A, Agosti M, Motta G, Mosca F: Effects of a dietary and environmental prevention programme on the incidence of allergic symptoms in high atopic risk infants: Three years follow-up. Acta Paediatr Suppl 1996;414:1–21.

Isolauri E, Walker WA (eds): Allergic Diseases and the Environment.
Nestlé Nutrition Workshop Series Pediatric Program, Vol. 53, pp. 27–32,
Nestec Ltd.; Vevey/S. Karger AG, Basel, © 2004.

Changing Definitions of Allergy

Carsten Bindslev-Jensen

Allergicentret, Odense Universitetshospital, Odense, Denmark

In the 1920's Coca and Cooke [1] introduced the term 'atopy' to designate some phenomena of hypersensitivity in man. They considered that heredity, association with immediate-type skin reactions, diseases such as hay fever and asthma, and the fact that the responses were limited to a small group of patients were prominent features.

The classical nomenclature for allergic reactions was introduced by Gell and Coombs [2] and in the 1970s Pepys [3] defined the term 'atopic allergy' as classical IgE-mediated reactions to inhalant allergens. Atopic diseases generally refer to asthma, rhinoconjunctivitis, gastrointestinal and characteristic skin reactions.

In 2001, a new nomenclature was proposed by the European Academy of Allergy and Clinical Immunology (EAACI) [4] in which hypersensitivity was defined as an umbrella term (fig. 1), atopy was defined as 'a familial or personal tendency to develop allergen-specific IgE on exposure to environmental allergens and to suffer from typical allergic symptoms', whereas the term 'allergy' should be reserved for clinical reactions in which an immunological mechanism can be proven or is strongly implicated'.

The EAACI Definitions

Hypersensitivity causes objectively reproducible symptoms or signs initiated by exposure to a defined stimulus at a dose tolerated by normal subjects.

Atopy is a personal or familial tendency to produce IgE antibodies in response to low doses of allergens, usually proteins, and to develop typical symptoms such as asthma, rhinoconjunctivitis, or eczema/dermatitis.

Allergy is a hypersensitivity reaction initiated by immunologic mechanisms.

As an example, according to this new definition asthma may be allergic or nonallergic and the allergic may further be subdivided into IgE-mediated and non-IgE-mediated (fig. 2).

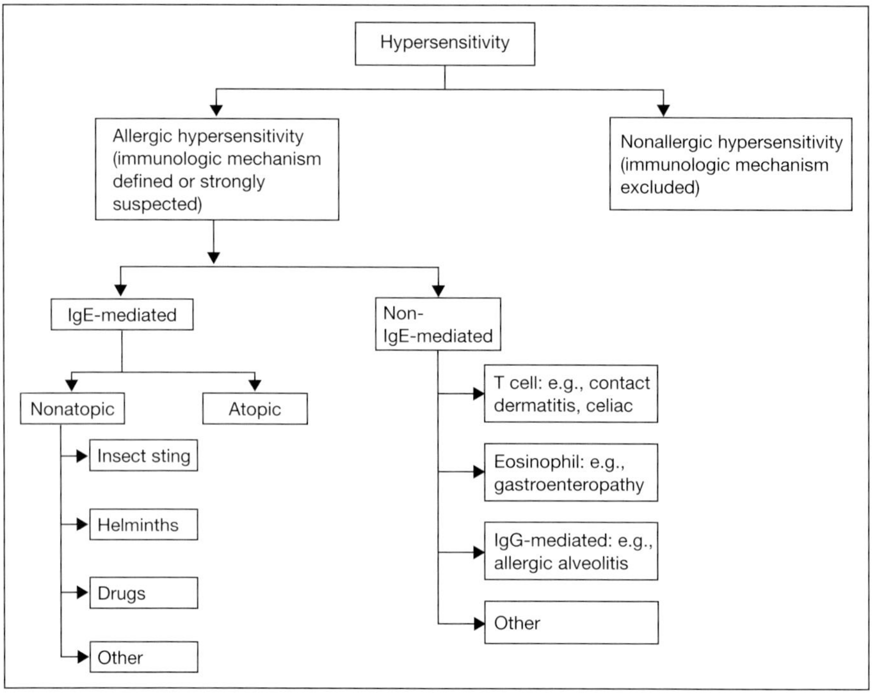

Fig. 1. The new nomenclature as proposed by the European Academy of Allergy and Clinical Immunology [4].

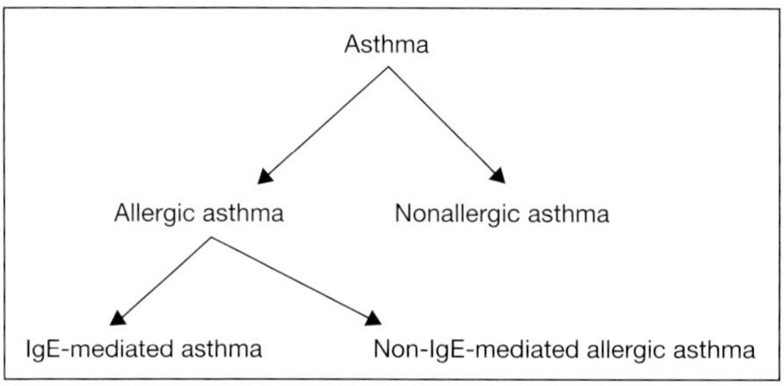

Fig. 2. An example taken from the new EAACI definitions, where asthma according to this new definition may be allergic or nonallergic, and allergic asthma may further be subdivided into IgE-mediated and non-IgE-mediated.

In the public perception, several other diseases are referred to as allergies or hypersensitivities; these syndromes, such as multiple chemical sensitivities [5] or electricity allergy [6], do not fit into these new definitions and should not at present be included in the hypersensitivity disorders.

The perhaps most important issue in the diagnostic work up of a patient is to determine the relative importance of an allergy to the patient's symptoms and signs. Sensitization does not imply clinical relevance and in many cases of, e.g., asthma in adults no allergies can be found, whereas sensitization is almost mandatory in pollen rhinoconjunctivitis.

The Relative Importance of Allergy in Various Atopic Diseases

Acute *urticaria* is often a feature elicited together with other signs from the airways and gastrointestinal tract upon exposure to, e.g., food, drugs or venom in sensitized patients. In this case, the urticaria is probably a Th2-related disease, but acute urticaria is also often elicited by infection, and in that case is probably not a Th2 disease. *Chronic urticaria(s)* is rarely associated with allergy [7] and has recently been demonstrated to be predominantly a Th0 disease [8]. On the other hand, in 30–40% of more severe cases of chronic urticaria, the presence of IgG antibodies directed against the Fc receptor on the mast cell or against IgE has been demonstrated [9], thus classifying this type of urticaria as 'non-IgE-mediated allergic urticaria'. It is important in this aspect to realize, however, that the pathophysiological significance of the antibodies remains to be established.

Following the proposed division of the atopic diseases into allergic and nonallergic, the term 'atopic dermatitis' was proposed by EAACI to be changed to 'atopic eczema/dermatitis syndrome' (AEDS). Also here we find allergic and nonallergic subtypes. The age of the patient with AEDS is important when looking at the frequency of allergic (IgE-mediated) AEDS: in more severe cases of AEDS in infants and children, sensitization and clinical allergy to foods such as egg, peanut or milk are often present, whereas in older children and adolescents sensitization seems to be associated with the patient's concomitant rhinoconjunctivitis and/or asthma [10]. Furthermore, a problem arises in defining patients with AEDS as allergic or nonallergic since in many cases of 'allergic AEDS', the patients, often adults, present with very high levels of IgE in serum but the physician fails to find a clinical correlate to the finding. The new EAACI nomenclature thus does not help the clinician in this situation in avoiding the term 'nonatopic atopic eczema'?

Again concerning *asthma* major differences emerge: most cases of recurrent wheezing in infants (asthmatic bronchitis) and small children are not allergic but due to viral infections and will not imply an increased risk of later development of asthma in the child, whereas allergic asthma to, e.g., house mites or cat is prevalent in later childhood and adolescence. In contrast in adults the relative role of sensitization seems to decline with age, where other substances such as tobacco smoke become important (as is in fact also the case in many cases of recurrent wheezing in infants.

In *food hypersensitivity* the role of nonallergic food hypersensitivity has been much overestimated and has attracted much attention by the public. Food allergy on the other hand is prevalent both in infants in whom sensitization to milk, egg and peanut/nuts predominates and in adults in whom cross-reactive IgE antibodies in pollen rhinitics elicit oral itching upon intake of fresh fruit and vegetables. Cross-reactions constitute a major problem in the diagnosis of food allergy, since many cross-reactive antibodies give rise to a significant response when measured in serum but do not elicit a clinical response when the incriminated food is ingested. This is the case in a proportion of patients with peanut allergy and serological cross-reaction to soy bean, where no more than 40% are clinically allergic to soy upon challenge [11], and even more obvious in Scandinavian patients with allergy to grass pollen, where a totally insignificant response to wheat in serum is found in many patients [12]. Knowledge of these cross-reactions and especially their clinical (in)significance is important in order to avoid unnecessary diets especially in children [13, 14].

In *drug hypersensitivity* the spectrum ranges from a classical IgE-mediated reaction to, e.g., penicillin over nonimmune-mediated but well-characterized reactions such as aspirin intolerance to diseases of unknown etiology, such as drug-induced erythema multiforme, fixed drug eruption or toxic epidermal necrolysis.

When trying to determine whether a given disease is allergic or nonallergic, the quality of the tests applied to the patient should also be taken into consideration. Normally, based on the physician's knowledge and experience, only a limited number of allergens are tested, and one must always bear in mind whether sensitization to other more exotic allergens or perhaps those found in the occupational field might be of importance. Furthermore, neither skin-prick testing nor measurement of specific IgE are perfect in the way of having a 100% sensitivity so false-negative test outcomes may result in misclassification of a given patient.

Does Sensitization Imply Clinical Relevance?

In many individuals, a positive skin-prick test to one or more allergens can be found, without the person ever having had an allergic disease [12]. This may be due to preclinical sensitization, i.e. the patient has been sensitized but has not yet developed clinical disease (sensitization to grass pollen in one season and development of rhinitis the next season), but may also be due to a very low clinical sensitivity to the allergen in question.

Assessment of the relative clinical importance of sensitization to an allergen should therefore also include an attempt to determine the clinical sensitivity of the actual patient to the allergen: many patients with pollen rhinitis only experience asthma symptoms in the peak pollen season in years with high pollen counts, whereas these patients normally have symptoms from the nose and eyes during every season. The sensitivity of the lungs in these cases are thus lower than the nose and eye, a phenomenon which cannot be exclusively attributed to exposure alone.

Another example is the search for safe levels of contaminating allergenic food (e.g. peanut or ground nut) in prepackaged foods, the no adverse effect level, (NOALL). The NOALL is important to the authorities in the risk-assessment procedure and therefore also to the manufacturer. An international approach to establish NOALLs for the most common food allergens has been made [15], but the outcome has been hampered by difficulties in comparing the procedures used for challenge, the preparation of food used, and differences between the patients. We took another approach, namely to try to develop a computer-based model on challenge data of various foods available from the world literature, and by doing so, we could come up with an attempt to establish threshold values [16]. NOALLs determine that the level of a given food is insufficient to cause a clinical reaction in even the most sensitive patient and is thus of mostly theoretical importance, whereas estimation of safe levels for, e.g., 95% of the susceptible population is much more operational.

Finally, the changing definitions of allergy should also address the public's perception of allergy, where several other disease entities are also included. Public perception of the frequency and clinical spectrum of hypersensitivity to milk in infants and to colorants and preservatives in children and adults differ dramatically from the findings in clinical investigations [17–20]. Furthermore, new life style diseases such as multiple chemical sensitivity or chronic fatigue syndrome are often referred to as being of hypersensitive origin [5] and the development of new allergens by genetic engineering may also attract attention in the future [21]. Therefore a mutual language is important and should be based on common standards for the diagnosis of allergic diseases.

References

1 Coca AF, Cooke RA: On the classification of the phenomena of hypersensitiveness. J Immunol 1923;8:163–182.
2 Gell PGH, Coombs RRA: Clinical Aspects of Immunology, ed 2. Oxford, Blackwell, 1968, pp 575–596.
3 Pepys J: Atopy; in Gell PGH, Coombs RRA, Lachmann PJ (eds): Clinical Aspects of Immunology, ed 3. Oxford, Blackwell Scientific, 1975, pp 877–902.
4 Johansson SGO, Hourihane JO, Bousquet J, et al: A revised nomenclature for allergy. An EAACI position statement from the EAACI nomenclature task force. Allergy 2001;56:813–824.
5 Buchwald D, Garrity D: Comparison of patients with chronic fatigue syndrome, fibromyalgia, and multiple chemical sensitivities. Arch Intern Med 1994;154:2049–2053.
6 Levallois P: Hypersensitivity of human subjects to environmental electric and magnetic field exposure: A review of the literature. Environ Health 2002;110(suppl 4):613–618.
7 Bindslev-Jensen C, Finzi A, Greaves M, et al: Chronic urticaria: Diagnostic recommendations. J Eur Acad Dermatol Venereol 2000;14:175–180.
8 Ferrer M, Luquin E, Sanchez-Ibarrola A, et al: Secretion of cytokines, histamine and leukotrienes in chronic urticaria. Int Arch Allergy Immunol 2002;129:254–260.

9 Greaves M: Autoimmune urticaria. Clin Rev Allergy Immunol 2002;23:171–183.
10 Mortz CG, Lauritsen JM, Bindslev-Jensen C, Andersen KE: Prevalence of atopic dermatitis, asthma, allergic rhinitis, and hand and contact dermatitis in adolescents. The Odense Adolescence Cohort Study on Atopic Diseases and Dermatitis. Br J Dermatol 2001;144:523–532.
11 Bernhisel-Broadbent J, Sampson HA: Cross-allergenicity in the legume botanical family in children with food hypersensitivity. J Allergy Clin Immunol 1989;83:435–440.
12 Mortz CG, Lauritsen JM, Andersen KE, Bindslev-Jensen C: Type I sensitization in adolescents: Prevalence and association with atopic dermatitis. Acta Derm Venereol 2003;83:1–8.
13 Ortolani C, Bruijnzeel-Koomen C, Bengtsson U, et al: Controversial aspects of adverse reactions to food. European Academy of Allergology and Clinical Immunology (EAACI) Reactions to Food Subcommittee. Allergy 1999;54:27–45.
14 Bruijnzeel-Koomen C, Ortolani C, Aas K, et al: Adverse reactions to food. European Academy of Allergology and Clinical Immunology Subcommittee. Allergy 1995;50:623–635.
15 Taylor SL, Hefle SL, Bindslev-Jensen C, et al: Factors affecting the determination of threshold doses for allergenic foods: How much is too much? J Allergy Clin Immunol 2002;109:24–30.
16 Bindslev-Jensen C, Briggs D, Osterballe M: Can we determine a threshold level for allergenic foods by statistical analysis of published data in the literature? Allergy 200;57:741–746.
17 Host A: Frequency of cow's milk allergy in childhood. Ann Allergy Asthma Immunol 2002; 89(suppl):33–37.
18 Fuglsang G, Madsen C, Saval P, Osterballe O: Prevalence of intolerance to food additives among Danish school children. Pediatr Allergy Immunol 1993;4:123–129.
19 Aardoom HA, Hirasing RA, Rona RJ, et al: Food intolerance (food hypersensitivity) and chronic complaints in children: The parents' perception. Eur J Pediatr 1997;156:110–112.
20 Young E, Stoneham MD, Petruckevitch A, et al: A population study of food intolerance. Lancet 1994;343:1127–1130.
21 Bindslev-Jensen C, Sten E, Earl LK, et al: Assessment of the potential allergenicity of ice structuring protein type III HPLC 12 using the FAO/WHO 2001 decision tree for novel foods. Chem Toxicol 2003;41:81–87.

Isolauri E, Walker WA (eds): Allergic Diseases and the Environment.
Nestlé Nutrition Workshop Series Pediatric Program, Vol. 53, pp. 33–51,
Nestec Ltd.; Vevey/S. Karger AG, Basel, © 2004.

The Changing Prevalence and Clinical Profile of Food Allergy in Infancy

David J. Hill, Ralf G. Heine and Clifford S. Hosking

Department of Allergy, Royal Children's Hospital, Melbourne, Australia

Introduction

It appears to be general consensus that the prevalence of food allergies and related atopic disorders is increasing in industrialized countries [1]. However, it has remained unresolved to what extent this represents a true prevalence increase or is attributable to an increasing awareness of the clinical manifestations of food allergy [2]. There are no population-based prevalence studies on food allergy that could provide firm evidence for or against this observation. Unfortunately, the few available prevalence studies cannot easily be compared due to differences in epidemiological methodology [3–9]. Another difficulty is the variation in the prevalence with age, as a significant proportion of food-allergic infants will develop tolerance during early childhood [10]. Finally, the prevalence of food allergy and the spectrum of food allergens may vary between countries due to differences in environmental and genetic factors [6, 11]. A summary of the main prevalence studies on food allergy is provided in table 1.

While many manifestations of food allergy are associated with IgE hypersensitivity, in approximately half of young children with challenge-proven food allergy an IgE-based mechanism cannot be demonstrated [12]. Previous prevalence studies have focused predominantly on IgE-mediated food allergy, and the non-IgE-mediated dermatological or gastrointestinal manifestations have often not been included. This is mainly due to the difficulty in making a definitive diagnosis of non-IgE food allergy without resorting to double-blind placebo-controlled food challenge, a resource-consuming procedure that is not suited for large population-based surveys.

Table 1. Prevalence studies on food allergies in infants and young children

Authors	Year of study	n	Age years	Prevalence food allergy	Comments
Jakobsson and Lindberg [3]	1979	1,079	<1	Cow's milk 1.9%	Swedish birth cohort
Høst and Halken [4]	1985	1,749	<1	Cow's milk 2.2%	Danish birth cohort
Schrander et al. [5]	1993	1,158	<1	Cow's milk 2.8%	Dutch birth cohort
Hill et al. [6]	1997	620	0–3	Cow's milk 2.0% Egg 3.2% Peanut 1.9%	Melbourne Atopy Cohort Study
Tariq et al. [7]	1989	1,218	4	Peanut 0.5%	Isle of Wight Birth Cohort Study
Grundy et al. [8]	1994–1996	1,246	4	Peanut 1.5%	Isle of Wight Birth Cohort Study (2nd cohort). Low recruitment rate (43%). Patients with convincing clinical reactions were not rechallenged
Sicherer et al. [9]	1999	12,032	Children and adults	Peanut 1.1%	Random digit telephone survey on peanut allergy in USA. Prevalence figure was corrected to include only typical immediate-type reactions (IgE-mediated)

The first part of this review will summarize the prevalence data on food allergy in infants and young children. In the second part, the changing clinical profile of food allergy in infancy will be described.

Definition

Adverse reactions to foods can be caused by several mechanisms, such as allergy, idiosyncrasy, toxins and metabolic diseases. They may involve either unwanted external agents, food additives or various molecular components of the food in question [13]. In this review, the term 'food allergy' will indicate an adverse clinical reaction attributed to the interaction of one or more food proteins with one or more immune mechanisms.

The Changing Prevalence of Food Allergy in Infancy

In principle, any food can cause an allergic reaction. However, a relatively small number of so-called 'major' food allergens account for the majority of food-allergic reactions (table 2). In a study of children with atopic dermatitis (AD), eight foods (cow's milk, egg, peanut, soy, wheat, tree nuts, fish and shellfish) caused 85% of food allergic reactions [14]. In adults, the allergen spectrum is quite different as a significant proportion of children with food allergies develop tolerance to some of these allergens. The main food allergens in adults are peanut, tree nuts, fish and shellfish [15]. In a study of 65 infants with AD, the comparison of 2 infant cohorts 10 years apart revealed no significant difference in the relative prevalence of the major food allergens [16]. New plant-origin food allergens derived from seeds (mustard, sesame and sunflower), chickpea, buckwheat, as well as those associated with the fruit-latex and *Prunoideae* groups, have recently been reviewed, reflecting an increased awareness of food hypersensitivity [17].

Cow's milk allergy (CMA) can be regarded as a model of food allergy as cow's milk is usually one of the first food proteins that infants are exposed to [18]. Furthermore, hypersensitivity to multiple food items is common in infants with CMA [2, 19]. Prevalence studies from Sweden [3], Denmark [4] and the Netherlands [5] demonstrated a prevalence for CMA of 1.9–2.8%. Prevalence figures from Australia were similar [6].

A recent random telephone survey of Americans revealed a self-reported prevalence of peanut allergy of 1.1% [9]. However, reliance on self-report may be prone to overestimate the true prevalence of food allergy [20]. Based on the Isle of Wight birth cohort studies, Grundy et al. [8] compared the prevalence of peanut allergy in 2 birth cohorts less than a decade apart. That study reported a significant increase in sensitization to peanut, from 1.1% in 1989 to 3.3% in 1994–1996 ($p = 0.001$). Of the 41 sensitized children, 10 had convincing

Table 2. Common food allergens [15]

Food item	Protein	Molecular mass, M_r
Cow's milk	Caseins	
	α_1-Casein	27,000
	α_2-Casein	23,000
	β-Casein	24,000
	κ-Casein	19,000
	γ-Casein	21,000
	Whey proteins	
	β-Lactoglobulin	36,000
	α-Lactalbumin	14,400
	Bovine serum albumin	69,000
Egg white	Ovomucoid (Gal d 1)	28,000
	Ovalbumin (Gal d 2)	45,000
	Ovotransferrin/conalbumin (Gal d 3)	77,000
	Lysozyme (Gal d 4)	14,300
Peanut	Vicilin (Ara h 1)	63,500
	Conglutin (Ara h 2)	17,500
	Glycinin (Ara h 3)	56,000
Soybean	Gly m 1	34,000
	Trypsin inhibitor	20,500

Modified from Burks et al. [15].

clinical reactions, 5 had no reaction on previous exposure, and 16 were tolerant on subsequent challenge. Only 8 of 24 children reacted clinically on food challenge. The prevalence of peanut allergy was 18/1,246 (1.5%), compared with 0.5% in the previous cohort [7]. This represents a significant prevalence increase ($p = 0.02$). These data, however, need to be interpreted cautiously as the 10 children with clinical reactions had not been rechallenged. Furthermore, the overall recruitment rate of 43% is relatively low, and patients with clinically evident peanut allergy may have been overrepresented due to selection bias. This highlights the importance of differentiating between IgE food sensitization (based on skin-prick test, SPT or radioallergosorbent test, RAST) and clinical hypersensitivity (based on food challenge). The reason for the 3-fold increase in sensitization is unclear; apart from a real prevalence increase, differences in methodology, such as an increased potency of SPT extracts or diagnostic sensitivity of food-specific IgE assays, should be considered.

The Changing Clinical Profile of Food Allergy

The Melbourne Milk Allergy Study (MMAS) described a diverse group of clinical symptoms and syndromes that could be demonstrated by dietary

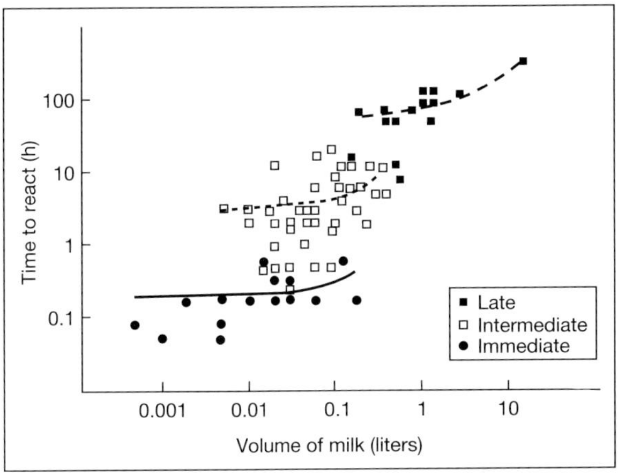

Fig. 1. Onset of reactions in CMA [2]. The time to onset of reactions is plotted against the volume of milk ingested. The 3 groups are indicated by the different symbols. The second-degree polynomial, the line of best fit for each of the groups, is shown. Reproduced with permission from Hill et al. [2].

challenge [12]. These ranged from anaphylaxis and urticaria occurring within minutes of challenge, to distress, vomiting and diarrhea within hours, and exacerbations of AD as well as gastrointestinal or respiratory symptoms occurring after 24 h of ingesting cow's milk. Analysis of these data identified 3 clinical groups with different immunological correlates (fig. 1).

The first group, the immediate reactors, developed acute skin rashes, including peri-oral erythema, facial angioedema, urticaria and pruritus at eczema sites, with or without signs of anaphylaxis. Patients in this group typically had high levels of cow's milk-specific IgE antibodies, detected either in vitro by RAST, or in vivo by SPT. The second, the intermediate reactors, group had reactions occurring from 1 to 24 h after ingestion of milk; they had predominantly gastrointestinal symptoms, including vomiting and diarrhea. As a group, these patients did not exhibit features of IgE sensitization. The third, late reactors, group developed symptoms from 24 h to 5 days after commencement of the challenge procedure; these patients presented with exacerbations of AD, cough, wheeze and/or diarrhea. Varying degrees of IgE sensitization were seen in those with AD. Subsequent studies have demonstrated that this group had greater levels of T-cell sensitization to milk than the immediate or intermediate reactors or control children [12, 21–23].

International agreement has been reached on a classification of gastrointestinal disorders due to adverse immune reactions to foods [24, 25] (table 3). This classification of food allergy syndromes was based on clinical

Table 3. Classification of gastrointestinal food hypersensitivity reactions [25]

IgE-mediated disorders
Immediate food hypersensitivity (IFS)
Oral allergy syndrome
Mixed IgE and non-IgE-mediated disorders
Allergic eosinophilic esophagitis, gastritis, enterocolitis
Non-IgE-mediated disorders
Dietary protein enterocolitis, dietary protein proctitis, dietary protein enteropathy

observations. In table 4, the relationship between the different clinical syndromes identified in the MMAS is shown in relation to the clinical syndromes described by the international group as well as various in vitro markers.

Since our initial studies, the clinical spectrum of CMA has been further expanded. First, Carroccio et al. [26] described a group of children presenting with very delayed reactions after challenge with cow's milk protein. In their cohort of 86 young children with CMA, 10 patients reacted 4–26 days after rechallenge with cow's milk. Symptoms included constipation, persistent wheeze or AD exacerbations [26]. Second, Caffarelli and Petroccione [27] reported on a small group of children with CMA who had apparent 'false-negative' immediate food challenges to cow's milk; however, on subsequent exposure on the day following their initial challenge they developed symptoms of immediate anaphylactic hypersensitivity. A similar phenomenon was observed in a small group of children in the MMAS [12].

CMA in infancy usually resolves around 12–24 months of age [18]. Høst and Halken [4] demonstrated the development of tolerance to cow's milk in 56% of infants with CMA at 1 year, 77% at 2 years, and 87% at 3 years. However, CMA may persist to adult life. Kokkonen et al. [28, 29] recently described a group of school-aged children with CMA in infancy in whom noncharacteristic gastrointestinal symptoms persisted to 10 years of age, suggestive of residual cow's milk-sensitive enteropathy. These patients may often tolerate small amounts of cow's milk protein but often limit their intake of dairy products. There was evidence of mucosal T-cell activation on small bowel biopsy [28]. The mechanisms leading to persistent non-IgE CMA hypersensitivity are poorly understood. Järvinen et al. [30] have hypothesized that sensitization to specific epitopes of several cow's milk proteins may be associated with long-term persistence of CMA.

The spectrum of immunological markers associated with CMA has been expanded. As mentioned above, non-IgE-mediated mechanisms may play an important pathophysiological role in infants with CMA [12], although some of these apparent non-IgE phenomena may be mucosal IgE- and eosinophil-driven [31]. In addition, eotaxin has recently been identified as an important

Table 4. The current spectrum of food allergy syndromes in relation to those identified by the Melbourne Milk Allergy Study

Challenge feature	Incidence	Clinical syndrome	In vitro association
Reaction time <1 h (immediate)			
Anaphylaxis	29	Immediate food hypersensitivity	IgE [1]
Urticaria	10		Histamine [1]
Angioedema	13		CLA + T cells [59]
Morbilliform eczematous eruptions	6		
Stridor	4		
Wheeze	29		
Perioral urticaria	26	Oral allergy syndrome	Mucosal IgE sensitization [1]
Reaction time 1–24 h (intermediate)			
Vomiting	41	Eosinophilic esophagitis, gastritis duodenitis	↑TNFα, ↓TGFβ [60]
Diarrhea	48	Enterocolitis (FPIES)	IgA deficiency, rotavirus infection [61]
Colitis	4		Enhanced T cell reactivity [13]
Perianal eruptions	1		
Functional intestinal obstruction	3		
Reaction time >24 h (late)			
Severe failure to thrive	22	Multiple food protein intolerance of infancy	Enhanced T-cell reactivity [13]
Gastroesophageal reflux (severe)	6	Gastroesophageal reflux disease	Patch test [58], Eotaxin, IL-5 [56]
Persistent crying/distress	14	Colic	Mucosal IgE sensitivity [62]
Atopic dermatitis	13	Atopic dermatitis	Patch test [23], CLA + T cells [63]

mediator in the induction of tissue eosinophilia in gastrointestinal food antigen-associated disorders, such as eosinophilic esophagitis [32]. Schade et al. [33] recently provided evidence of T-cell activation in infants with CMA and AD. Infants with AD had evidence of specific T-helper (Th) cell reactivity to major cow's milk proteins. However, infants with AD and CMA showed a Th2-predominant cytokine profile (high levels of interleukin (IL)-4, IL-5 and IL-13) whereas those without CMA had a Th1-skewed response with high levels of interferon-γ (IFN-γ), as well as low levels of IL-4, IL-5 and IL-13. That study inferred that antigen-specific Th2 cells mediate the skin manifestations of AD in children with CMA [33].

Multiple Food Protein Intolerance of Infancy

Over a 10-year period, the Melbourne Food Allergy Study identified 60 infants allergic to cow's milk, soy and extensively hydrolyzed formula, as well as to several other major food allergens, including egg, wheat, peanut and fish. A significant clinical problem of these infants was the difficulty in maintaining adequate nutrition because of their intolerance to multiple food proteins. We called this syndrome 'multiple food protein intolerance of infancy' [34]. These infants need to be distinguished from infants with 'oligo-food hypersensitivity' who may be intolerant to common food proteins but usually tolerate soy and extensively hydrolyzed formulae.

In our initial study which defined multiple food protein intolerance, patients presented with symptoms of irritability (colic), vomiting and distress (reflux esophagitis), AD and growth failure which persisted despite trials of hypoallergenic formulae [34]. All infants had remained symptomatic while ingesting soy, extensively hydrolyzed casein-based (EHCF) or extensively hydrolyzed whey-based formula (EHWF). In 16, symptoms developed while being exclusively breast-fed. Remission of symptoms occurred within 2 weeks of commencing an amino acid-based formula. Hypoallergenic solids, including rice, potato, pumpkin, zucchini, apple, pear, chicken and lamb were sequentially added to the diet at 2- to 4-week intervals. On subsequent double-blind placebo-controlled food challenge, 12 infants were found intolerant to EHCF (n = 4), EHWF (n = 2) or soy (n = 6). Of these 12 intolerant infants, 2 developed immediate hypersensitivity reactions to soy which they previously appeared to tolerate while suffering severe AD. The remaining 10 patients developed slowly evolving reactions over 4–7 days. In 6 infants, food challenges demonstrated the development of tolerance to soy milk (n = 1), cow's milk (n = 1), EHCF (n = 2) and EHWF (n = 2).

One surprising feature was the reported frequency of adverse reactions to a number of low-allergen foods, including rice, vegetables, fruits, chicken and lamb. On average, adverse reactions to 6 of 10 low-allergen foods were documented for each patient. Follow-up to the age of 3 years has shown that most of the patients tolerated these low-allergen foods by the age of 2 years, and by the age of 3 years only 3 required ongoing nutritional support with amino acid-based formula [35]. Vanderhoof et al. [36] and de Boissieu et al. [37] have reported similar data for infants with this disorder.

Infantile Colic

Infantile colic, i.e. unexplained paroxysms of crying or fussing, affects between 15 and 40% of infants in the first 4 months of life. The role of dietary factors in colic is controversial. In our initial study, the effect of dietary change was prospectively evaluated in 38 bottle-fed and 77 breast-fed 'colicky' infants, referred from community-based pediatric facilities [38]. Bottle-fed infants were assigned to either casein hydrolysate (EHCF) or cow's milk formula. All mothers of breast-fed infants were started on an artificial color-free, preservative-free, additive-free diet and, in addition, randomized to either a low-allergen diet (milk-, egg-, wheat-, and nut-free) or a control diet.

The response to diet was assessed on day 1 and day 8 using a previously validated infant distress chart on which parents recorded distress levels [39]. If a successful outcome was defined as a reduction in distress of 25% or more, infants on active diet had a significantly higher rate of improvement than those on the control diet (OR = 2.32; 95% CI 1.07, 5.0; p = 0.03). Analysis of the day 8/day 1 distress ratio, showed infants on the active diet reduced distress by 39% (95% CI 26, 50) compared with 16% (95% CI 0, 30) for those on the control diet (p = 0.012). The treatment effect was greatest in breast-fed infants less than 6 weeks of age.

In order to examine the role of dietary change in infants with colic under 6 weeks of age, an open pilot study was conducted [40]. Mothers of 17 breast-fed colicky infants less than 6 weeks of age were commenced on low-allergen diets for 2 weeks. The low-allergen diet had previously been used in the Melbourne Colic Study, but in order to ensure a sufficient maternal energy and protein intake, the diet was supplemented by an amino acid-based preparation, Elemental 028 (SHS, Liverpool, UK). Of 17 patients, 13 reduced distressed behavior by more than 25% over the 2-week study period. Seven of them demonstrated relapse of distressed behavior within 24 h of the maternal diet being normalized. The significance of these findings has now been tested prospectively (personal observation, unpublished data).

Atopic Dermatitis

AD is a chronic relapsing inflammatory disease of the skin associated with increased serum IgE levels, allergen sensitization and a family history of atopy [41]. Based on data generated from the Melbourne Atopy Cohort Study (MACS), we estimated that 27% of infants will develop AD, and 9.4% of infants have at least moderately severe disease. The role of hypersensitivity to dietary antigens in the induction and maintenance of this chronic inflammatory response is controversial. An expert panel of American pediatric dermatologists recently concluded, 'food allergy affects only a minority of AD patients' [42]. Hanifin [43] estimated that only 10% of children with AD have food allergy contributing to their disease, whereas Sampson [44] reported that 74% of highly selected children with AD deteriorated on formal food challenge. This association has been dismissed as reflecting patient selection bias [45].

In the MACS birth cohort of 620 children with a positive family history of atopy, we prospectively investigated the association between the level of sensitization to common food allergens (cow's milk, egg, peanut) and the presence of AD [46]. In addition, we compared the frequency of IgE food allergy and AD in the MACS children with AD (MACS AD+), without AD (MACS AD−) and in a group of consecutively referred infants of similar age

Table 5. Frequency of IgE-mediated food allergy in infants with and without atopic dermatitis (AD)

Number of food items subjects were allergic to[a]	6 months of age						12 months of age					
	MACS AD−[b]		MACS AD+[b]		severe AD[c]		MACS AD−[b]		MACS AD+[b]		severe AD[c]	
	n	%	n	%	n	%	n	%	n	%	n	%
0	382	95	97	78	7	17	350	89	77	64	10	35
1	16	4	24	19	13	32	31	8	31	26	10	34
2	4	1	3	2	13	32	13	3	11	9	5	17
3	0		1	1	8	20	0		2	2	4	2
Total	20	5	28	22	34	83	44	11	44	37	19	65
Cases in total	402		125		41		394		121		29	

Reproduced with permission from Hill et al. [2].
[a] IgE-mediated food allergy (SPT >3+) to 1, 2 or 3 foods.
[b] MACS = Melbourne Atopy Cohort Study subjects.
[c] This represents a separate group of infants with severe atopic dermatitis treated in a tertiary referral hospital outpatient clinic.

with severe AD (table 5). IgE-food allergy to egg, milk and peanut was diagnosed by measuring SPT wheal diameters to extracts of these substances and selecting the 'derivative gold standard' wheal diameter associated with 100% specificity for a positive challenge reaction [47].

For the MACS AD+ cohort, IgE-food allergy to cow's milk, egg or peanut was significantly more prevalent than for those without AD (MACS AD−), both at 6 months (22 vs. 5%, RR 4.5 (95% CI 2.8, 7.3) $p < 10^{-6}$) and 12 months of age (35 vs. 11%, RR 3.1 (95% CI 2.4, 4.4) $p < 10^{-6}$). The calculated attributable risk percent for IgE-mediated food allergy as a cause of AD was 65% (95% CI 53, 74) and 62% (95% CI 49, 72), respectively. In the separate group of infants with severe AD, the equivalent degree of IgE-food allergy was 83% at 6 months, and 65% at 12 months. In addition, table 5 demonstrates the number of children in each group who were allergic to 1, 2 or 3 of the food items cow's milk, egg or peanut. As the severity of AD increased across the groups so did the number of these 3 foods to which children showed IgE-mediated food allergy, i.e. the more severe the AD the greater the number of foods to which the children showed IgE-food allergy.

The probability that the association between IgE-mediated food allergy and AD was due to chance was calculated to be less than one in a million and could not be attributed to a number of putative confounding factors previously implicated in the development of atopic diseases in childhood [46]. A strength of association of this magnitude, taken together with evidence from studies showing an improvement in AD with food avoidance and exacerbations with relevant food exposure [44], and an animal model of low-dose food antigen-induced eczematous eruptions with immunological features resembling human AD [48], further supports such a causal relationship. Based on these results, most infantile eczema is due to an IgE-mediated adverse reaction to foods. Management of infantile AD at both the individual and community level should incorporate appropriate diagnostic and dietary strategies.

Gastroesophageal Reflux and Esophagitis

The term gastroesophageal reflux (GER) describes the involuntary passage of gastric contents above the lower esophageal sphincter. GER is common during infancy and is considered pathological if it causes esophagitis, failure to thrive or respiratory symptoms. The majority of infants outgrow GER by 12–18 months of age. GER has traditionally been considered a primary motility disorder. Several recent studies have suggested a causal relationship between CMA and GER in infancy [49]. In a large study involving 204 infants with GER and esophagitis, more than 40% of the patients had evidence of CMA and improved symptomatically on hydrolyzed formula [50]. Electrophysiological studies in infants with CMA have demonstrated gastric motility disturbances following ingestion of cow's milk [51], making an association of food allergies and GER plausible.

It is commonly assumed that esophagitis is the direct result of acid-peptic injury due to prolonged acid exposure to the distal esophagus. In a recent study, however, we found only poor diagnostic agreement between esophageal histological findings and distal esophageal acidification, as measured by esophageal 24-hour pH monitoring. This suggested a non-acid-peptic etiology of esophagitis in some of these infants [52, 53]. In 2 previous studies we have demonstrated that esophagitis, gastritis and duodenitis were common in infants with food intolerances [52, 53]. Esophagitis in infancy may therefore be part of an allergic upper gastrointestinal inflammatory reaction.

In older children and adults with eosinophilic esophagitis who had failed to respond to standard antireflux medication or fundoplication, treatment with amino acid-based formula [54] or corticosteroids was effective in reducing symptoms and histological findings [55]. Butt et al. [56] have recently demonstrated a lymphocytic infiltrate and upregulated mucosal expression of eotaxin in children with cow's milk-associated eosinophilic esophagitis. Similarly, Straumann et al. [57] found evidence of Th2 lymphocyte activation in patients with eosinophilic esophagitis, suggestive of underlying allergies. Recent studies by Spergel et al. [58] have also suggested that allergies to cow's milk, egg, and wheat, as detected by SPT or patch testing, were common in children with eosinophilic esophagitis. Of 24 patients with eosinophilic esophagitis, 18 had a complete and 6 a partial resolution of their symptoms after allergen elimination.

Conclusion

Although it has been suggested that the prevalence of food allergies is increasing in industrialized countries, there are currently no population-based studies available to firmly assess a change in prevalence. This is mainly due to the significant methodological difficulties in performing prevalence studies on IgE and non-IgE-mediated food allergies. There is some recent evidence of an increase in the prevalence of peanut allergy. In general, the spectrum of the major food allergens in childhood seems to have remained unchanged over the past decade. However, several new plant-origin food allergens have recently been reported, probably reflecting an increased awareness of food allergic manifestations. Our understanding of the immunology and clinical presentations of food allergies is evolving. Apart from the 'classic' IgE-mediated immediate-type manifestations, including urticaria and angioedema, a spectrum of delayed-onset, non-IgE-mediated manifestations of food allergy has been recognized. In infancy, these delayed-onset manifestations may be mediated via antigen-specific activated T-helper cells. The exact mechanisms require further investigation. Common pediatric presentations, such as AD, infantile colic and gastroesophageal reflux are closely associated with food hypersensitivity and respond to dietary elimination. These manifestations from the expanded spectrum of food allergies may affect up to 30% of infants and call for a public health approach in the prevention and treatment of food allergy in infancy. Education of health professionals and parents about the spectrum of food allergic disorders will facilitate the early diagnosis and appropriate management of these conditions and may provide significant cost savings to the health care budget.

References

1 Kay AB: Allergy and allergic diseases. First of two parts. N Engl J Med 2001;344:30–37.
2 Hill DJ, Hosking CS, Heine RG: Clinical spectrum of food allergy in children in Australia and South-East Asia: Identification and targets for treatment. Ann Med 1999;31:272–281.
3 Jakobsson I, Lindberg T: A prospective study of cow's milk protein intolerance in Swedish infants. Acta Paediatr Scand 1979;68:853–859.
4 Høst A, Halken S: A prospective study of cow milk allergy in Danish infants during the first 3 years of life. Clinical course in relation to clinical and immunological type of hypersensitivity reaction. Allergy 1990;45:587–596.
5 Schrander JJP, van den Bogart JPH, Forget PP, et al: Cow's milk protein intolerance in infants under 1 year of age: A prospective epidemiological study. Eur J Pediatr 1993;152:640–644.
6 Hill DJ, Hosking CS, Zhie CY, et al: The frequency of food allergy in Australia and Asia. Environ Toxicol Pharmacol 1997;4:101–110.
7 Tariq SM, Stevens M, Matthews S, et al: Cohort study of peanut and tree nut sensitisation by age of 4 years. BMJ 1996;313:514–517.
8 Grundy J, Matthews S, Bateman B, et al: Rising prevalence of allergy to peanut in children: Data from 2 sequential cohorts. J Allergy Clin Immunol 2002;110:784–789.
9 Sicherer SH, Muñoz-Furlong A, Burks AW, Sampson HA: Prevalence of peanut and tree nut allergy in the US determined by a random digit dial telephone survey. J Allergy Clin Immunol 1999;103:559–562.

10 Bock SA: Prospective appraisal of complaints of adverse reactions to foods in children during the first 3 years of life. Pediatrics 1987;79:683–688.
11 Shek LP, Lee BW: Food allergy in children – the Singapore story. Asian Pac J Allergy Immunol 1999;17:203–206.
12 Hill DJ, Firer MA, Shelton MJ, Hosking CS: Manifestations of milk allergy in infancy: Clinical and immunologic findings. J Pediatr 1986;109:270–276.
13 Sampson HA: Food allergy. Part 1: Immunopathogenesis and clinical disorders. J Allergy Clin Immunol 1999;103:717–728.
14 Sampson HA, McCaskill CC: Food hypersensitivity and atopic dermatitis: Evaluation of 113 patients. J Pediatr 1985;107:669–675.
15 Burks W, Helm R, Stanley S, Bannon GA: Food allergens. Curr Opin Allergy Clin Immunol 2001;1:243–248.
16 Ellman LK, Chatchatee P, Sicherer SH, Sampson HA: Food hypersensitivity in two groups of children and young adults with atopic dermatitis evaluated a decade apart. Pediatr Allergy Immunol 2002;13:295–298.
17 Pastorello EA, Pravettoni V, Calamari AM, et al: New plant-origin food allergens. Allergy 2002; 57(suppl 72):106–110.
18 Heine RG, Elsayed S, Hosking CS, Hill DJ: Cow's milk allergy in infancy. Curr Opin Allergy Clin Immunol 2002;2:217–225.
19 Zeiger RS, Sampson HA, Bock SA, et al: Soy allergy in infants and children with IgE-associated cow's milk allergy. J Pediatr 1999;134:614–622.
20 Eggesbø M, Botten G, Halvorsen R, Magnus P: The prevalence of CMA/CMPI in young children: The validity of parentally perceived reactions in a population-based study. Allergy 2001; 56:393–402.
21 Firer MA, Hosking CS, Hill DJ: Humoral immune response to cow's milk in children with cow's milk allergy. Relationship to the time of clinical response to cow's milk challenge. Int Arch Allergy Appl Immunol 1987;84:173–177.
22 Hill DJ, Ball G, Hosking CS, Wood PR: Gamma-interferon production in cow milk allergy. Allergy 1993;48:75–80.
23 Isolauri E, Turjanmaa K: Combined skin prick and patch testing enhances identification of food allergy in infants with atopic dermatitis. J Allergy Clin Immunol 1996;97:9–15.
24 Sampson HA, Sicherer SH, Birnbaum AH: AGA technical review on the evaluation of food allergy in gastrointestinal disorders. American Gastroenterological Association. Gastroenterology 2001; 120:1026–1040.
25 Sampson HA, Anderson JA: Summary and recommendations: Classification of gastrointestinal manifestations due to immunologic reactions to foods in infants and young children. J Pediatr Gastroenterol Nutr 2000;30(suppl):S87–S94.
26 Carroccio A, Montalto G, Crusto N, et al: Evidence of very delayed clinical reactions to cow's milk in cow's milk-intolerant patients. Allergy 2000;55:574–579.
27 Caffarelli C, Petroccione T: False-negative food challenges in children with suspected food allergy. Lancet 2001;358:1871–1872.
28 Kokkonen J, Haapalahti M, Laurila K, et al: Cow's milk protein-sensitive enteropathy at school age. J Pediatr 2001;139:797–803.
29 Kokkonen J, Tikkanen S, Savilahti E: Residual intestinal disease after milk allergy in infancy. J Pediatr Gastroenterol Nutr 2001;32:156–161.
30 Järvinen K-M, Chatchatee P, Bardina L, et al: IgE and IgG binding epitopes on alpha-lactalbumin and beta-lactoglobulin in cow's milk allergy. Int Arch Allergy Immunol 2001;126:111–118.
31 Caffarelli C, Romanini E, Caruana P, et al: Clinical food hypersensitivity: The relevance of duodenal immunoglobulin E-positive cells. Pediatr Res 1998;44:485–490.
32 Hogan SP, Foster PS, Rothenberg ME: Experimental analysis of eosinophil-associated gastrointestinal diseases. Curr Opin Allergy Clin Immunol 2002;2:239–248.
33 Schade RP, Ieperen-Van Dijk AG, Van Reijsen FC, et al: Differences in antigen-specific T-cell responses between infants with atopic dermatitis with and without cow's milk allergy: Relevance of TH2 cytokines. J Allergy Clin Immunol 2000;106:1155–1162.
34 Hill DJ, Cameron DJ, Francis DE, et al: Challenge confirmation of late-onset reactions to extensively hydrolyzed formulas in infants with multiple food protein intolerance. J Allergy Clin Immunol 1995;96:386–394.
35 Hill DJ, Heine RG, Cameron DJ, et al: The natural history of intolerance to soy and extensively hydrolyzed formula in infants with multiple food protein intolerance. J Pediatr 1999;135:118–121.

36 Vanderhoof JA, Murray ND, Kaufman SS, et al: Intolerance to protein hydrolysate infant formulas: An underrecognized cause of gastrointestinal symptoms in infants. J Pediatr 1997; 131:741–744.
37 de Boissieu D, Matarazzo P, Dupont C: Allergy to extensively hydrolyzed cow milk proteins in infants: Identification and treatment with an amino acid-based formula. J Pediatr 1997;131: 744–747.
38 Hill DJ, Hudson IL, Sheffield LJ, et al: A low allergen diet is a significant intervention in infantile colic: Results of a community-based study. J Allergy Clin Immunol 1995;96:886–892.
39 Hill DJ, Menahem S, Hudson I, et al: Charting infant distress: An aid to defining colic. J Pediatr 1992;121:755–758.
40 Hill DJ, Hosking CS: Infantile colic and food hypersensitivity. J Pediatr Gastroenterol Nutr 2000;30(suppl):S67–S76.
41 Leung DY, Bieber T: Atopic dermatitis. Lancet 2003;361:151–160.
42 Halbert AR, Weston WL, Morelli JG: Atopic dermatitis: Is it an allergic disease? J Am Acad Dermatol 1995;33:1008–1018.
43 Hanifin JM: Atopic dermatitis in infants and children. Pediatr Clin North Am 1991;38:763–789.
44 Sampson HA: Food sensitivity and the pathogenesis of atopic dermatitis. J R Soc Med 1997; 90(suppl 30):2–8.
45 Hanifin JM: Critical evaluation of food and mite allergy in the management of atopic dermatitis. J Dermatol 1997;24:495–503.
46 Hill DJ, Sporik R, Thorburn J, Hosking CS: The association of atopic dermatitis in infancy with immunoglobulin E food sensitization. J Pediatr 2000;137:475–479.
47 Sporik R, Hill DJ, Hosking CS: Specificity of allergen skin testing in predicting positive open food challenges to milk, egg and peanut in children. Clin Exp Allergy 2000;30:1540–1546.
48 Li XM, Kleiner G, Huang CK, et al: Murine model of atopic dermatitis associated with food hypersensitivity. J Allergy Clin Immunol 2001;107:693–702.
49 Salvatore S, Vandenplas Y: Gastroesophageal reflux and cow milk allergy: Is there a link? Pediatrics 2002;110:972–984.
50 Iacono G, Carroccio A, Cavataio F, et al: Gastroesophageal reflux and cow's milk allergy in infants: A prospective study. J Allergy Clin Immunol 1996;97:822–827.
51 Ravelli AM, Tobanelli P, Volpi S, Ugazio AG: Vomiting and gastric motility in infants with cow's milk allergy. J Pediatr Gastroenterol Nutr 2001;32:59–64.
52 Hill DJ, Heine RG, Cameron DJ, et al: Role of food protein intolerance in infants with persistent distress attributed to reflux esophagitis. J Pediatr 2000;136:641–647.
53 Heine RG, Cameron DJS, Chow CW, et al: Esophagitis in infants with persistent distress: Poor diagnostic agreement between pH monitoring and histopathological findings. J Pediatr 2002; 140:14–19.
54 Kelly KJ, Lazenby AJ, Rowe PC, et al: Eosinophilic esophagitis attributed to gastroesophageal reflux: Improvement with an amino acid-based formula. Gastroenterology 1995;109:1503–1512.
55 Liacouras CA, Wenner WJ, Brown K, Ruchelli E: Primary eosinophilic esophagitis in children: Successful treatment with oral corticosteroids. J Pediatr Gastroenterol Nutr 1998;26:380–385.
56 Butt AM, Murch SH, Ng CL, et al: Upregulated eotaxin expression and T cell infiltration in the basal and papillary epithelium in cows' milk associated reflux oesophagitis. Arch Dis Child 2002;87:124–130.
57 Straumann A, Bauer M, Fischer B, et al: Idiopathic eosinophilic esophagitis is associated with a TH2-type allergic inflammatory response. J Allergy Clin Immunol 2001;108:954–961.
58 Spergel JM, Beausoleil JL, Mascarenhas M, Liacouras CA: The use of skin prick tests and patch tests to identify causative foods in eosinophilic esophagitis. J Allergy Clin Immunol 2002; 109:363–368.
59 Beyer K, Castro R, Feidel C, Sampson HA: Milk-induced urticaria is associated with the expansion of T cells expressing cutaneous lymphocyte antigen. J Allergy Clin Immunol 2002;109: 688–693.
60 Chung HL, Hwang JB, Park JJ, Kim SG: Expression of transforming growth factor beta1, transforming growth factor type I and II receptors, and TNF-alpha in the mucosa of the small intestine in infants with food protein-induced enterocolitis syndrome. J Allergy Clin Immunol 2002;109:150–154.
61 Firer MA, Hosking CS, Hill DJ: Possible role for rotavirus in the development of cows' milk enteropathy in infants. Clin Allergy 1988;18:53–61.

62 Chung HL, Hwang JB, Kwon YD, et al: Deposition of eosinophil-granule major basic protein and expression of intercellular adhesion molecule-1 and vascular cell adhesion molecule-1 in the mucosa of the small intestine in infants with cow's milk-sensitive enteropathy. J Allergy Clin Immunol 1999;103:1195–1201.
63 Abernathy-Carver KJ, Sampson HA, Picker LJ, Leung DY: Milk-induced eczema is associated with the expansion of T cells expressing cutaneous lymphocyte antigen. J Clin Invest 1995;95: 913–918.

Discussion

Dr. Bindslev-Jensen: I think you demonstrated very beautifully that when you really try to dig down into what the patients present with, then you come up with different fingerprints or phenotypes or whatever. I still have a problem with these late-phase reactors. Could you clarify when you define patients with cow's milk allergies as late-phase reactors? Are they those who only react on the 3rd day of challenge but perhaps 1 h after you gave the last challenge? So they are the least sensitive patients. The way I interpret your data is that you have a scheme where you start on day 1 with minute amounts and then you increase over the next 2 days until the top dose of normal daily feeding has been reached. Those you call late reactors are the patients who are the least sensitive, meaning that they only react to the dose given on the 3rd day, which means 3 days after commencement of challenges but perhaps 1 or 2 h after the last dose given. So they react acutely within 1 or 2 h but 3 days after challenge was started.

Dr. Hill: The patients who reacted within 1 or 2 hours of cow milk challenge but after continuing ingesting cow milk for 3 days were classified as late reactors. This phenomenon of acute urticaria after ingesting a food for several days has been attributed to priming [1]. It is not uncommon.

Dr. Bindslev-Jensen: But then the late reactors have time to react, 100 h. Is that 100 h after the last dose given?

Dr. Hill: No. In this study reactions were timed from the first dose challenge on Day 1.

Dr. Bindslev-Jensen: So it is 100 h from start. They might react 2 h after the last dose given. They are still very slightly sensitive, but acute phase reactors.

Dr. Hill: Yes. Children who reacted within minutes or hours, particularly with urticaria, several days after repeatedly ingesting the food, are demonstrating the priming phenomenon described by Caffarelli [1].

It is important to understand that our initial classification of immediate, intermediate and late reactors to cow milk was based on a statistical analysis which used a K-means algorithm to group patients with common clinical features [2]. In many other classifications of food reactions, i.e. IgE-mediated and non-IgE mediated, are based on a mechanistic approach [3]. During my presentation I tried to relate the findings and classification of our initial studies on cow milk allergy, which were statistically based, with the more recent international classification of adverse reactions to foods based largely on clinical data [4].

Dr. Guesry: I would like to come back to the colic issue because obviously you think that colic is an allergic disease. Your results are very convincing, particularly the one dealing with the change of diet in the mother, because in the first study the extensive hydrolysate of casein is also lactose-free. I don't mean that lactose is responsible for colic, but lactose could make some symptoms more severe in an intestine that has already been irritated. But if it is an allergic disease, it is very different from the other one because sensitization will take place in fully breast-fed babies with a minute quantity of different types of allergens and, usually without changing anything, within a few weeks, 12–16 weeks, the disease disappears, much faster than for other types of allergic disease.

Dr. Hill: I think you are right. We hypothesize that in a significant number of infants colic is the result of transient food protein intolerance. Several studies have documented levels of dietary proteins in breast milk. These appear capable of eliciting adverse symptoms in sensitized infants. For example, the levels of betalactoglobulin in breast milk in mothers ingesting normal volumes of cow milk are comparable to the levels of betalactoglobulin in extensively hydrolysed casein and whey preparations [5].

Dr. Guesry: I agree with you. I was perhaps on the wrong concept that you need more allergens to sensitize than to start a reaction in an already sensitized baby. That may be wrong, but that is what we have been told for many years. In that case we speak of sensitization because colic starts usually very early in life, so we are still in the period of sensitization.

Dr. Hill: I agree. The process of sensitization probably does require more total antigen exposure (over a prolonged period) than the amount of antigen required to elicit an immediate hypersensitivity reaction. We have in the past attempted to calculate the estimated loading dose of common antigens during the putative period of sensitization. Colic infants appear to have an entirely non-IgE associated disorder and developed symptoms within days of delivery. By contrast, breast fed eczematous infants are usually not distressed, become IgE sensitized and present with symptoms later, i.e. after several weeks if breast fed. Presumably the loading dose of antigen sensitization is less in colic infants than in eczematous infants.

Dr. Szajewska: Can you explain how you define colic in your study?

Dr. Hill: In our initial study we followed the international definition for colic as 3 or more hours of distressed behaviour for more than 3 days per week for more than 3 weeks. However in our recently completed study (the preliminary data was presented today), we were investigating breast fed infants of less than 6 weeks of age. We defined colic as distressed behaviour for more than 3 hours per day for more than 3 days in the week prior to presentation. Data not presented today demonstrated that most of these infants had colic for at least 3 weeks before we saw them. Our initial studies suggested the former definition had a specificity of 80% when validated against parent recorded distressed charts [6].

Dr. Vandenplas: How long does it take for allergens to disappear from mother's milk?

Dr. Hill: I have not conducted studies on that point.

Dr. Isolauri: There have been studies [2–4] demonstrating that if you put the mother on an elimination diet you cannot achieve a zero level with, for instance, antigenic β-lactoglobulin in breast milk. Our data show that maybe other components in breast milk, like fatty acids and so on, play a role there, and since these are accumulated also during pregnancy, doing anything for the breast-feeding mother might be unhelpful.

Dr. Vandenplas: Which fatty acids?

Dr. Isolauri: I will present these data in my talk. For instance the levels of n-3 and n-6 fatty acids and their proportions are important in the risk of developing atopic disease in the infant, and these concentrations are not necessarily associated with the diet of the mother at that time because most of these are derived from the mother's stores which accumulate during pregnancy, only 10, 20, or 30% of the fatty acids are derived from the diet.

Dr. Lack: There is a big debate as to the role of food allergy in eczema and its relative contribution at different ages. You showed this very interesting association with increasing odds ratios between the severity of eczema and food allergy. I think you made the implication that food allergy is a major cause of eczema in the first year of life. I just wanted to point out that one could say the opposite: perhaps it is the eczema that is leading to food allergy, or both might be manifestations of a very abnormal host immune response. Eczema often precedes the development of food allergy and starts at a few months of age. I am not sure one can actually make the assumption that one is causing the other.

Dr. Hill: I am not aware of the data. Are you suggesting challenging an infant at risk of eczema before he shows eczema? He might not have food allergy.

Dr. Lack: I am only saying that just because you show a high association between eczema and food allergy, it doesn't allow us to necessarily conclude that food allergy in the 1st year of life is the main cause of eczema.

Dr. Hill: You are correct. In epidemiological studies we cannot show causation. We can only show strength of association between atopic dermatitis and IgE food allergy. However, if one takes into account DBPC food challenges which have demonstrated relapse of eczema, and recent animal models of food allergy induced eczema, together with our findings, they are sufficient to suggest causation.

Dr. Vandenplas: I have a second question regarding your group of esophagitis patients. How many of those patients have esophagitis as a single manifestation or do most of them have multiple system involvement? Have they also got eczema or other manifestations? If I understand you, most of them have eosinophil infiltration, and therefore it is no longer reflux by definition.

Dr. Hill: The oesophagitis patients did not have multi-system disease. As a group they were non-atopic. The data relating to reflux oesophagitis and eosinophilic oesophagitis is based on report by Heine et al [7]. Re-analysing his data, there was no association between reflux, measured by pH monitoring and eosinophils in the oesophagus.

Dr. Vandenplas: So it is the infiltration with eosinophils which is of major importance, not the reflux time? It is in fact the histological reaction and not the severity of the reflux that you are measuring.

Dr. Hill: To summarise the preliminary findings from our second study on reflux oesophagitis and distressed infants (2003): the infants who had eosinophilic oesophagitis did not respond to the L-amino acid formula diet program as did the other infants. However in this second study of reflux oesophagitis the distressed infants received no medication. By contrast, in our first study [8] all the patients responded to L-amino acid formula; however most were also being treated at the same time with prokinetic agents and/or H2 antagonists.

Dr. Neijens: Can I bring up the issue of the expression of food allergy in the respiratory system? I am thinking about asthma in which food allergy plays an important role. Is this a kind of special disease, can you recognize it, can you diagnose it, if you challenge those patients do you get reactions in the bronchial tree, eosinophilia, etc.; what do we know about the treatment of these children with certain diets, etc?

Dr. Hill: Wheezing in the first 12 months of life is usually not due to food allergy. In 5% of children in the Melbourne Milk Allergy Study respiratory symptoms was the sole manifestation of their milk allergy on challenge. But your question has raised another interesting point. I presented data which examined the relationship of sensitization to cow milk, egg and peanut in the first 12 months of life, to eczema severity. If you look at the level of sensitization to house dust mite, grass pollen and cat dander in the same patients in the first 12 months of life, there is a very good correlation between the level of sensitization to these inhalant allergens and eczema severity. We calculated that for infants who had IgE food allergy to cow milk, egg or peanut and eczema at 12 months, the risk of them having "doctor-diagnosed" asthma at the age of 5 years is increased 5-fold (unpublished data).

Dr. Neijens: But are there children aged 6 or 8 years or in puberty who have severe reactions to food allergens whether or not they are induced by exercise reactions? This seems to be a special group.

Dr. Hill: I understand that you are seeing children with severe reactions to food presenting for the first time in an older age-group. In our studies it is uncommon to see children develop hypersensitivity reactions to foods regularly in the past without difficulty. However several studies have reported older children developing the first manifestations of the oral allergy syndrome associated with hypersensitivity to fruits and vegetables in late adolescence; some of these reactions may be exacerbated by birch pollen and rag weed pollen seasons. We have not had experience with wheat allergy-induced exercise anaphylaxis in our children.

Dr. Marini: From an epidemiological point of view, why have we seen colic more frequently in the first-born child and males? If it is an allergic disease I would expect both, male and female. The second point is, do you have any experience in dosing gastrointestinal hormones in these cases? We have found that, from an allergic point view, the administration of hydrolysate is able to lower the levels of neurotensin and motilin which might explain why these babies do better.

Dr. Hill: I don't have data on the effect of diet exclusion on motilin. Your comments are of other interest; Lothe [9] documented high motilin levels at birth in infants who subsequently developed colic as well as those who had colic at the time of presentation. They documented resolution of colic when their infants were commenced on extensively hydrolysed casein formula but I am not aware of whether they measured motilin levels after remission of colic.

Dr. Marini: We have experience showing that this kind of diet, for instance giving hydrolysate to the mother or the baby, lowers the level of gastrointestinal hormones. So the babies feel well because they have less constriction on the gut.

Dr. Suyoko: My question is from a clinical point of view as a pediatrician. In our daily practice we see patients with infantile colic and gastroesophageal reflux that we think are caused by food allergy or something else. Are there specific food allergy symptoms that these patients suffer from?

Dr. Hill: There are no specific features about the pattern of distress in breast fed colic infants or in infants with gastro-oesophageal reflux which suggested food allergy as the cause of their distress. At a clinical level, if an infant is thriving but demonstrated significant clinical distress, i.e. more than 3 hours of distress per 24 hours, and this is documented on validated infant distress charts, we would be prepared to implement a trial of a low allergen diet program for a breast feeding mother or a L-amino acid formula for a bottle fed infant. Where the infant responds it is critical the child and mother be seen by a nutritionalist to ensure adequate nutrition during the period of diet exclusion.

Dr. Murch: I would argue against the straightforward observations about studies and biopsies. When you use impedance analysis you find that about 80% of the reflux episodes of infants in these age groups are in fact non-acid, and that in the great majority of these you can't exclude ongoing reflux. The second thing is that the advantages themselves may be superficial. Ferruto showed that, in children with eosinophilic esophagitis, when you look at T cells they are actually beneath the epithelium, in the subepithelial stroma, and that of course is where the plexus is going to be situated. A superficial biopsy may look normal, but there may well be significant T-cell-mediated responses going on subjacent to the way you are looking. So in many cases there is no cause to rule allergy in or out.

Dr. Hill: The diagnosis of food allergy depends on the outcome of appropriate double-blind placebo-controlled challenges. I have drawn on your own groups work on eotaxin deposition and note you comment with interest. Perhaps eotaxin mediated activation of eosinophils might be more important to the manifestation and development of food allergy than just the mere presence of eosinophils.

Dr. Murch: Can I just point out also that eosinophils are very pH dependent and there is a 10-fold drop in the pH from 7.6 to 7.0. What is the effect of acid reflux?

Dr. Hill: Clearly this subject needs further investigation.

Dr. Sorensen: Is it known whether the amount of cow's milk that a mother intakes influences the likelihood of the baby becoming sensitized? I ask you this because we are going to discuss oral tolerance, and perhaps the way cow's milk protein in the mother's milk is presented to the baby is similar to partial hydrolysate. It might be important to understand the amount of cow's milk that gets into the mother's milk. When we say stop taking milk, should we not be telling the mother to take more milk, and see if we can brake the cycle of sensitization and induce tolerance?

Dr. Hill: Your question is whether we can induce tolerance to cow's milk in infants by asking mothers to ingest substantial volumes of milk. I am not aware of studies which have examined high dose milk antigen ingestion in mothers influencing subsequent milk allergy in their infants. However there are data suggesting giving babies high dose antigen exposure to milk following delivery did not influence subsequent development of milk allergy and others claiming an adverse effect of such exposure.

References

1 Caffarelli C, Petroccione T: False-negative food challenges in children with suspected food allergy. Lancet 2001;358:1871–1872.

2 Hill DJ, Firea MA, Shelton MJ, Hosking CS: Manifestations of milk allergy in infancy: clinical and immunological findings. J Pediatr 1986;109:270–276.

3 Bruijnzeel-Koomen C, Ortalani C, Aas K et al: Adverse reactions to food. Allergy 1995;50: 623–638.

4 Sampson HA, Anderson JA. Classification of gastrointestinal disease of infants and children due to adverse immunologic reactions to foods. J Pediatr Gastroenterol Nutr 2000; 30 (Supp 1):S87–94.

5 Sorva R, Makinen-Kiljunen S, Juntunen-Backman K: β-Lactoglobulin secretion in human milk varies widely after cow's milk ingestion in mothers of infants with cow's milk allergy. J Allergy Clin Immunol 1994;93:787–792.

6 Hill DJ, Menahem S, Hudson I et al: Charting infant distress: an aid to defining colic. J Pediatr 1992;121:755–758.

7 Heine RG, Cameron DJ, Chow CW, Hill DJ, Catto-Smith AG: Oesophagitis in distress of infants: poor correlation between oesophageal pH monitoring and histological findings. J Pediatr 2002;140:14–19.

8 Hill DJ, Heine RG, Cameron DJ et al: Role of food protein intolerance in infants with persistent distress attributed to reflux oesophagitis. J Pediatr 2000;136:641–647.

9 Lothe L, Ivarsson A, Lindberg T: Motilin, vasoactive intestinal peptide and gastrin in infantile colic. Acta Pediatr Scand 1987;76:316–320.

Isolauri E, Walker WA (eds): Allergic Diseases and the Environment.
Nestlé Nutrition Workshop Series Pediatric Program, Vol. 53, pp. 53–68,
Nestec Ltd.; Vevey/S. Karger AG, Basel, © 2004.

The Hygiene Hypothesis: Modulation of the Atopic Phenotype by Environmental Microbial Exposure

P.G. Holt

Telethon Institute for Child Health Research, and Centre for Child Health Research, Faculty of Medicine and Dentistry, University of Western Australia, Perth, Australia

Introduction

The hygiene hypothesis was first proposed in its present form by Strachan [1] in a landmark publication in 1989, as an explanation for the apparent inverse relationship between family size and/or hygiene, and susceptibility to allergic disease. The subjects studied in this report were from a First-World European country, and hallmark differences were observed between different social groups within the Caucasian population. In particular, low socioeconomic class and large family size was associated with reduced risk for allergic disease. The general mechanism proposed to explain these differences in disease prevalence was based on the supposition that overall levels of microbial exposure were highest amongst the lower socioeconomic groups in the study population. Additionally, the hypothesis proposes that increased microbial exposure during childhood amongst the less affluent population groups, in particular increased exposure to pathogens, serves to divert the attention of the immune system from nonpathogenic environmental allergens, resulting in lower levels of allergic sensitization.

Essentially the same conclusions had been drawn 13 years previously in a study of an indigenous Indian population (the Métis) living under the equivalent of Third-World conditions in northern Canada. Gerrard et al. [2] reported that serum IgE levels were lower in an adjacent white community than within the Métis community, but that expression of allergic disease was much less frequent amongst the Métis. In contrast, severe viral and bacterial infections and parasitism was much more common in the Indian community.

Gerrard et al. [2] presciently suggested that 'atopic disease is the price paid by some members of the white community for their relative freedom from diseases due to viruses, bacteria and helminths'.

Indirect supporting evidence for a protective role for infections in the development of atopy has been provided from epidemiological studies amongst pediatric populations, initially comparing First- and Second-World populations in Europe [3]. However, the potential role of infections, in particular respiratory infections, in this context, is complicated by findings indicating that viruses can play a positive role in triggering exacerbations of allergic diseases (such as atopic asthma) in previously sensitized individuals [4], and in some cases may also promote allergic sensitization. The organism most frequently quoted in this context is respiratory syncytial virus (RSV), the most common respiratory pathogen affecting First-World infants [5], which has also been suggested to selectively boost allergy-associated T-helper type-2 (Th2) immunity via a variety of 'bystander' mechanisms [6, 7].

An alternative suggestion is that the principal microbial drive for stimulation of resistance to allergic sensitization comes not from pathogens, but from the normal commensal flora of the gastrointestinal tract [8]. This suggestion, which derives from a long history of studies comparing physiological (including immunological) functions in germ-free versus microbiologically conventional animals, is discussed in more detail below.

Setting the Scene: The Immunological Basis for Allergic Disease

Current perceptions of the cellular and molecular mechanisms underlying atopy derive from earlier studies in the mouse by Mosmann and Coffman [9], which were subsequently translated into human systems [10, 11]. The key discovery was the existence of reciprocally polarized subpopulations of CD4+ (and subsequently CD8+) Th cells which, after differentiation, become committed to secretion of one of two major combinations of cytokines. These respectively constitute Th1 cells secreting interferon-γ (IFNγ), tumor necrosis factor-α (TNFα) and interleukin (IL)-2, which are predominantly associated with cell-mediated immunity, and Th2 cells secreting IL-4, IL-5, IL-9 and IL-13, which drive humoral immunity. High production of these four Th2 cytokines in allergen-specific recall responses is associated respectively with activation of IgE B cells, eosinophils and tissue mast cells, and IL-13 with effects upon goblet cells and bronchial smooth muscle cells.

The immunological basis for the 'allergen non-responder' phenotype expressed by nonatopics is still a matter of intense debate, and appears to involve both high zone tolerance and low zone tolerance mechanisms. It is clear, however, that for many allergens, unresponsiveness does not equate to 'immunological ignorance', for example by deletional tolerance, as cognate immunity to inhalant allergens such as house dust mite (HDM) is common amongst nonatopics as shown in T-cell cloning studies [10, 11] and in short-term bulk culture studies [12, 13] demonstrating low level Th1-like responses in these subjects.

Initiation of Allergic Sensitization in Early Life

The central issue in understanding the etiology of atopy is how these two contrasting patterns of allergen-specific Th-cell memory, i.e. the Th1 versus Th2 cytokine phenotype, are initially programmed into the naive immune system. Based on the collective experience of many researchers working in animal model systems, it appeared likely to many in this field (including my group), that this programming process was likely to be initiated in early life, when the immature immune system is first confronted with environmental allergens [14]. The question of when that first occurs, at least in an immunologically productive sense, is becoming increasingly complex.

In particular, there is a wide body of data from a growing number of independent laboratories [14–19] which demonstrate the presence in cord blood of T cells which proliferate and/or produce cytokines, in response to coculture with inhalant and food allergens. Moreover, cloning studies on these allergen-responsive cord T cells and subsequent DNA typing of the clones have confirmed the fetal origin of the responder cells [20]. These findings have been widely interpreted, including by our group [15], as supporting the possibility that transplacental transport of environmental allergen, perhaps carried via IgG, may weakly prime the fetal immune system. This possibility is further supported by the demonstration of transplacental allergen 'leakage' in ex vivo perfusion models [21, 22].

However, alternative interpretations are possible, and this question merits further investigation in light of the demonstration of the apparent lack of correlation between maternal exposure to indoor allergens and subsequent sensitization of their offspring [23]. Ongoing experiments in our laboratory (Jones and Holt, to be published) indeed suggest that the responding T cells in these cultures do not mature into conventional CD45RO+ Th-memory cells, and their role may be restricted to acute, short-term cytokine responses to allergen challenge during infancy. Nevertheless, it is also evidence that regardless of the precise nature of these early immune responses, the period between birth and 2 years is one during which major changes occur with respect to T-cell immunity to environmental allergens, and in which immune response patterns are established which appear to determine long-term clinical phenotypes. In particular, responses to inhalant allergens such as HDM progressively increase in magnitude in virtually all children, but at the same time appear to diverge in relation to cytokine production, consolidating into a Th2-like pattern in infants who develop clinical symptomatology versus a more Th1-like pattern in those who remain symptom free [24]. These response patterns, at the population level, suggest the underlying operation of 'low zone tolerance' mechanisms. In contrast, responses to dietary allergens such as ovalbumin (OVA), both at the level of overall proliferation in response to whole OVA and in regard to the number of OVA-specific T-cell epitopes recognized [24, 25], typically decrease rapidly during infancy. This latter pattern is consistent with regulation of responses to dietary allergens via 'high zone tolerance' mechanisms, presumably involving variable combinations of T-cell deletion and T-cell anergy induction.

By the end of the preschool years, the sequelae of these two classes of regulatory processes within the population at large are readily evident from the results of large birth cohort studies. One example of such a study is one involving approximately 2,500 children followed in Perth by our group and our collaborators. By age 6 years, reactivity to dietary allergens such as OVA is restricted to a small group of skin-prick test (SPT) positive atopics which comprise <2% of the population, in contrast to SPT responsiveness to inhalants which is observed in approximately 40% of children [26, 27]. In detailed studies on HDM responses we have demonstrated that cytokine production patterns in these 6-year-olds are of the classical mixed Th1/Th2 (or Th0) type [28], typical of that observed in the majority of atopic adults, whereas those in nonatopics involve a modified form of Th1 immunity comprising low-level production of IFNγ and IL-10.

We have also shown that the size of the HDM-induced skin-prick wheal in HDM-SPT+ atopic 6-year-olds is inversely related to the magnitude of the IL-10 component of their in vitro Th0 responses, which is consistent with a 'feedback inhibitory' role for this anti-inflammatory cytokine [28]. We postulate that production of IL-10 in the Th1-like responses of the nonatopics may be one reason why the IFNγ component of their responses does not result in sufficient inflammation to trigger delayed-type hypersensitivity.

Thus, our findings [20, 25, 26, 28], and those from others in this field [29–31], suggest that long-term sensitization to the clinically most important group of allergens, the inhalants, results from a predilection to development of Th2-polarised immunity to these agents during infancy and/or early childhood. Moreover, risk for development of this form of allergen-specific T-cell memory is highest amongst children with a positive atopic family history (AFH+) [26], indicating the importance of genetic background.

Genetic Risk for Atopy: A Transient Developmental Deficiency in Th1 Function?

T-cell cloning studies from our group in the early 1990s have supplied one plausible mechanism which appears to contribute significantly to genetic risk for early sensitization to inhalants. Notably, it has been recognized for many years that the fetal T-cell system is deficient (relative to adults) in capacity to secrete all classes of cytokines [32, 33], and more recent studies indicate that Th1 cytokine production is preferentially downregulated resulting in a 'Th-2-like state' at the fetomaternal interface [34]. Our cloning studies on infants (mean age 18 months) indicate firstly that this fetal state persists into postnatal life, and moreover that it is exaggerated in AFH+ children who display decreased capacity to mount CD4+ Th-cell cytokine response of both the Th1 and Th2 phenotype, the deficiency being most marked for Th1 cytokines, resulting in an overall 'Th2-skewing' of their immune responses [35]. It is noteworthy that this skewing amongst AFH+ children also occurs in initial immune responses to vaccine antigens such as DTPa [36]. These findings have been independently confirmed by several independent laboratories and extended to studies on cord blood cells [24, 30, 31, 37–40].

The mechanism for this postnatal persistence of the fetal 'Th2-skew' is incompletely understood, and is likely to involve several sets of regulatory factors. Firstly, at the level of the T-cell system, we have recently shown that an important mechanism for negative regulation of the principal Th1 cytokine gene IFNγ during the neonatal period involves hypermethylation of CpG sites in the proximal promoter of this gene [41]. This mechanism in humans is highly selective for CD4+ Th cells [41], and ongoing studies in our laboratory are investigating possible differences between AFH− and AFH+ children.

A second major possibility involves the activity of cells of the innate immune system, in particular the principal antigen-presenting cells which are the dendritic cells (DC). In animal models [42] and in humans [13, 43] DC are known to be deficient in capacity to express Th1-stimulatory cytokine signals during the early postnatal period, which is likely to contribute to the tendency to default to Th2 immunity during this life phase. It is also pertinent to note that DC populations in the airway mucosa (the site of 'sampling' of inhalant allergens) are very slow to develop postnatally, and require environmental stimulation to acquire full competence [for further discussion see, 44].

A third possibility, discussed in more detail below, involves the attenuation in some subjects of a capacity to respond to environmental signals responsible for stimulation of postnatal maturation of Th1 function.

Postnatal Maturation of Adaptive Immune Function: The Role of Microbial Stimuli in Establishing the Th1/Th2 Balance

As noted earlier [8], a long history of careful research in the 1960s–1980s on immune function in germ-free animals has established that postnatal exposure to microbial stimuli, in particular the commensal flora of the gastrointestinal tract, is essential in order to drive the final stages of maturation of 'adult-equivalent' immune competence. It is now clear from experimental studies on expression of immunity at the fetomaternal interface [34] and upon development of tolerance to antigens during early infancy [42, 45] that this late-stage maturation involves preferential upregulation of Th1 function in order to achieve the necessary Th1/Th2 balance.

It has been suggested that a quantitative and/or qualitative reduction in microbial stimulation, involving both commensal flora and pathogens, has occurred in First-World countries over time (i.e. since the 1950s–1960s), and has been sufficient to attenuate (in particular to delay) postnatal maturation of immune function in a subset of 'susceptible' individuals. In particular, improved public health and hygiene practices, especially those which impact upon young children during the period in which their immune systems are developing allergen-specific Th memory, may have reduced overall immune stimulation to levels which (in some cases) are below the critical threshold needed to optimally drive Th1 maturation. This may in turn increase the risk for compartmentalization of allergen-specific Th-memory responses into the Th2-cytokine phenotype in this susceptible subgroup [8, 46–48].

Indirect evidence in support of this general hypothesis has been provided by a series of recent epidemiological studies. Of particular note are studies on the children of northern European farmers who are exposed to very high levels of airborne microbial breakdown products during infancy, and who manifest relative 'resistance' to allergic disease [49], and studies demonstrating an inverse relationship between microbial exposure during infancy in household dust and allergic sensitization [50]. In both cases, microbial exposure was associated with more robust cytokine responsiveness.

Further confirmatory support comes from studies focusing on polymorphisms in genes associated with a capacity to respond to environmental microbial stimuli. In particular, polymorphisms in CD14 [51] and TLR-2 [52], which are likely to reduce responsiveness to microbial stimulation, have been associated with increased susceptibility to severe atopic disease. It is of interest to note in this context that CD14 and the TOLL genes have traditionally been considered to encode receptors which are specific to bacteria. However, recent evidence suggests that several of these receptors also recognize virus-specific motifs, for example one associated with RSV [53]. This latter finding provides direct support for the suggested Th1-stimulatory (and hence atopy-sparing) effects of viral infection in early childhood [3]. However, there is an important caveat which should be applied to this argument, notably the growing evidence that severe respiratory viral infections during infancy may deleteriously influence early postnatal growth and differentiation of lung and airway tissues, producing changes in airway function which can interact synergistically with inhalant allergy later in life, to trigger severe asthma [54, 55]. In this latter scenario, the same genetic predisposition to 'slow postnatal maturation of

Th1 function' which increases risk for allergy, also increases risk for RSV infection [36, 54, 55].

Exploitation of Hygiene Hypothesis Principles for Allergy Prophylaxis: A Potential Double-Edged Sword?

An obvious extrapolation from the findings reviewed above is the possibility for reducing risk of allergy by enhancing levels of early postnatal microbial stimulation, thus boosting/accelerating maturation of Th1 functions. Ongoing studies in many centers employing probiotics [56] or vaccination with nonspecific microbial adjuvants [57] are two high-profile examples of this approach.

While endorsing these approaches, I feel it is necessary to add a note of caution, which is well understood by researchers active in this area but less so by observers from other fields. Notably, while Th1 cytokines play a key role in antagonizing the initial development of Th2-polarized memory, once Th-memory development progresses beyond the early stages, it is common to observe co-expression of both Th1 and Th2 cytokines [28]. Moreover, Th1 cytokines (in particular IFNγ and TNFα) are also potentially highly toxic, and if produced in excessive levels at the 'wrong sites' can contribute to disease pathogenesis. A notable example is autoimmune disease(s) in which pathogenesis is almost invariably Th1-mediated. Moreover, several murine models have been described in which local airway mucosal expression of Th1 immunity to inhaled allergens can trigger a disease which appears identical to atopic asthma [58–60]. Furthermore, evidence from several laboratories suggests that hyperproduction of IFNγ is a hallmark of a significant proportion of atopic children [61–63]. Accordingly, studies involving early boosting of Th1 immunity in infants by any means should include careful monitoring of T-cell function to detect any possible overshoot.

Conclusions

The hygiene hypothesis, in its modern form, has survived as an increasingly viable theory for over a decade [48]. While the precise mechanism(s) underlying the protective effects of microbial agents in relation to the susceptibility to allergy remain to be elucidated, it appears highly plausible that their major effects are likely to be mediated in the developmental context illustrated in figure 1. Thus, the primary targets for microbial stimulation are likely to be cells within the innate immune system such as DC, which require inductive signals via specific receptors such as CD14 and TLR-2 to mature functionally. These cells in turn develop the capacity to 'instruct' the immature T-cell system to efficiently generate

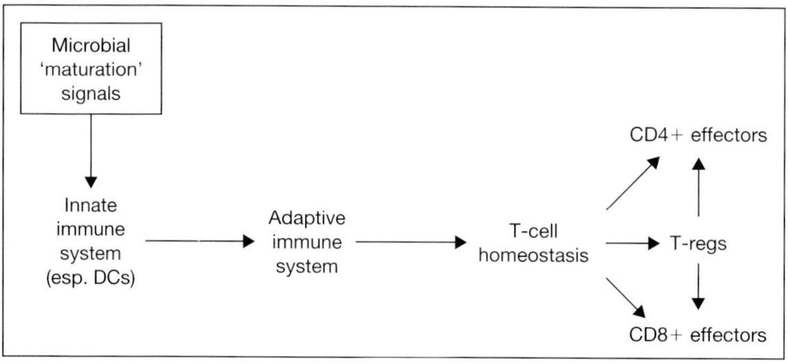

Fig. 1. Sequential microbial-induced maturation of cellular functions in the innate and adaptive arms of the immune system as the mechanistic basis for the hygiene hypothesis.

specific CD4+ and CD8+ Th-memory effector cells required for immune defense, as well as a range of cytokine-secreting T-regulatory cells which maintain an appropriate balance between different effector T-cell subsets in immune responses, hence maintaining overall T-cell homeostasis.

References

1 Strachan DP: Hay fever, hygiene, and household size. BMJ 1989;299:1259–1260.
2 Gerrard JW, Geddes CA, Reggin PL, et al: Serum IgE levels in white and Metis communities in Saskatchewan. Ann Allergy 1976;37:91–100.
3 Martinez FD: Role of viral infections in the inception of asthma and allergies during childhood: Could they be protective? Thorax 1994;49:1189–1191.
4 Johnston SL, Pattemore PK, Sanderson G, et al: The relationship between upper respiratory infections and hospital admissions for asthma: A time-trend analysis. Am J Respir Crit Care Med 1996;154:654–660.
5 Hall CB: Respiratory syncytial virus and parainfluenza virus. N Engl J Med 2001;344:1917–1928.
6 Sparer TE, Matthews S, Hussell T, et al: Eliminating a region of respiratory syncytial virus attachment protein allows induction of protective immunity without vaccine-enhanced lung eosinophilia. J Exp Med 1998;187:1921–1926.
7 Welliver RC, Duffy L: The relationship of RSV-specific immunoglobulin E antibody responses in infancy, recurrent wheezing, and pulmonary function at age 7–8 years. Pediatr Pulmonol 1993;15:19–27.
8 Holt PG: Environmental factors and primary T-cell sensitisation to inhalant allergens in infancy: Reappraisal of the role of infections and air pollution. Pediatr Allergy Immunol 1995;6:1–10.
9 Mosmann TR, Coffman RL: TH1 and TH2 cells: Different patterns of lymphokine secretion lead to different functional properties. Annu Rev Immunol 1989;7:145–173.
10 Romagnani S: Human TH1 and TH2 subsets: Doubt no more. Immunol Today 1991;12:256–257.
11 Wierenga EA, Snoek M, de Groot C, et al: Evidence for compartmentalization of functional subsets of CD4+ T lymphocytes in atopic patients. J Immunol 1990;144:4651–4656.

12 Imada M, Estelle F, Simons R, et al: Allergen-stimulated interleukin-4 and interferon-1 production in primary culture: Responses of subjects with allergic rhinitis and normal controls. Immunology 1995;85:373–380.
13 Upham JW, Lee PT, Holt BJ, et al: Development of interleukin-12-producing capacity throughout childhood. Infect Immun 2002;70:6583–6588.
14 Holt PG: Primary allergic sensitisation to environmental antigens: Perinatal T-cell priming as a determinant of responder phenotype in adulthood. J Exp Med 1996;183:1297–1301.
15 Holt PG, O'Keeffe PO, Holt BJ, et al: T-cell 'priming' against environmental allergens in human neonates: Sequential deletion of food antigen specificities during infancy with concomitant expansion of responses to ubiquitous inhalant allergens. Pediatr Allergy Immunol 1995;6:85–90.
16 Kondo N, Kobayashi Y, Shinoda S, et al: Cord blood lymphocyte responses to food antigens for the prediction of allergic disorders. Arch Dis Child 1992;67:1003–1007.
17 Miles EA, Warner JA, Jones AC, et al: Peripheral blood mononuclear cell proliferative responses in the first year of life in babies born to allergic parents. Clin Exp Allergy 1996;26: 780–788.
18 Piastra M, Stabile A, Fioravanti G, et al: Cord blood mononuclear cell responsiveness to beta-lactoglobulin: T-cell activity in 'atopy-prone' and 'non-atopy-prone' newborns. Int Arch Allergy Immunol 1994;104:358–365.
19 Piccinni M-P, Mecacci F, Sampognaro S, et al: Aeroallergen sensitization can occur during fetal life. Int Arch Allergy Immunol 1993;102:301–303.
20 Prescott SL, Macaubas C, Holt BJ, et al: Transplacental priming of the human immune system to environmental allergens: Universal skewing of initial T-cell responses towards the Th-2 cytokine profile. J Immunol 1998;160:4730–4737.
21 Loibichler C, Pichler J, Gerstmayr M, et al: Materno-fetal passage of nutritive and inhalant allergen across placentas of term and pre-term deliveries perfused in vitro. Clin Exp Allergy 2002;32:1546–1551.
22 Szépfalusi Z, Loibichler C, Pichler J, et al: Direct evidence for transplacental allergen transfer. Pediatr Res 2000;48:404–407.
23 Custovic A, Simpson BM, Simpson A, et al: Effect of environmental manipulation in pregnancy and early life on respiratory systems and atopy during first year of life: A randomised trial. Lancet 2001;358:188–193.
24 Prescott SL, Macaubas C, Smallacombe T, et al: Development of allergen-specific T-cell memory in atopic and normal children. Lancet 1999;353:196–200.
25 Yabuhara A, Macaubas C, Prescott SL, et al: Th-2-polarised immunological memory to inhalant allergens in atopics is established during infancy and early childhood. Clin Exp Allergy 1997;27:1261–1269.
26 Oddy WH, Holt PG, Sly PD, et al: Association between breast feeding and asthma in 6 year old children: Findings from a prospective birth cohort study. BMJ 1999;319:815–819.
27 Oddy WH, de Klerk NH, Sly PD, Holt PG: The effects of respiratory infections, atopy, and breastfeeding on childhood asthma. Eur Respir J 2002;19:899–905.
28 Macaubas C, Sly PD, Burton P, et al: Regulation of T-helper cell responses to inhalant allergen during early childhood. Clin Exp Allergy 1999;29:1223–1231.
29 Piccinni M-P, Beloni L, Giannarini L, et al: Abnormal production of T helper 2 cytokines interleukin-4 and interleukin-5 by T cells from newborns with atopic parents. Eur J Immunol 1996;26:2293–2298.
30 van der Velden VHJ, Laan MP, Baert MRM, et al: Selective development of a strong Th2 cytokine profile in high-risk children who develop atopy: Risk factors and regulatory role of IFN-, IL-4 and IL-10. Clin Exp Allergy 2001;31:997–1006.
31 Williams TJ, Jones CA, Miles EA, et al: Fetal and neonatal IL-13 production during pregnancy and at birth and subsequent development of atopic symptoms. J Allergy Clin Immunol 2000; 105:951–959.
32 Holt PG: Postnatal maturation of immune competence during infancy and early childhood. Pediatr Allergy Immunol 1995;6:59–70.
33 Holt PG, Jones CA: The development of the immune system during pregnancy and early life. Allergy 2000;55:688–697.
34 Wegmann TG, Lin H, Guilbert L, Mosmann TR: Bidirectional cytokine interactions in the maternal-fetal relationship: Is successful pregnancy a Th2 phenomenon? Immunol Today 1993;14:353–356.

35 Holt PG, Clough JB, Holt BJ, et al: Genetic 'risk' for atopy is associated with delayed postnatal maturation of T-cell competence. Clin Exp Allergy 1992;22:1093–1099.
36 Rowe J, Macaubas C, Monger T, et al: Heterogeneity in diphtheria-tetanus-acellular pertussis vaccine-specific cellular immunity during infancy: Relationship to variations in the kinetics of postnatal maturation of systemic Th1 function. J Infect Dis 2001;184:80–88.
37 Liao SY, Liao TN, Chiang BL, et al: Decreased production of IFN3 and increased production of IL-6 by cord blood mononuclear cells of newborns with a high risk of allergy. Clin Exp Allergy 1996;26:397–405.
38 Martinez FD, Stern DA, Wright AL, et al: Association of interleukin-2 and interferon-3 production by blood mononuclear cells in infancy with parental allergy skin tests and with subsequent development of atopy. J Allergy Clin Immunol 1995;96:652–660.
39 Rinas U, Horneff G, Wahn V: Interferon-gamma production by cord-blood mononuclear cells is reduced in newborns with a family history of atopic disease and is independent from cord blood IgE-levels. Pediatr Allergy Immunol 1993;4:60–64.
40 Warner JA, Miles EA, Jones AC, et al: Is deficiency of interferon gamma production by allergen triggered cord blood cells a predictor of atopic eczema? Clin Exp Allergy 1994;24: 423–430.
41 White GP, Watt PM, Holt BJ, Holt PG: Differential patterns of methylation of the IFNγ promoter at CpG and non-CpG sites underlie differences in IFNγ gene expression between human neonatal and adult CD45RO– T-cells. J Immunol 2002;168:2820–2827.
42 Ridge JP, Fuchs EJ, Matzinger P: Neonatal tolerance revisited: Turning on newborn T cells with dendritic cells. Science 1996;271:1723–1726.
43 Lee SM, Suen Y, Chang L, et al: Decreased interleukin-12 (IL-12) from activated cord versus adult peripheral blood mononuclear cells and upregulation of interferon-gamma, natural killer, and lymphokine-activated killer activity by IL-12 in cord blood mononuclear cells. Blood 1996;88:945–954.
44 Nelson DJ, McMenamin C, McWilliam AS, et al: Development of the airway intraepithelial dendritic cell network in the rat from class II MHC (Ia) negative precursors: Differential regulation of Ia expression at different levels of the respiratory tract. J Exp Med 1994;179: 203–212.
45 Sudo N, Sawamura S-A, Tanaka K, et al: The requirement of intestinal bacterial flora for the development of an IgE production system fully susceptible to oral tolerance induction. J Immunol 1997;159:1739–1745.
46 Björkstén B, Sepp E, Julge K, et al: Allergy development and the intestinal microflora during the first two years of life. J Allergy Clin Immunol 2001;108:516–520.
47 Matricardi PM, Rosmini F, Riondino S, et al: Exposure of foodborne and orofecal microbes versus airborne viruses in relation to atopy and allergic asthma: Epidemiological study. BMJ 2000;320:412–417.
48 Strachan DP: Family size, infection and atopy: The first decade of the 'hygiene hypothesis'. Thorax 2000;55(suppl 1):S2–S10.
49 Von Ehrenstein OS, Von Mutius E, Illi S, et al: Reduced risk of hay fever and asthma amongst children of farmers. Clin Exp Allergy 2000;30:187–193.
50 Gereda JE, Leung DYM, Thatayatikom A, et al: Relation between house-dust endotoxin exposure, type 1 T-cell development, and allergen sensitisation in infants at high risk of asthma. Lancet 2000;355:1680–1683.
51 Baldini M, Lohman IC, Halonen M, et al: A polymorphism in the 5′-flanking region of the CD14 gene is associated with circulating soluble CD14 levels with total serum IgE. Am J Respir Cell Mol Biol 1999;20:976–983.
52 Lauener RP, Birchler T, Adamski J, et al: Expression of CD14 and Toll-like receptor 2 in farmers' and non-farmers' children. Lancet 2002;360:465–466.
53 Kurt-Jones EA, Popova L, Kwinn L, et al: Pattern recognition receptors TLR4 and CD14 mediate response to respiratory syncytial virus. Nat Immunol 2000;1:398–401.
54 Holt PG, Sly PD: Interactions between RSV infection, asthma, and atopy: Unraveling the complexities. J Exp Med 2002;196:1271–1275.
55 Holt PG, Sly PD: Interactions between respiratory tract infections and atopy in the aetiology of asthma. Eur Respir J 2002;19:538–545.
56 Kalliomäki M, Salminen S, Arvilommi H, et al: Probiotics in primary prevention of atopic disease: A randomised placebo controlled trial. Lancet 2001;357:1076–1079.

57 Arkwright PD, David TJ: Intradermal administration of a killed *Mycobacterium vaccae* suspension (SRL 172) is associated with improvement in atopic dermatitis in children with moderate-to-severe disease. J Allergy Clin Immunol 2001;107:531–534.
58 Hessel EM, Van Oosterhout AJM, Van Ark I, et al: Development of airway hyperresponsiveness is dependent on interferon-γ and independent of eosinophil infiltration. Am J Respir Cell Mol Biol 1997;16:325–334.
59 Randolph DA, Stephens R, Carruthers CJL, Chaplin DD: Cooperation between Th1 and Th2 cells in a murine model of eosinophilic airway inflammation. J Clin Invest 1999;104:1021–1029.
60 Randolph DA, Carruthers CJL, Szabo SJ, et al: Modulation of airway inflammation by passive transfer of allergen-specific Th1 and Th2 cells in a mouse model of asthma. J Immunol 1999; 162:2375–2383.
61 Holt PG, Rudin A, Macaubas C, et al: Development of immunologic memory against tetanus toxoid and pertactin antigens from the diphtheria-tetanus-pertussis vaccine in atopic versus nonatopic children. J Allergy Clin Immunol 2000;105:1117–1122.
62 Magnan AO, Mely LG, Camilla CA, et al: Assessment of the Th1/Th2 paradigm in whole blood in atopy and asthma. Increased IFN-gamma-producing CD8(+) T cells in asthma. Am J Respir Crit Care Med 2000;161:1790–1796.
63 Smart JM, Kemp AS: Increased Th1 and Th2 allergen-induced cytokine responses in children with atopic disease. Clin Exp Allergy 2002;32:796–802.

Discussion

Dr. Zakiudin Munasir: I want to ask you about the role of the immunomodulator in the prevention of allergic disease, especially in the first 6 months of life.

Dr. Holt: The potential use of immunomodulators to prevent allergic disease is a very valid approach. I think the problem we face at the moment is that we only have a rough snapshot of what is going on in terms of the maturation of the immune system. We know that there are maturational problems and that maturation needs to be accelerated, but the problem at the moment is that we don't know how to control that process. So to use powerful immunomodulators at this point wouldn't be defensible because we know that excessive Th1 immunity can potentially be pathogenic. Like many groups, we are doing things with probiotics, which is a very gentle way to start this process along, but I think at the moment the safety issues of going beyond using gentle immunomodulators is such that in most countries it would be very difficult to get these approaches through ethics committees.

Dr. Guesry: In many countries poor hygiene is linked not only to bacterial infection but also parasitic infection. You have mentioned bacterial infection as a way to set the system toward Th1, but parasitic infection may result in a Th2 setting. So what is your interpretation of that?

Dr. Holt: That was really the reason for the last slide I put up. We believe that just upstream from the point at which the immune system makes the Th1–Th2 decision, there is another set of information translation which is handled by cells of the innate immune system. The postnatal maturation of these cells is clearly regulated by the totality of the organism's stimulation from the outside environment. This stimulation can come either from parasites or from viruses or bacteria. There is a set of stimulation events that occurs at this upstream point even before the rest happens. So to some extent that is why we are making dendritic cells our major research target in trying to sort out these mechanisms.

Dr. Lack: Allergy is an antigen-specific disease, so if you take a child of 7 with house dust mite allergy you will have Th2 linked to house dust mite but not to normal responses to other antigens. The same is true in younger children with egg allergy; although they show a Th2-skewed response to egg protein but Th0 or Th1 responses to other food proteins. You discussed here a generalized maturational problem in the neonate with perhaps an exaggeration in atopics. How does this translate into an allergen-specific disease as opposed to an across the board phenomenon?

Dr. Holt: I agree, but what we are looking at is the product of gene by environment interactions. So there is clearly a genotype in there that has got a certain phenotype as far as immune response capacity is concerned, and requires a particular collection of environmental exposures to turn that immunophenotype into an allergy phenotype. The reality is that what we see is a spectrum. We see some children that are sensitized to 10 different allergens, some sensitized to 9, and some sensitized to 1, in fact that is probably most common. Because the ones with multiple sensitizations are relatively uncommon, I guess this is telling us that all of the regulatory mechanisms that are built into the immune system to try to stop this happening are actually efficient. So there is only a sneak through of a few allergen specificities and that is where I think the environment comes in. It won't be as simple as just having high concentrations of allergens such as house dust mite. Other factors are needed that might have something to do, for example, with the barrier function of the epithelium because we still don't know how these high molecular weight allergens, like the house dust mite allergens which have a molecular weight of 100,000, can get through the mucosa. We have no idea how that happens.

Dr. Isolauri: Thank you very much for this very clear presentation, and I fully agree with that general idea. I just have one question about the last slide. You mentioned that mucosally processed protein favors the Th2 type.

Dr. Holt: No, I am sorry, this is not what I meant. I meant that the environmental proteins that cause allergic disease enter through the mucosal surfaces, whereas endogenous antigens come through a different route and can cause Th1 responses. What I did not mean to say was that the mucosa is always preferentially Th2, although we actually know that at baseline it is, but that is another story.

Dr. Isolauri: Yes, that is another story. I want to make the point that if we think of gastrointestinal mucosa, dietary antigens are modified to a much different peptide that can induce suppression as studied by Sütas et al. [1]. Such processing decreases the antigen load and the antigenicity of the protein. Our chairman has nicely shown that specific strains of gut microbiota can mount suppressive (anti-inflammatory) cytokines towards dietary antigens. There is also research on feeding encapsulated antigens which abrogate this tolerance unlike mucosally processed antigens. I think that the clinical correlate of these pieces of information is clearly that when the dietary antigens are transferred and modulated by the mother, they are different in breast milk. We understand that gastrointestinal mucosa is a strong suppressor modulating antigens towards tolerogens.

Dr. Holt: It is interesting, the default response in the gastrointestinal tract is actually still Th2-polarized, the same as that in the respiratory tract. But as you say there is layer upon layer of protection that comes in to push gently in the other direction.

Dr. Isolauri: Probably because it includes this anti-inflammatory response.

Dr. Schiffrin: I wanted to ask you about the factors produced by the placenta to inhibit fetal reactivity. First of all I haven't seen transforming growth factor-β (TGF-β) because I think it was formerly postulated that the amniotic fluid contained TGF-β. Then if the babies at risk can already prenatally be exposed to lower levels of these regulatory factors, they can already be said to have higher activity.

Dr. Holt: We have a study, which has recently been published [3], that was trying to address some of those issues, but we could not get directly into that tissue compartment. We thought it might be useful to just have a look at the cytokine levels of cord blood which we had stored at –85°C from one of our large cohorts, and see if there was anything predictive about asthma and allergy outcomes at age 6, and very interestingly we had very strong signals. The phenotype that we see in the T-cell system in babies at high risk of allergy, which is lower IL-4 and lower interferon-γ, is reflected in the cord serum samples from the same children, yet we know that the principle source of those cytokines is not T cells but placental trophoblasts. So there are regulatory processes that work in the whole fetal compartment, including presumably the placenta, which are influencing what we see postnatally. Perhaps the operation of this regulatory mechanism in infants represents a hangover from something that should really have stayed in the placental compartment.

Dr. Sorensen: In your early slides about lymphocyte proliferation you seem to have worked with only one allergen or antigen dose. I presume that prior to that you did extensive dose-response curves. If you did, then my question is, did you check if different antigen concentrations may have induced different cytokine patterns?

Dr. Holt: We spent a lot of time mainly with house dust mite allergens trying to sort that out because we were very struck by the amount of work that has been done in the mouse showing that at both ends of the dose-response spectrum you can differentially stimulate Th1 and Th2 responses. But we were disappointed that this did not seem to be the case in the human in vitro PBMC cultures. We have seen this in in vitro systems with mature T-cell clones, so it is possible that the stage of maturation of an immune response in an individual is what determines the sensitivity of their particular T-cell clones to that kind of control. It worked so well in the mouse, and we have seen this in other models so that we believe it operates in humans but is not something that happens in all immune responses. We don't know yet what the rules are that determine which immune responses are susceptible.

Dr. Marini: In your study on cord blood, did you have babies born by elective cesarean section and, if so, did they behave the same as the other ones?

Dr. Holt: We tried the best we could to control for that, but we don't have really definite information except in a large cohort study. We have now 2,500 children and they are a mixture of elective cesarean section and all manners of births. As part of looking at multiple logistic regressions, we put them in as confounding factors, and certainly at about the age of 5 there is no signal there. We suspect that some of the early immune responses in the first 6 months may well be influenced and we intend to look at this issue in some of the newer cohort studies that we are doing. The problem is that our cohorts tend to come from the higher end of the socioeconomic spectrum and the frequency of elective cesarean sections tends to be somewhat higher than for the rest of the population.

Dr. Neijens: First of all I would like to thank you for the beautiful way in which you presented your work and for giving an enormous insight into the modulation of the immune system, which fits the clinical and epidemiological observations quite well. That brings me to a practical question, what we really do need are risk factors. You emphasize genetic risk factors; however, we don't have very precise genetic risk factors yet, and those we have don't predict outcome precisely later on, so we need additional ones. Taking all this work on modulation of the immune system into account, is it possible that several factors might function as risk factors in combination with genetic factors such as soluble receptors or responses? They are needed for early prevention programs and good therapy and risk assessment. What is your opinion?

Dr. Holt: I agree. The future to us involves bringing together immunology, respiratory physiology and genetics so that we can accurately divide pediatric populations into the different disease phenotypes, because the bigger the data sets are, the more heterogeneity we can find in these human populations. It is becoming very clear that we are dealing with a whole series of overlapping diseases in allergy. This was discussed this morning very elegantly by Dr. Bindslev-Jensen. There are so many phenotypes there at the moment that I think it is right to scratch our heads, but all of those phenotypes have been defined thus far on clinical criteria. What we need to do now is to match those up with large population studies where we can get big immunology data sets and big clinical data sets and see how they all fit together. There are a number of studies around that are trying to do that. In the study I described on 12-year-olds, this is precisely what we want to do and we want to see exactly how far this whole issue of immunophenotyping the population can be pushed to identify these different subtypes, and then see if there is any clinical sense in it or not.

Dr. Neijens: What do you presently consider as good candidates for immunological markers? Have you an explanation?

Dr. Holt: At the moment the kind of approach that we are using is to look at as many cytokines as we can in these immune responses, 20 or 30 at the moment, and we have a microarray program going on to try and broaden this. Eventually the sort of technique that you would use at the population level would probably be a microchip-type approach. There are some sensitivity issues which I think will be resolved as this technology grows in the next couple of years, and I think we are not too far away from being able to do this. We have a dream that when the child walks into the physician's room that a little bit of blood will be taken and processed in a sophisticated machine which will provide a genetic profile and an immunological profile which, with the use of the right sort of algorithm, will tell us a lot more than we currently know about the clinical phenotype and how that child should be optimally treated. I think this is a few years down the line, but I don't think it is too far away because there is considerable research ongoing into this issue in different parts of the world.

Dr. Walker: I have two questions. One, you emphasized that the allergy-prone infant takes a longer period of time to balance the Th2–Th1 response than does the nonallergy-prone child. Do you have any bias or any thoughts about why that occurs?

Dr. Holt: Two thoughts, we have some initial information that there is some level of control that works either directly or indirectly on the methylation profile of the interferon-γ gene, but we don't know whether that is primary or secondary. It will obviously be part of the process, and we are starting to spot some differences among children. But my guess is that there is another set of regulatory mechanisms that has exclusively to do with the antigen-presenting cell compartment, particularly those in the monocyte and dendritic cell lineage. Probably part of that will involve receptors such as CD14 and the Toll family which are all to do with recognizing the microbial environment. It is not a coincidence that the cells that actually transduce those recognition signals are these same cells that I am talking about, and they are the same cells that are instructing the T-cell system on whether to make an immune response or whether to make an allergic response or how long that antiviral response should be. So to me they are the prime candidates.

Dr. Walker: So it could very well be the genetic basis for how microbes interact with a lot of lymphoid elements that are the actual bottom line factors. I think that is what you are suggesting.

Dr. Holt: I am suggesting that is likely to be one of the very important factors. I am very nervous about single bottom lines because biological systems have got so many full-back positions, but I think it is going to be one of the most powerful factors.

Dr. Walker: They are not necessarily all coming from the same perspective. I mean there could be multiple stimuli environmental changes. But the other question I have is the timing during which the balance occurs. From Martinez and others it sounds as if there is a finite period where the balance can be established and will prevent long-term disease.

Dr. Holt: I think this is one of the most important issues. I showed one set of data on a cohort of 130 children, and we could see that this maturational defect was very strong at 6 and 12 months, and by 18 months the whole thing had turned over on its head and the initial group that were immunocompromised now had excessive Th1 function. During the period in which the life-long immunological memory is being programmed, which is typically in the first 12 months, that is when Th1 functional capacity is most important. If you want to do something about memory to allergens you have to accurately identify that programming period and do the manipulation during that window period. At the population level the other thing we don't know is how long that window operates for individuals. These were population data and we know that the standard deviations are large. But the other side of the coin is that some of these children are going to continue on until they are nearly 4 or 5 years of age and still be in the lower 25th percentile for Th1 function. But it looks as though the most common window period is very early postnatally. Then again we don't know what the consequences are of aggressively driving this maturation process. We must not lose sight of the fact that evolution has conserved this immunosuppression in the early postnatal period. Evolution doesn't typically make mistakes so therefore it is likely to confer a survival advantage. This may be relevant to what happened with the old respiratory syncytial virus vaccine, which was probably a strong Th1 immunostimulant, but was given to subjects who were too young to handle it adequately, because all of the regulatory mechanisms that are necessary to control the intensity of immune reactions are also going through the same functional transition during this life phase. As we work through these processes the thing that we have to ensure is that we don't try and push too fast in relation to immunostimulation in infancy. The credibility of pediatric medicine relies absolutely on safety issues being the very first concern during the development of new therapies.

Dr. Al-Malik: How would you explain the development of severe atopic dermatitis in patients with severe combined immune deficiency where there are no T cells available?

Dr. Holt: Very good point. I think one of the things that has come out from what Dr. Bindslev-Jensen was saying and some of the earlier discussion is that atopic dermatitis is a disease about which we know very little. It is clearly mislabeled because a very high proportion of the dermatitis has got absolutely nothing to do with atopy. We have just concluded a big survey on our 12-year-olds, and although we get very strong associations with respect to allergen-specific Th2 cytokine production in allergic rhinitis and atopic asthma, we saw a very poor relationship with what was diagnosed as atopic dermatitis. So there are several other phenotypes. One of those we are interested in is related to microbial pressure, in particular to the kind of super antigens that are made by staphylococci. This sort of stimulus from microbial sources amongst skin commensals is probably indicative of a whole range of similar molecules, that we know little about.

Dr. Papageorgiou: From all you told us, I would like you to comment on whether conventional immunotherapy with peptides or modified allergens stimulating IL-10 and TGF and suppressing both Th1 and Th2 may be finally preferable over DNA immunization?

Dr. Holt: We are not fans of DNA immunization at this stage because we don't believe it can be controlled in that context. So we are not even considering that. But we are considering early immunotherapy in pediatrics involving high-risk children as young as perhaps 18 months to 2 years in the ultra high-risk group. At the moment we are trying to get trials involving European and Australian sites to try out this principle. We suspect that this approach will play a part in prophylactic treatment, not only therapeutic treatment.

Dr. Murch: Twice this morning we heard the unexplained facts that allergy is more common in boys, or certain types are more common in boys, and that maternal inheritance is dominant. Do you see a difference in interferon-γ methylation depending on maternal inheritance, and do you see a difference between boys and girls?

Dr. Holt: We do see gender-related differences in interferon-γ response maturation and that was published by Prescott et al. [2] in *Allergy* maybe about 18 months ago from their cohort study. It was very clear that the maturation defect in interferon-γ function was strongly associated with maternal transmission. But the problem is the low power of that study: because it was relatively small, virtually all of the symptomatic children had maternal inheritance. So the groups weren't balanced although the statisticians said it was fine, and if you look it up you can draw your own conclusions. But it is quite clear that this is something we do see, but I have no explanation for it. The precise relationship between low interferon-γ production and interferon-γ promoter methylation has not yet been determined.

Dr. Rijntjes: My question is about what happens in utero. With the IgE syndrome there is a lack especially of Th1 cytokines and not too much Th2, so the allergens presenting to the mucosa in particular are driven to keep the Th2 response. Is it possible that the amount of allergens the child swallows in utero is the reason why the dendritic cells are stressed to develop Th cells so that they don't become tolerant and remain so after birth until new allergens are presented to the child? Particularly, how much allergen does the child swallow during pregnancy?

Dr. Holt: If those exposures were generating immune responses we might hope that we would see some evidence of positive immunity in cord blood. We have had to revise all of our notions about what those immune responses are because very clearly the responding cord blood cells are not conventional memory cells. So there could be regulatory processes going on in utero, perhaps involving deletion of responsive cells, but if so it is a covert process and we haven't seen any definite evidence of it yet. We can't dismiss the fact that this might be occurring and we need to address this issue in more detail. We need to get these new data published and then all the cord blood response data can be seen and evaluated. At the moment our conclusion is that these are not memory responses because the main result is apoptosis, and so virtually all of the cells that respond to the antigen die in these cultures, unlike what we see in cultures from older subjects. So there is some other process that is happening in the cord blood responses and we don't have a complete explanation for it yet, but we no longer believe that it is just simply that the mother eats allergen, allergen crosses the placenta, primes the memory cells and the baby is born with allergen-specific memory cells. We now don't subscribe to that idea for peanut or for any allergen because the responsive cells in cord blood don't have the genuine memory phenotype.

References

1 Sütas Y, Soppi E, Korhonen H, et al: Suppression of lymphocyte proliferation in vitro by bovine caseins hydrolysed with *Lactobacillus* GG-derived enzymes. J Allergy Clin Immunol 1996;98: 216–224.
2 Prescott SL, Holt PG, Jenmalm M, Bjorksten B: Effects of maternal allergen-specific T-cell immunity. Allergy 2000;55:470–475.
3 Macaubas C, de Klerk NH, Holt BJ, et al: Association between antenatal cytokine production and the development of atopy and asthma at age 6 years. Lancet 2003;362:1192–1197.

Isolauri E, Walker WA (eds): Allergic Diseases and the Environment.
Nestlé Nutrition Workshop Series Pediatric Program, Vol. 53, pp. 69–95,
Nestec Ltd.; Vevey/S. Karger AG, Basel, © 2004.

Allergy: Is It a Th2-Predominant Disease? Pro

Sergio Romagnani

Section of Clinical Immunology, Allergy, and Respiratory Diseases,
Department of Internal Medicine, University of Florence, Florence, Italy

Introduction

The history of discoveries on the pathogenesis of atopic allergy can be divided into two main phases. The first phase, which started in 1879 when Ehrlich [1] first described mast cells and eosinophils, includes the discovery of reagins by Prausnitz and Kustner [2] in 1921, and ended in 1967 with the identification of the IgE nature of reaginic antibodies, independently performed by Ishizaka and Ishizaka [3] and Johansson [4]. At the end of this phase, the allergic reaction emerged as a form of inflammatory process mainly sustained by mediators released by mast cells following the interaction between common environmental allergens and specific IgE antibodies bound to IgE receptors present on the surface of these cells. The second phase started in 1986 with the discovery of T-cell-derived cytokines that regulate the IgE antibody production by B cells, performed by Coffman and Carty [5] in mice, and by Del Prete et al. [6] and Pene et al. [7] in humans, and includes the description of type-1 T helper (Th1) and type-2 Th (Th2) lymphocytes by Mosmann et al. [8] in mice and by Del Prete et al. [9] in humans, and is still going on.

Currently, because of many other discoveries not mentioned above, the allergic reaction appears to be the result of a Th2 lymphocyte response to one or more common environmental allergens. The allergen-specific Th2 response indeed represents the triggering event for the recruitment and involvement of all other cell types, as well as of a large number of soluble factors and adhesion molecules, thus resulting in an inflammatory cascade of unequaled complexity. On the basis of these findings, atopic allergy may presently be defined as a ‘Th2-driven hypersensitivity to innocuous antigens (allergens) of complex genetic and environmental origins’. In recent years, the ‘Th2 hypothesis in allergy’ has become a dogma since an impressive series of experimental findings have supported the assumption initially based only on conceptual remarks that atopic diseases are the result of Th2-dominated responses.

The Concept of Th1/Th2 Polarization

Th1 and Th2 cells do not represent distinct subsets, but polarized forms of the CD4+ Th cell-mediated immune response which occur under particular experimental or pathophysiological conditions. Th1 responses are characterized by the prevalent production of interleukin (IL)-2, interferon (IFN)-γ, and tumor necrosis factor (TNF)-β, without IL-4, IL-5, IL-9, and IL-13 production. By contrast, Th2 responses are characterized by the prevalent production of IL-4, IL-5, IL-9, and IL-13 in the absence of IFN-γ and TNF-β production. The Th cell responses characterized by the conjunct production of Th1 and Th2 cytokines are commonly defined as type-0 Th (Th0) responses. Th1/Th2 polarization is clear-cut in murine models based on artificial immunization, whereas it is usually less restricted among human Th cell-mediated responses [10, 11]. In general, Th1-polarized responses are highly protective against infections by the majority of microbes, especially intracellular parasites, because of the ability of Th1-type cytokines to activate phagocytes and promote the production by B lymphocytes of opsonizing and complement-fixing antibodies (phagocyte-dependent host defense). However, when the microbe is not rapidly removed from the body, the Th1 response may become dangerous for the host, because of the strong and chronic inflammatory reaction evoked. By contrast, cytokines produced by Th2 cells induce the differentiation, activation, and in situ survival of eosinophils (through IL-5), promote the production by B lymphocytes of high amounts of antibodies, including IgE (through IL-4 and IL-13), as well as the growth and degranulation of mast cells and basophils (through IL-4 and IL-9). Moreover, IL-4 and IL-13 inhibit several macrophage functions and IL-4 can suppress the development of Th1 cells. Thus, the phagocyte-independent Th2 response is usually less protective than the Th1 response against the majority of infectious agents, with the exception of some gastrointestinal nematodes [12]. In addition to their protective activity against some nematodes, Th2 cells probably also play a regulatory role in the immune system, because a switch from Th1 to Th2 may provide a protective effect when the Th1 response threatens to become a dangerous event for the host [10, 11].

Besides the selective production of IL-4, IL-5, IL-6, IL-9, and IL-13, human Th2 cells also exhibit the preferential release of leukemia inhibitory factor (LIF), which is very important for egg implantation and, therefore, for successful pregnancy [13]. Moreover, human Th2 cells exhibit the preferential expression of some surface molecules, such as CD30, CCR4, CCR8, and chemoattractant receptor of Th2 cells (CRTH2) [14], whereas human Th1 cells preferentially express the lymphocyte activation gene-3, CXCR3, and CCR5 [14]. The chemoattractant receptors prevalently expressed on the surface of Th1 or Th2 cells are important for the recruitment and homing in target tissues of one or the other type of effector Th cells.

Mechanisms Responsible for the Th1/Th2 Polarization

In the last few years, the factors responsible for the polarization of specific immune responses into a predominant Th1 or Th2 pathway have been extensively investigated. Clear evidence suggests that Th1 and Th2 cells develop from the same Th cell precursor under the influence of both environmental and genetic factors acting at the level of antigen presentation. Among the environmental factors, a role for the route of antigen entry, the physical form of immunogen, the type of adjuvant, and the dose of antigen have been suggested [10, 11]. The genetic mechanisms that concur in controlling the type of Th cell differentiation still remain elusive. Independently or in association, genetic and environmental factors can influence a series of modulatory factors that include: (i) the ligation of T-cell receptor (TCR); (ii) the activation of costimulatory molecules, such as B7/CD28, OX40/OX40L, LAF-3/ICAM-1, and (iii) the predominance of a given cytokine in the microenvironment of the responding Th cell, such as IL-4, IL-12, IL-18, IFN-γ and IFN-α [10, 11].

While the role of contact-dependent factors is still controversial, it is generally accepted that early IL-4 expression during an immune response is critical for the development of Th2 cells, whereas the early expression of IL-12 and IFNs favors the development of Th1 cells. Naïve Th cells themselves are able to produce small amounts of IL-4 from their initial activation, and the concentration of IL-4 that accumulates at the level of the Th cell response increases with increasing lymphocyte activation. The inducing effect of IL-4 dominates over other cytokines so that, if IL-4 levels reach a necessary threshold, differentiation of the Th cell into the Th2 phenotype occurs [14]. Other possible sources of early IL-4 production may be natural killer (NK) T cells, basophils, mast cells and eosinophils. However, IL-4 produced by these cells may be more important in the amplification rather than in the initiation of a Th2 response [14]. In contrast to IL-4, the early production of IL-12, IL-18, and IFNs (γ and α) favors the development of Th1 cells. IL-12, which is the most powerful Th1-inducing agent, is mainly produced by dendritic cells (DCs) under the stimulation provided by exogenous signals and is upregulated by both CD40L/CD40 interaction and the presence of IFN-γ. Of interest, IFN-γ, but not IFN-α, promotes Th1 differentiation in mice, whereas both IFN-γ and IFN-α play an important role in humans, IFN-α upregulating the expression of the IL-12 receptor (IL-12R) β chain [14].

Signals through contact molecules, as well as through cytokine receptors, elicit a complex series of molecular interactions that culminate in the binding of cell-type-specific transcription factors to multiple regulatory elements in the promoters and subsequent activation of cytokine genes. Even these signal transduction cascades have emerged as important regulators of Th1 or Th2 differentiation because of their possible antagonism. At least 5 groups of transcription factors play an important role in the Th2 differentiation. The interaction of IL-4 with its receptor on the surface of the naïve Th cell results in the activation of the signal transducer and activator of transcription (STAT) 6. Proteins of the nuclear factor of activated T cell family are also involved, since they bind specifically to the promoter region of the IL-4 gene and cooperate with activator protein factors, like Fra and Jun, to induce IL-4 transcription. However, the nuclear factor of activated T cells and activator protein are expressed in both Th1 and Th2 cells and their role in the selective Th-cell differentiation appears to be very complex. By contrast, the protooncogene, c-Maf, is specifically expressed by Th2 but not Th1 cells and binds to a maf response element within the IL-4 proximal promoter. Mice deficient in c-Maf have impaired IL-4 production, but do not exhibit changes in the other Th2 cytokines, like IL-5 and IL-13. Moreover, c-Maf is specific for IL-4 and is critical for high levels of IL-4 production, but is not sufficient for the initiation of IL-4 transcription. An even more important transcription factor for Th2 differentiation is GATA-3 which is undetectable in Th1 cells. GATA-3 inhibits the production of IFN-γ, increases the transactivation of the IL-4 promoter, and also directly regulates IL-5 and IL-13 expression. Thus, the fact that GATA-3 not only plays a more global role in upregulating Th2 cytokines, but also concomitantly inhibits Th1 development, suggests that this transcription factor has a key role in determining the fate of Th2 [15].

While the binding of IL-4 to its receptors induces the STAT6 activation, the IL-12/IL-12R interaction results in the activation of STAT4. This transcription factor as well as IFN-regulatory factor-1 have been implicated in Th1 differentiation because mice deficient for each of these factors lack Th1 cells, but the exact roles that these factors play in Th1 generation are unclear. A substantial advance in elucidating Th1 lineage commitment and IFN-γ gene expression has been provided with the isolation of the protein T box expressed in T cells (T-bet). T-bet expression strongly correlates with IFN-γ expression; it is specifically upregulated in primary Th cells differentiated along the Th1 but not the Th2 pathway; its transduction into fully polarized Th2 cells converts them into IFN-γ-producing Th1 cells and simultaneously represses the Th2 cytokines IL-4 and IL-5 [15]. Thus, a model for Th1/Th2 polarization that involves a balance between the Th1-specific T-bet and the Th2-specific GATA3 transcription factors may presently be envisaged (fig. 1).

The Th cell fate is not only regulated by differentiating signals delivered by early produced cytokines, contact-dependent factors, as well as the antagonism of transcription factors, but is also dependent upon cell cycle

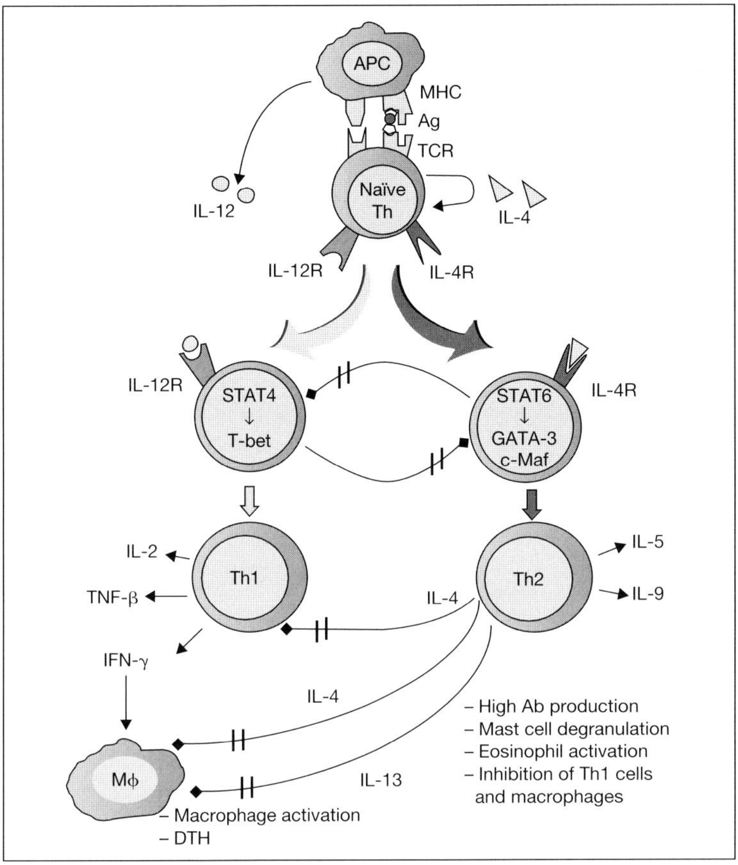

Fig. 1. Mechanisms involved in Th1/Th2 polarization. Signals through the T-cell receptor (TCR) and costimulatory molecules of naïve T-helper (Th) cell in the presence of interleukin (IL)-12 produced by the antigen-presenting cell (APC) favor the activation of signal transducer and activation of transcription (STAT)4, that in turn results in the activation of the T box expressed in T cells (T-bet), which promotes type-1 Th (Th1) lineage commitment. By contrast, signals that favor the activation of STAT6 via the early IL-4 production induce GATA-3 activation, thus leading to the Th2 differentiation. The proto-oncogene c-Maf is then upregulated, which results in increased IL-4 production and Th2 polarization. The mutually exclusive expression pattern of the T box expressed in T cells (T-bet) and GATA-3 may reflect the ability of these transcription factors to antagonize each other. Therefore, the relative predominance of T-bet or GATA-3 may determine Th1 or Th2 polarization, respectively. Th1 cells produce IL-2, tumor necrosis factor (TNF)-β, and interferon (IFN)-γ, and are responsible for macrophage activation and delayed-type hypersensitivity (DTH) responses. Th2 cells produce IL-4, IL-5, IL-9, and IL-13, which are responsible for high antibody production including IgE, mast cell degranulation, and eosinophil activation. Moreover, IL-4 has a regulatory effect on the development of Th1 cells and both IL-4 and IL-13 inhibit several macrophage (Mr) activities. Thus, Th2 cells also regulate the Th1 response when it becomes dangerous for the host.

expression, i.e. the number of post-activation cell divisions. Several studies suggest that there is an opportunity for a Th cell to initiate cytokine gene expression at each cell division and that the probability for this event varies between cytokines. It is of interest that these division relationships and probabilities of expression appear not to be heavily dependent upon the genetic background of the T cells, but rather on epigenetic events that may control cytokine gene accessibility. Thus, in addition to a deterministic process related to the above-mentioned factors, a probabilistic process may concur to influence the final choice in the cytokine pattern during the specific Th-cell response [14].

Data Suggesting that Atopic Allergy Is a Th2-Predominant Disorder

Since several components of the Th1 or Th2 response have been clearly elucidated at both the cellular and molecular level, it is relatively easy to establish whether a given disease is characterized by the predominance of one or the other type of Th-cell polarization. The presence in atopic allergy of a Th2 predominance has been demonstrated by assessing the type of cytokines, chemokines, and transcription factors expressed in the target organs of allergic patients and by comparing these patterns with those found in experimental animal models of allergy and asthma.

Detection of Cytokines, Chemokines, and Transcription Factors in Subjects Suffering from Atopic Disorders

Cytokines

The initial demonstration that in atopic subjects allergens mainly induce Th2 responses was initially provided by cloning peripheral blood T cells. Following polyclonal stimulation, the majority of allergen-specific CD4+ T-cell clones from allergic donors produced IL-4 and IL-5, but little or no IFN-γ, whereas virtually all T-cell clones specific for bacterial antigens, such as purified protein derivative, generated from the same donors, produced high concentrations of IFN-γ, but little if any IL-4 [16]. Although some authors argued that these data could result from an in vitro artifact, similar findings have recently been obtained by using a more reproducible and reliable technique than T-cell cloning, such as intracytoplasmic cytokine detection performed at the single cell level by flow cytometry. The majority of peripheral blood CD4+ T cells from *Dermatophagoides pteronyssinus* group 1 (Der p 1)- or penicillin G-sensitive donors produced high amounts of IL-4, IL-5, and IL-13 and little or no IFN-γ when they were expanded for a few days in vitro with Der p 1 or penicillin, whereas virtually all CD4+ T cells from the same donors stimulated under the same experimental conditions with the bacterial antigen streptokinase produced a high IFN-γ concentration, but little or no IL-4, IL-5, and IL-13 [17]. By contrast, no differences in the pattern of cytokine production between Der p 1- and streptokinase-specific T cells obtained from the peripheral blood of nonatopic donors were observed (fig. 2). Concomitant with the initial description of the Th2-polarized phenotype of allergen-specific T-cell clones generated from the peripheral blood of allergic donors, the presence of IL-4 but not IFN-γ mRNA-expressing T cells was demonstrated using in situ hybridization on bronchial biopsy specimens of patients suffering from allergic asthma [18]. This finding was confirmed by generating T-cell clones from bronchial biopsy specimens of allergic asthmatics challenged with the specific allergen. A number of allergen-specific CD4+ T-cell clones could be generated from these biopsies which appeared to be clearly Th2-polarized [19]. More recently the same finding was reported using a highly sensitive and sophisticated technique: confocal microscopy combined with in situ hybridization. IL-4- and IL-5- but not IFN-γ-producing T cells were observed in the bronchial biopsy specimens of allergic asthmatics, whereas under the same experimental conditions IFN-γ- but neither IL-4- nor IL-5-producing T cells were observed in bronchial biopsies of patients with chronic obstructive pulmonary diseases [20]. Finally, T cells expressing intracellular IL-4 were significantly higher in the bronchoalveolar lavage fluid of subjects with asthma [21], and increased IL-4 was observed in the exhaled breath condensate of asthmatic children [22]. With regard to other Th2 cytokines, a highly significant difference in the expression of IL-9 mRNA and protein was detected in the airways of asthmatic subjects compared with those of nonatopic subjects or subjects suffering from sarcoidosis [23]. Likewise, an increased expression of IL-13 mRNA has been reported in both atopic and nonatopic asthma [24, 25]. Moreover, increased numbers of IL-13 mRNA and immunoreactive protein cells were detected 24 h after segmental allergen challenge [26, 27].

By contrast, expression of Th1 cytokines is depressed in peripheral blood and exhaled breath condensate of asthmatics [22, 28], and DCs from atopic subjects produce lower quantities of IL-12 compared with those from normal donors [29]. Moreover, resolution of asthma was found to be associated with normalization in polyclonal and allergen-induced IFN-γ responses by peripheral blood lymphocytes [28]. Successful specific immunotherapy has also been associated in different studies with a shift of the allergen-specific response from Th2 to Th1 [30–32], as well as with the increase in the number of IL-12 mRNA-expressing cells at the cutaneous level [33].

Chemoattractants

As mentioned above, the recruitment of Th1 or Th2 cells in inflamed tissues results from the local production of chemoattractants which interact with their receptors, prevalently or selectively expressed by effector Th cells

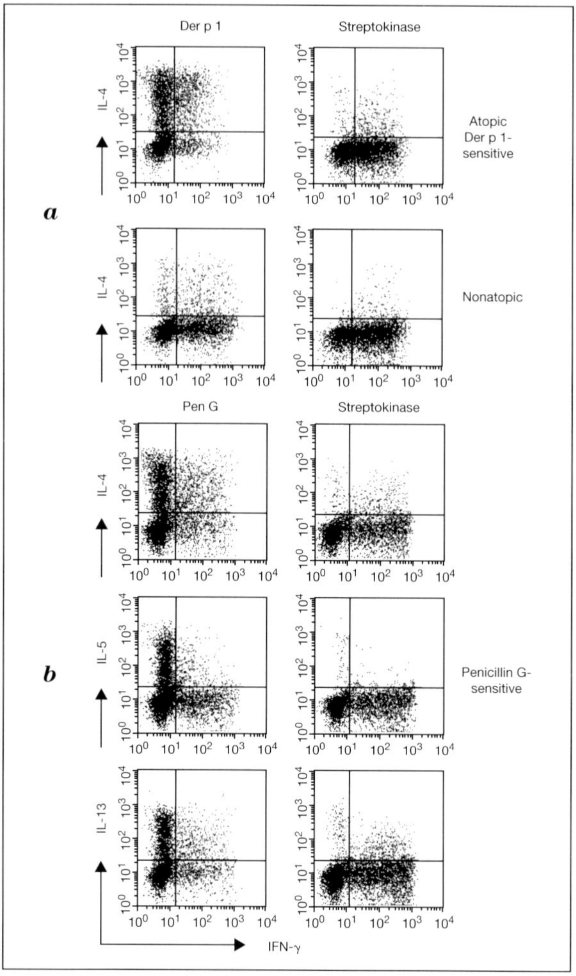

Fig. 2. Th2 predominance in the allergen-specific response of atopic, but not nonatopic, subjects and in the drug-specific response of drug-sensitive individuals. ***a*** Detection by flow cytometry of intracytoplasmic synthesis of IL-4 and IFN-γ produced by single peripheral blood T cells from 1 atopic *Dermatophagoides pteronyssinus* group 1 (Der p 1)-sensitive subject and 1 nonatopic individual. T cells were expanded for 7 days with the bacterial antigen streptokinase or the purified allergen Der p 1 and then assessed for cytokine production in response to stimulation with phorbol myristate acetate (PMA) plus ionomycin. Most Der p 1-specific T cells from the atopic donor produce IL-4 alone or IL-4 plus IFN-γ, whereas virtually all Der p 1-specific T cells from the nonatopic donor and streptokinase-specific T cells from both donors produce IFN-γ, but no IL-4. ***b*** Detection under the same experimental conditions as IL-4, IL-5, IL-13, and IFN-γ production by T cells from 1 penicillin G (pen G)-sensitive donor. T cells were expanded in vitro for 7 days with pen G or streptokinase. The great majority of pen G specific CD4+ T cells produce IL-4, IL-5, and IL-13, but not IFN-γ, whereas virtually all streptokinase-specific T cells from the same donor produce IFN-γ but no Th2 cytokines.

following their polarization. Since Th1 cells mainly express CXCR3 (the receptor for CXCL9, CXCL10 and CXCL11) and CCR5 (the receptor for CCL3, CCL4 and CCL5), they are attracted into inflamed sites where these chemokines are produced [14]. By contrast, Th2 cells mainly express CCR4 (the receptor for CCL17 and CCL22), CCR8 (the receptor for CCL1) and CRTH2 (one of the receptors for PGD_2), which can presently be considered as the only selective marker of human Th2 cells [14]. Contrary to an initial report [34], the presence of CCR3 in human Th2 cells is negligible, this chemokine receptor being mainly expressed by eosinophils, basophils, and mast cells [35]. Therefore, the presence of CCR4, CCR8, and CRTH2 in CD4+ T cells of tissues showing allergic inflammation, as well as the increase in the expression of Th2-attracting factors in the blood and/or target tissue of subjects suffering from allergic disorders, has to be expected. Indeed, CCR4 and CCR8 have been shown to identify airway T cells of allergen-challenged atopic asthmatics [20] and the percentage of CCR4+ cells in CD4+ CD45RO+ T cells from atopic dermatitis (AD) patients was significantly higher than that in healthy controls [36]. In addition, the numbers of CD4+ CRTH2+ cells were found to be elevated in the circulation of subjects with AD [37] and an elevation in PGD_2 levels was observed in allergic diseases, such as asthma, hay fever, as well as in atopic subjects [38, 39]. High levels of CCL22 were found in the serum of AD subjects and CCL22 production by both T cells and DCs was observed in the skin of the same subjects [40]. Elevated plasma concentrations of CCL17 have been observed in childhood asthma [41]. More importantly, CCL17 and CCL22 expression was strongly upregulated on airway epithelial cells of asthmatic subjects following allergen-challenge [20]. By contrast, CXCL10 (a Th1-attracting chemokine) markedly upregulated environmental allergen-driven human IFN-γ but not IL-4 synthesis [42]. Furthermore, plasma CXCL10 levels in nonatopic donors immediately following the grass pollen season fell to within the same range as the recombinant CXCL10 levels yielding a maximum impact in vitro on the antigen-driven IFN-γ response [42]. These data suggest a potential role for IP-10 in maintaining the default Th1-like responses to environmental allergens, thus preventing atopic disease [43]. Therefore, even studies on chemoattractants and their receptors in humans point out the promoting role of Th2 cells and the protective role of Th1 cells in the development of allergic disorders.

Transcription Factors

Th1 and Th2 cells not only exhibit the production of distinct cytokines and the prevalent expression of some chemoattractant receptors, but also the expression of selective transcription factors. Th2 cells express STAT6, c-Maf and GATA-3, whereas T-bet appears to be specific for Th1 cells [15]. So far, a few studies have investigated the expression of these factors in target tissues of subjects with allergic disorders. However, GATA-3 mRNA expression was significantly increased in the airways of asthmatic subjects compared with those of normal control subjects. Cells expressing GATA-3 were mainly CD3+ T cells and the density of GATA-3 mRNA+ cells in asthmatic airways correlated significantly with the numbers of cells expressing IL-5 mRNA [44]. More importantly, GATA-3 expression was increased after allergen challenge even in the absence of de novo inflammatory cell recruitment in the inferior turbinate biopsy specimens of patients with allergic rhinitis [45], as well as in peripheral blood CD4+ CD45RO+ T cells from atopic subjects during allergen-specific reactivation [46]. Accordingly, reduced expression of the specific Th1 transcription factor T-bet was observed in T cells from airways of patients with asthma compared with that in T cells from airways of nonasthmatic subjects [47]. These findings provide evidence even at the molecular level on the Th2 predominance in allergic disorders.

Dominant Role of Th2 Cells in Experimental Models of Allergy and Asthma

The experimental animal models of allergy and asthma based on the transfer of Th1 or Th2 cells have provided controversial results. In some studies, transfer of Th2 but not of Th1 cells into recipient mice induced airway eosinophilia, mucus hypersecretion, and airway hyper-responsiveness (AHR) [48, 49]. Other studies, however, found that transfer of Th1 cells not only fails to counterbalance Th2-induced airway hyper-reactivity, but may even cooperate with Th2 cells in promoting inflammation, particularly in the initial phases [50–52]. However, data obtained in both gene-deficient and transgenic mice provide clear and undoubtable evidence on the critical role of Th2 cells and their cytokines in the pathogenesis of allergy and asthma. Allergy and asthma cannot be induced or are less severe in animals in which the genes involved in the development of Th2 responses, such as CD4+ T cell, major histocompatibility complex, IL-4, IL-5 or IL-13, have been targeted [53–56]. Targeting GATA-3 (a Th2-specific transcription factor) severely attenuated all key features of asthma, such as airway eosinophilia, mucus production and IgE synthesis [57]. Accordingly, the failure of STAT6 (another Th2-selective transcription factor)-deficient mice to develop airway eosinophilia and AHR [58] could only be overcome by IL-5 injection [59]. Likewise, mice with JunB-deficient CD4+ T cells exhibited a strong reduction in IL-4 and IL-5 production, as well as impaired allergen-induced airway inflammation [60]. By contrast, T-bet (a Th1-specific transcription factor)-deficient mice spontaneously demonstrated multiple physiological and inflammatory features characteristic of asthma [47]. Consistent with the critical role of Th2 responses in allergy and asthma are also the observations that transgenic mice overexpressing Th2 cytokines in the airway epithelium exhibit the main pathophysiological features of allergic asthma, such as airway eosinophilia, mucus hyper-production, AHR, and airway remodeling [61–65]. The findings supporting the Th2 predominance in atopic allergy and in experimental animal models of allergy and asthma are summarized in table 1.

Table 1. Data suggesting that allergy is a Th2-dominated disorder

In humans

- Common environmental allergens expand Th2 cells in atopics, but not in nonatopics [16, 17, 19, 109]
- T cells expressing Th2 cytokines are present in the bronchial biopsy specimens [18, 20, 23, 26, 27], in the bronchoalveolar lavage [21], and in the exhaled breath condensate [22] of allergic asthmatics
- Expression of Th1 cytokines is depressed in the blood [28] and in the exhaled breath condensate [22] of asthmatics and DCs from atopic donors produce lower quantities of IL-12 (a powerful Th1-inducing cytokine) than those from normal subjects [29]
- Successful specific immunotherapy is associated with shifting from Th2 to Th1 [30–32], as well as with the increase in the number of IL-12-expressing cells at cutaneous level [33]
- T cells from bronchial biopsies of allergic asthmatics express CCR4 and CCR8 [20] and the production by epithelial cells from the same specimens of CCR4-binding chemokines, CCL17 and CCL22 (which mainly attract Th2 cells), is upregulated by allergen challenge [20]
- Elevated levels of CCL22 are present in the serum of AD patients [40] and elevated levels of CCL17 are present in childhood asthma [41], whereas CXCL10 (which mainly attracts Th1 cells) upregulates allergen-driven IFN-γ and plasma CXCL10 levels in nonatopic subjects fall following the grass pollen season [43]
- Expression of GATA-3 (a Th2-specific transcription factor) by T cells is upregulated in the airways of asthmatics [44] and it is increased following allergen challenge or reactivation [45, 46]
- Expression of T-bet (a Th1-specific transcription factor) is downregulated in T cells present in the airways of asthmatics [47]

In experimental animal models

- Allergic inflammation and asthma cannot be induced in mice made deficient of genes that are required for Th2 differentiation or Th2 effector function [53–60], whereas T-bet-deficient mice spontaneously undergo multiple physiological and inflammatory features characteristic of asthma [47]
- Transgenic mice overexpressing Th2 cytokines in the airway epithelium exhibit the main pathophysiological features of allergic asthma [61–65]

Th2 Responses Account Directly or Indirectly for Virtually All Pathophysiological Manifestations of Allergy and Asthma

Th2 responses can account directly or indirectly for the great majority of pathophysiological manifestations of allergic patients (fig. 3). Besides, to be critical for the differentiation of naïve Th cells into Th2 cells (fig. 1), IL-4 is indeed able to induce the rolling on and adhesion to endothelial cells of circulating eosinophils [66], which can then be attracted into target tissues by both IL-5 and some chemokines. Besides the induction of IgE switching, IL-13 also promotes hypersecretion and induces metaplasia of mucus cells [67].

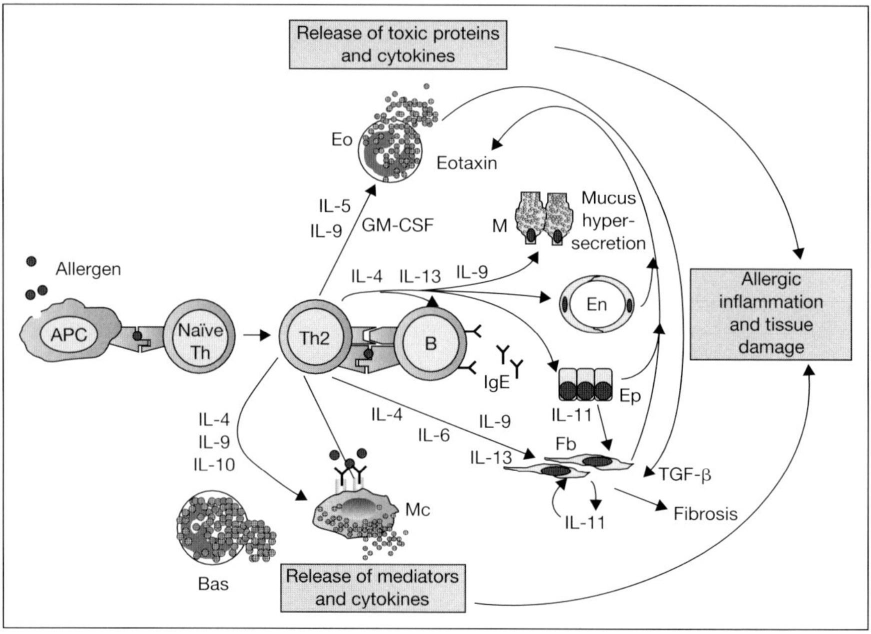

Fig. 3. Allergen-specific Th2 responses to allergens can account directly or indirectly for virtually all pathophysiological manifestations of allergic inflammation and asthma. APC = Antigen-presenting cell; Th = T helper; Th2 = type-2 Th; IL = interleukin; GM-CSF = granulocyte macrophage-colony stimulatory factor; E = eosinophil; B = B lymphocyte; Mc/B = mast cell/basophil; En = endothelial cell; Ep = epithelial cell; TGF = transforming growth factor. See the text for explanations.

IL-13 can cause AHR by directly acting on epithelial cells and smooth muscle cells [68]. IL-9 is also able to induce mucus hypersecretion. By testing lavage fluids from the airways of allergen-challenged dogs and by assessing the activity of asthmatic airway fluids on cultured airway epithelial cells, it was found that IL-9 can account for as much as 50–60% of the mucin-stimulating activity [69]. Both IL-4 and IL-13 stimulate fibroblast growth and chemotaxis, as well as the synthesis of extracellular matrix proteins [70]. However, subepithelial fibrosis in asthma seems mainly to result from the activity of transforming growth factor (TGF)-β, produced by T cells, eosinophils and fibroblasts, IL-11 produced by epithelial cells, as well as IL-6 produced by several cell types, including Th2 cells themselves [67, 71]. Accordingly, engineering of Th2 cells to produce latent TGF-β1 reverted allergen-induced AHR and inflammation, which supports the concept that TGF-β1-producing T cells may play an important regulatory role in asthma [72], and suggests that airway fibrosis and remodeling may be the final consequence of chronic or repeated TGF-β production. Taken all together, these findings indicate that

Th2 cytokines, either directly or indirectly, can account for all the hallmarks of allergic inflammation, including airway remodeling in asthma. It is of note that Th2 cells responsible for experimental allergic asthma persist as long-lived Th2 memory after animal recovery from acute disease and are involved in the generation of allergic asthma upon antigen reexposure [73].

However, it should be noted that at least some pathophysiologic consequences of allergic reactions may occur even in the absence of IgE and mast cell responses. Indeed, B-cell-, IgE-, CD40- or mast cell-deficient mice can still develop asthma [56]. Moreover, at least in a minor proportion of allergic asthmatics, short allergen-derived peptides were found to directly initiate a major histocompatibility complex-restricted, T-cell-dependent, late asthmatic reaction without the requirement for an early IgE/mast cell-dependent response [74], or the production of Th2 cytokines [75]. Thus, at least in a proportion of asthmatics, T-cell-mediated responses may be responsible for the pathophysiological manifestations of asthma even in the apparent absence of the production of Th2 cytokines.

The Role of Environmental Factors in Determining the Th2 Predominance in Allergic Subjects

It is well known that the expression of the allergic phenotype is dependent on two major factors: a genetic predisposition, and the environmental interactions. The pattern of allergic inheritance does not follow the Mendelian concepts usually associated with single-gene diseases. Rather, the pattern of inheritance is that of a complex polygenic disorder. This is consistent with the fact that the development of a prevalent Th2 response is up- and downregulated by the activity of a series of cytokines, cytokine receptors, and transcription factors. Therefore, alterations may be localized in atopic individuals on multiple genes and may differ in different subjects. This makes it difficult to identify major common genetic alterations responsible for atopic allergy, despite the present availability of new powerful technologies.

Environmental Factors Acting before Birth

Environmental factors may influence the differentiation of allergen-specific T cells into a prevalent Th2 phenotype and therefore the development of atopic allergy by acting both before and after birth. Some years ago, we showed that the immune response to Der p begins during fetal life [76], a finding that has since been confirmed by others [77, 78]. In pregnancy a Th2-skewed priming probably occurs in all cases because of the maternal environment. Successful pregnancy may indeed be characterized by a switch from Th1 to Th2 at the maternal–fetal interface to reduce the reactivity of the maternal immune system against the fetal allograft. Accordingly, at the concentrations present at the fetal–maternal interface, progesterone favors the development of T cells into IL-4-producing cells [79]. Moreover, T-cell clones generated from the decidua of women with unexplained recurrent abortions showed significantly reduced production of IL-4, IL-10, and leukemia inhibitory factor in comparison with T-cell clones generated from the decidua of women with underlying voluntary abortion (normal gestation) [80]. More recently, by staining with the Th2-specific marker CRTH2, Th2 cells were found to be significantly increased at the maternal–fetal interface (implantation site) in the decidua [81]. The accumulation of Th2 cells could be explained by the demonstration of PGD_2 synthase in the trophoblast, uterine epithelium and endometrial glands, PGD_2 being a strong chemoattractant for cells expressing CRTH2 [81]. Thus the pregnancy-related environment may favor a weak Th2-skewed priming to transplacental allergens, which is obviously enhanced under the influence of an 'atopic' genetic background.

Environmental Factors Acting after Birth: The 'Hygiene Hypothesis'

Environmental factors acting after birth are certainly more important in influencing the individual outcome in the Th-cell response to ubiquitous allergens and can account for the increased prevalence of allergy over the last decades in Western countries. Indeed, a genetic mechanism with steep changes in gene frequency is highly unlikely in the absence of extraordinary mutation rates or very powerful Darwinian selection. More important, we know that after the occurrence of random TCR rearrangements and the processes of positive and negative selection in the thymus, the educational process of the immune system continues in the periphery, especially in the first years of life, throughout repeated interactions with infectious agents, 'innocuous antigens', and the commensal flora. This process results in both a fine tuning of the TCR repertoire and the progressive shifting of the T-cell effector balance from Th2 to Th1. At the beginning of the 1990s, data from my laboratory showed that, at least in vitro, cytokines (IL-12 and IFNs) produced by cells of 'natural immunity', such as macrophages, DCs, and NK cells, were able to shift the development of allergen-specific T cells from the Th2 or Th0 to the Th1 profile in response to *Mycobacterium tuberculosis* or its components [82–84]. Based on these data and in contrast with the dogma prevailing at that time that pollution was responsible for the increasing prevalence of allergy in developed countries, I hypothesized that this phenomenon could rather be related to changes that have occurred in the infectious environment of children since the Second World War [85]. Since then, several epidemiologic studies (table 2) have clearly shown that changes in the infectious environment and in the pattern of microbial exposure of children, associated with Westernization, are critical factors underlying the rising severity and prevalence of atopic disorders over the last decades in developed countries. This possibility is presently known as the 'hygiene hypothesis'. The 'hygiene hypothesis' has recently been substantiated

Table 2. Main epidemiological findings supporting the validity of the 'hygiene hypothesis'

• Inverse association between tuberculin responses and atopic disorders [86, 88]
• Inverse association between past hepatitis A virus infection and risk for atopy [87]
• Reduced prevalence of atopy in children from anthroposophic families [89]
• Farm environment in childhood prevents the development of allergies [89–92]

by several epidemiological and molecular findings showing that increased exposure to endotoxins is a major protective factor for the development of atopy [93], possibly by upregulating CD14 (the acceptor site for lipopolysaccharide) and Toll-like receptor-2 (which recognizes bacterial lipoprotein and leptospiral lipopolysaccharide) [94]. Of note, the existence of a polymorphism in the CD14 gene [95] suggests a possible molecular model of gene-by-environment interaction in the regulation of Th2 development against allergens during childhood.

If the 'hygiene hypothesis' is now generally accepted as the most reasonable explanation for the 'allergy epidemics', the mechanisms by which the reduced exposure to pathogenic and nonpathogenic microbes during childhood and therefore the reduced stimulation of the innate immunity determines an increased prevalence of Th2 responses to innocuous environmental antigens (allergens) are more controversial. As an alternative to the initial hypothesis of a shift of allergen-specific responses from Th1 to Th2, the importance of reduced suppression of immune responses (both of Th1- and Th2-type) mainly due to a decrease in the production of IL-10 and TGF-β by the immune system has been suggested [97–99]. The last view is based on two major points: (a) allergic diseases have a low prevalence in world areas characterized by diffuse and chronic helminthic infections, which induce strong and persistent Th2 responses, but also high production of IL-10 and TGF-β [97], and (b) the prevalence of insulin-dependent diabetes mellitus (IDDM), an autoimmune disorder which is thought to be characterized by a Th1 predominance, has also increased in the last decades in developed countries [100].

However, I believe that both these points represent wrong checkpoints and, therefore, they can generate rough oversimplifications. Helminth infestation was indeed a rare condition in industrialized countries even when the prevalence of allergy was lower and it is presently absent amongst children from Estonia [101] where prevalence of allergy is as low as in world areas characterized by diffuse and chronic helminthic infestation. This simple remark is sufficient to exclude the possibility that a reduced immune suppression due to the absence of helminthic infestations may cause the increase in the prevalence of atopic allergy in developed countries. The equalization between the increased prevalence of allergy and IDDM is also inappropriate. Atopic allergy is indeed a chronic and often systemic inflammatory process, which affects a high proportion of the population (10–25%), whereas IDDM is a rare (0.0001–0.001%), short-lasting, inflammatory disorder limited to the pancreatic β cells which rapidly ends with their destruction. In addition, it has recently been pointed out that 'initial hopes for a simple Th1-based model to explain the immunopathogenesis of IDDM appear unrealistic' [102]. Thus, based on such a wrong comparison, it is not correct to suggest that both Th1- and Th2-dominated diseases are increased since IDDM cannot be considered as an opposite pole to allergy. In my opinion, there are much more meaningful epidemiological observations showing that subjects with multiple sclerosis, a clearly Th1-polarized and chronic autoimmune disorder, are virtually free from allergic disorders and this is associated with enhanced IL-12 production [103, 104]. Likewise, it is noteworthy that rheumatoid arthritis, another chronic and systemic Th1-mediated disorder, is characterized by a strong reduction in atopic disorders [105]. However, the opponents to the Th1/Th2 switch, as an explanation for the increased prevalence of allergy due to the low burden of infections in childhood, usually neglect both these epidemiological findings. Finally, a series of cellular and molecular findings point out the differences between atopic and nonatopic subjects in terms of Th2 or Th1 polarization in response to allergens and provide evidence that many microbial substances are able, at least in vitro, to induce a switch from Th2 to Th1 in the response to common environmental allergens in atopic subjects. For example, atopic subjects exhibit defective expression of T-bet, a transcription factor essential for Th1 development, whereas nonallergic subjects do not [47]. Microbial oligodeoxynucleotides and synthetic adjuvants, such as imidazoquinolines, which induce high IL-12 production by DCs and IFN-γ production by NK cells, as the majority of microbes do, shift the in vitro allergen-specific T-cell responses from Th2 to Th1 [106, 107]. Recently, it has been reported that children who grew up in Eastern Germany had a marked bias towards Th0/Th1 responsiveness, regardless of whether they were atopic or not, whereas the children of Western Germany, particularly when they were atopic, showed Th2 polarization [108]. Finally and most importantly, although nonallergic subjects exhibit allergen-specific Th1 responses (production of IFN-γ but not IL-4) at the clonal level [109], and as detected by flow cytometry [17] (fig. 2), they have neither allergic symptoms nor any type of inflammatory response to allergen challenge. Taken all together and because of the reduction in the severity and chronicity of infectious diseases during childhood, these findings suggest that the Th1 to Th2 switch represents a more likely explanation for the increased prevalence of allergy which occurred in the last decades in industrialized countries than the reduction in immunosuppressive responses (table 3). Thus, both mechanisms

Table 3. Data suggesting that immune deviation from Th1 to Th2 is a more important mechanism than reduced immune suppression to explain the 'hygiene hypothesis'

Reduced immune suppression

Pro

- High pathogen (viruses, bacteria, helminths) burden results in the production of high concentrations of suppressive cytokines (IL-10, TGF-β)
- Prevalence of allergy is low in world areas characterized by diffuse and chronic helminthic infestations that induce strong Th2 responses
- Prevalence of IDDM (thought to be Th1-predominant inflammatory disorders) is also increasing in developed countries

Contra

- Prevalence of allergy is low even in children from Estonia, where there is no helminthic infestation
- Allergy is a chronic, often systemic, inflammatory disorder, whereas IDDM is a short-lasting inflammation limited to pancreatic β cells, which ends with their destruction

Th1/Th2 switch

Pro

- Subjects with multiple sclerosis, a chronic autoimmune disorder associated with enhanced IL-12 production, are virtually free of atopic disorders
- Subjects with rheumatoid arthritis, a chronic and systemic autoimmune disorder, exhibit a strong reduction in atopic disorders
- Atopic subjects exhibit detective expression of T-bet, a Th1-specific transcription factor that exerts antagonism on the differentiation of Th2 cells
- Many microbial substances or synthetic adjuvants inducing high production of IL-12 and IFNs shift the allergen-specific response from Th2 to Th1
- Children from western Germany (high prevalence of allergy) show major Th2 polarization than children from eastern Germany (low prevalence of allergy)
- Nonallergic subjects exhibit Th1 responses against allergens, as detected both at clonal level and at single cell level by flow cytometry

may be operating, but certainly there is no evidence to point out, as has been done [97], that shifting allergen-specific T-cell responses from Th2 to Th0/Th1 for prevention and/or cure of allergic diseases may be useless or even dangerous.

Conclusions

During the past 10 years, strong evidence has been provided to suggest that Th2-cell responses to 'innocuous' environmental antigens (allergens) play a critical triggering role in the development of allergic inflammation. Th2 cells are not only an explanation for the joint involvement of IgE-producing B cells (via IL-4 and IL-13), mast cells (via IL-4 and IL-9) and eosinophils (via IL-5) in the allergic inflammatory processes, but also account for other pathophysiological features of both allergy and asthma. IL-4, IL-9 and IL-13 can indeed induce mucus hypersecretion and together with IL-5 contribute to the increase in AHR, and together with TGF-β, IL-6 and IL-11 to airway remodeling. More recently, the important role of chemokines in the inflammatory network responsible for allergy and asthma has also been discovered. Chemokines can directly cause cellular activation and inflammatory mediator release by eosinophils and basophils, and can promote the selective recruitment of different effector cell subsets, including Th2 cells, in the inflamed tissue. On the other hand, IL-4 and IL-13 are able to increase the production of the chemokines, such as CCL1, CCL17 and CCL22, that are responsible for Th2 recruitment, whereas IFN-γ produced by Th1 cells stimulates the release of CXCL10, a chemokine that rather favors the development of beneficial allergen-specific T-cell responses. Accordingly, increased levels of Th2 cytokines, Th2-attracting chemokines, as well as transcription factors specific for Th2-cell differentiation have been observed in the target organs of allergic inflammation, whereas the expression of Th1 cytokines, Th1-attracting chemokines, and Th1-specific transcription factors is normal or reduced in the same subjects in comparison with nonatopic individuals. Furthermore, the great majority of experimental animal models of allergy and asthma support the concept of Th2 predominance in the pathogenesis of these disorders.

The demonstration that dominant Th2 responses are responsible for inflammation in atopic individuals can also explain the increased prevalence of allergy and asthma that has occurred during the past few decades in developed countries. Several epidemiological studies suggest that this increase may depend on either the altered balance between Th1 and Th2 responses or the reduction in suppressive mechanisms due to the dramatic change that has occurred in the microbial environment during childhood: the 'hygiene hypothesis'.

References

1 Ehrlich P: Ueber die spezifischen Granulationen des Blutes. Arch Anat Physiol Lpz Physiol Abt 1879;3:571.

2 Prausnitz C, Kustner H: Studien über die Ueberempfindlichkeit. Zbl Bakt Abt I 1921;86:160.

3 Ishizaka K, Ishizaka T: Identification of gamma-E-antibodies as a carrier of reaginic activity. J Immunol 1967;99:1187–1198.

4 Johansson SG: Raised levels of a new immunoglobulin class (IgND) in asthma. Lancet 1967;ii: 951–953.

5 Coffman RL, Carty J: A T cell activity that enhances polyclonal IgE production and its inhibition by interferon-gamma. J Immunol 1986;136:949–954.

6 Del Prete G, Maggi E, Parronchi P, et al: IL-4 is an essential factor for the IgE synthesis induced in vitro by human T cell clones and their supernatants. J Immunol 1988;140: 4193–4198.

7 Pene J, Rousset F, Briere F, et al: IgE production by normal human B cells induced by alloreactive T cell clones is mediated by IL-4 and suppressed by IFN-gamma. J Immunol 1988;141: 1218–1224.

8 Mosmann TR, Cherwinski H, Bond MW, et al: Two types of murine T cell clone. I: Definition according to profiles of lymphokine activities and secreted proteins. J Immunol 1986;136: 2348–2357.
9 Del Prete GF, De Carli M, Mastromauro C, et al: Purified protein derivative of *Mycobacterium tuberculosis* and excretory-secretory antigen(s) of *Toxocara canis* expand in vitro human T cells with stable and opposite (type 1 T helper or type 2 T helper) profile of cytokine production. J Clin Invest 1991;88:346–350.
10 Abbas AK, Murphy K, Sher A: Functional diversity of helper T lymphocytes. Nature 1996;383: 787–793.
11 Romagnani S: Lymphokine production by human T cells in disease states. Annu Rev Immunol 1994;12:227–257.
12 Finkelman FD, Shea-Donohue T, Goldhill J, et al: Cytokine regulation of host defense against parasitic gastrointestinal nematodes: Lessons from studies with rodent models. Annu Rev Immunol 1997;15:505–533.
13 Chen JR, Cheng JG, Shatzer T, et al: Leukemia inhibitory factor can substitute for nidatory estrogen and is essential to inducing a receptive uterus for implantation but is not essential for subsequent embryogenesis. Endocrinology 2000;141:4365–4372.
14 Romagnani S: T-cell subsets (Th1 versus Th2). Ann Allergy Asthma Immunol 2000;85:9–18.
15 Rengarajan J, Szabo SJ, Glimcher LH: Transcriptional regulation of Th1/Th2 polarization. Immunol Today 2000;21:479–483.
16 Parronchi P, Macchia D, Piccinni M-P, et al: Allergen- and bacterial antigen-specific T-cell clones established from atopic donors show a different profile of cytokine production. Proc Natl Acad Sci USA 1991;59:3768–3773.
17 Romagnani S: The Th2 hypothesis in allergy. 'Eppur si muove'. ACI Intern 1998;10:158–165.
18 Robinson DS, Hamid Q, Ying S, et al: Predominant Th2-like bronchoalveolar T-lymphocyte population in atopic asthma. N Engl J Med 1992;326:298–304.
19 Del Prete G, De Carli M, D'Elios MM, et al: Allergen exposure induces the activation of allergen-specific Th2 cells in the airway mucosa of patients with allergic respiratory disorders. Eur J Immunol 1993;23:1445–1449.
20 Panina-Bordignon P, Papi A, Mariani M, et al: The C-C chemokine receptors CCR4 and CCR8 identify airway T cells on allergen-challenged atopic asthmatics. J Clin Invest 2001;107: 1357–1364.
21 Brigtling CE, Symon FA, Birring SS, et al: Th2 cytokine expression in bronchoalveolar lavage fluid T lymphocytes and bronchial submucosa is a feature of asthma and eosinophilic bronchitis. J Allergy Clin Immunol 2002;110:899–905.
22 Shahid SK, Kharitonov SA, Wilson NM, et al: Increased interleukin-4 and decreased interferon-gamma in exhaled breath condensate of children with asthma. Am J Respir Crit Care Med 2002;165:1290–1293.
23 Shimbara A, Christodoulopoulos P, Soussi-Gounni A, et al: IL-9 and its receptor in allergic and nonallergic lung disease: Increased expression in asthma. J Allergy Clin Immunol 2000;105: 108–115.
24 Naseer T, Minshall EM, Leung DY, et al: Expression of IL-12 and IL-13 mRNA in asthma and their modulation in response to steroid therapy. Am J Respir Crit Care Med 1997;155:845–851.
25 Humbert M, Durham SR, Kimmitt P, et al: Elevated expression of messenger ribonucleic acid encoding IL-13 in the bronchial mucosa of atopic and nonatopic subjects with asthma. J Allergy Clin Immunol 1997;99:657–665.
26 Huang SK, Xiao HQ, Kleine-Tebbe J, et al: IL-13 expression at the sites of allergen challenge in patients with asthma. J Immunol 1995;155:2688–2694.
27 Kroegel C, Jiulius P, Matthys H, et al: Endobronchial secretion of interleukin-13 following local allergen challenge in atopic asthma: Relationship to interleukin-4 and eosinophil counts. Eur Respir J 1996;9:899–904.
28 Smart JM, Horak E, Kemp AS, et al: Polyclonal and allergen-induced cytokine responses in adults with asthma: Resolution of asthma is associated with normalization of IFN-gamma responses. J Allergy Clin Immunol 2002;110:450–456.
29 Reider N, Reider D, Ebner S, et al: Dendritic cells contribute to the development of atopy by an insufficiency in IL-12 production. J Allergy Clin Immunol 2002;109:89–95.
30 Secrist H, Chelen CJ, Wen Y, et al: Allergen immunotherapy decreases interleukin 4 production in CD4+ T cells from allergic individuals. J Exp Med 1993;178:2123–2130.

31 McHugh SM, Deighton J, Stewart AG, et al: Bee venom immunotherapy induces a shift in cytokine responses from a Th2 to a Th1 dominant pattern: Comparison of rush and conventional immunotherapy. Clin Exp Allergy 1995;25:828–838.
32 Jutel M, Pichler WJ, Skrbic D, et al: Bee venom immunotherapy results in decrease of IL-4 and IL-5 and increase of IFN-γ secretion in specific allergen-stimulated T cell cultures. J Immunol 1995;54:4187–4194.
33 Hamid QA, Schotman E, Jacobson MR, et al: Increases in IL-12 messenger RNA+ cells accompany inhibition of allergen-induced late skin responses after successful grass pollen immunotherapy. J Allergy Clin Immunol 1997;99:254–260.
34 Sallusto F, Mackay CR, Lanzavecchia A: Selective expression of the eotaxin receptor CCR3 by human T helper 2 cells. Science 1997;277:2005–2007.
35 Romagnani P, De Paulis A, Beltrame C, et al: Tryptase-chymase double-positive human mast cells express the eotaxin receptor CCR3 and are attracted by CCR3-binding chemokines. Am J Pathol 1999;155:1195–1204.
36 Okazaki H, Kakurai M, Hirata D, et al: Characterization of chemokine receptor expression and cytokine production in circulating CD4+ T cells from patients with atopic dermatitis: Up-regulation of C-C chemokine receptor 4 in atopic dermatitis. Clin Exp Allergy 2002;32: 1236–1242.
37 Cosmi L, Annunziato F, Iwasaki M, et al: CRTH2 is the most reliable marker for the detection of circulating human type 2 Th and type cytotoxic cells in health and disease. Eur J Immunol 2000;30:2972–2979.
38 Barr RM, Koro O, Francis DM, et al: The release of prostaglandin D_2 from human skin in vivo and in vitro during immediate allergic reactions. Br J Pharmacol 1988;94:773–780.
39 Pienkowski MM, Adkinson NF, Plaut M, et al: Prostaglandin D_2 and histamine during the immediate and late-phase components of allergic cutaneous responses. J Allergy Clin Immunol 1988;82:95–100.
40 Galli G, Chantry D, Annunziato F, et al: Macrophage-derived chemokine production by activated human T cells in vitro and in vivo: Preferential association with the production of type 2 cytokines. Eur J Immunol 2000;30:204–210.
41 Leung TF, Wong CK, Chan IH, et al: Plasma concentration of thymus and activation-regulated chemokine is elevated in childhood asthma. J Allergy Clin Immunol 2002;110:404–409.
42 Gangur V, Simons ER, Hayglass KT: Human IP-10 selectively promotes dominance of polyclonally activated and environmental antigen-driven IFN-gamma over IL-4 responses. FASEB J 1998;12:705–713.
43 Gangur V, Oppenheim JJ: Are chemokines essential or secondary participants in allergic responses. Ann Allergy Asthma Immunol 2000;84:569–581.
44 Nakamura Y, Ghaffar O, Olivenstein R, et al: Gene expression of the GATA-3 transcription factor is increased in atopic asthma. J Allergy Clin Immunol 1999;103:215–222.
45 Nakamura Y, Christodoulopoulos P, Cameron L, et al: Upregulation of the transcription factor GATA-3 in upper airway mucosa after in vivo and in vitro allergen challenge. J Allergy Clin Immunol 2000;105:1146–1152.
46 Macaubas C, Lee PT, Smallacombe TB, et al: Reciprocal patterns of allergen-induced GATA-3 expression in peripheral blood mononuclear cells from atopic vs. non-atopics. Clin Exp Allergy 2002;32:97–106.
47 Finotto S, Neurath MF, Glickman JN, et al: Development of spontaneous airway changes consistent with human asthma in mice lacking T-bet. Science 2002;295:336–338.
48 Cohn L, Tepper JS, Bottomly K: IL-4-independent induction of airway hyperresponsiveness by Th2, but not Th1, cells. J Immunol 1998;161:3813–3818.
49 Cohn L, Homer RJ, Niu N, Bottomly K: T helper 1 cells and interferon regulate allergic airway inflammation and mucus production. J Exp Med 1999;190:1309–1317.
50 Randolph DA, Stephens R, Carruthers CJL, Chaplin DD: Cooperation between Th1 and Th2 cells in a murine model of eosinophilic airway inflammation. J Clin Invest 1999;104:1021–1029.
51 Randolph DA, Carruthers CJ, Szabo SJ, et al: Modulation of airway inflammation by passive transfer of allergen-specific Th1 and Th2 cells in a mouse model of asthma. J Immunol 1999; 162:2375–2383.
52 Hansen G, McIntire JJ, Yeung P, et al: CD4+ T helper cells engineered to produce latent TGF-β1 reverse allergen-induced airway hyperreactivity and inflammation. J Clin Invest 2000; 105:61–70.

53 Corry DB, Grunig G, Hadeiba H, et al: Requirements for allergen-induced airway hyperreactivity in T and B cell-deficient mice. Mol Med 1998;4:344–355.
54 Schmitz J, Thiel A, Kuhn R, et al: Induction of interleukin 4 (IL-4) expression in T helper (Th) cells is not dependent on IL-4 from non-Th cells. J Exp Med 1994;179:1349–1354.
55 Matthaei KI, Foster P, Young IG: The role of interleukin-5 (IL-5) in vivo: Studies with IL-5-deficient mice. Mem Inst Oswaldo Cruz 1997;92(suppl 2):63–68.
56 Ray A, Cohn L: Th2 cells and GATA-3 in asthma: New insights into the regulation of airway inflammation. J Clin Invest 1999;104:995–1006.
57 Zhang DH, Yang L, Cohn L, et al: Inhibition of allergic inflammation in a murine model of asthma by expression of a dominant-negative mutant of GATA-3. Immunity 1999;11:473–482.
58 Miyata S, Matsuyama T, Kodama T, et al: STAT6 deficiency in a mouse model of allergen-induced airways inflammation abolishes eosinophilia but induces infiltration of CD8+ T cells. Clin Exp Allergy 1999;29:114–123.
59 Tomkinson A, Kanehiro A, Rabinovitch N, et al: The failure of STAT6-deficient mice to develop airway eosinophilia and airway hyperresponsiveness is overcome by interleukin-5. Am J Respir Crit Care Med 1999;160:1283–1291.
60 Hartenstein B, Teurich S, Hess J, et al: Th2 cell-specific cytokine expression and allergen-induced airway inflammation depend on JunB. EMBO J 2002;21:6321–6329.
61 Zhu Z, Homer RJ, Wang Z, et al: Pulmonary expression of interleukin-13 causes inflammation, mucus hypersecretion, subepithelial fibrosis, physiologic abnormalities, and eotaxin production. J Clin Invest 1999;103:779–788.
62 Temann UA, Geba GP, Rankin JA, Flavell RA: Expression of interleukin 9 in the lungs of transgenic mice causes airway inflammation, mast cell hyperplasia, and bronchial hyperresponsiveness. J Exp Med 1998;188:1307–1320.
63 Rankin JA, Picarella DE, Geba GP, et al: Phenotypic and physiologic characterization of transgenic mice expressing interleukin-4 in the lung: Lymphocytic and eosinophilic inflammation without airway hyperreactivity. Proc Natl Acad Sci USA 1996;93:7821–7825.
64 Lee NA, McGarry MP, Larson KA, et al: Expression of IL-5 in thymocytes/T cells leads to the development of a massive eosinophilia, extramedullary eosinophilopoiesis, and unique histopathologies. J Immunol 1997;158:1332–1344.
65 Elias JA, Zhu Z, Chupp G, Homer RJ: Airway remodelling in asthma. J Clin Invest 1999;104: 1001–1006.
66 Bochner BS, Schleimer RP: The role of adhesion molecules in human eosinophils and basophils recruitment. J Allergy Clin Immunol 1994;94:427–438.
67 Zhu Z, Lee GG, Zheng T, et al: Airway inflammation and remodelling in asthma. Lessons from interleukin 11 and interleukin 13 transgenic mice. Am J Respir Crit Care Med 2001;164: S67–S70.
68 Kuperman DA, Huang X, Koth LL, et al: Direct effects of interleukin 13 on epithelial cells cause airway hyperreactivity and mucus hyperproduction in asthma. Nat Med 2002; 8:885–889.
69 Longphre M, Li D, Gallup M, et al: Allergen-induced IL-9 directly stimulates mucin transcription in respiratory epithelial cells. J Clin Invest 1999;104:1375–1382.
70 Doucet C, Brouty-Boye D, Pottin-Clemenceau C, et al: Interleukin (IL) 4 and IL-13 on human lung fibroblasts. Implication in asthma. J Clin Invest 1998;101:2129–2139.
71 Ohno I, Nitta Y, Yamauchi K, et al: Transforming growth factor-β (TGF-β) gene expression by eosinophils in asthmatic airway inflammation. Am J Respir Crit Care Med 1996;15:404–409.
72 Hansen G, McIntire JJ, Yeung VP, et al: CD4+ T helper cells engineered to produce latent TGF-beta1 reverse allergen-induced airway hyperreactivity and inflammation. J Clin Invest 2000;105:61–70.
73 Mojitabavi N, Dekan G, Stingl G, Epstein MM: Long-lived Th2 memory in experimental allergic asthma. J Immunol 2002;169:4788–4796.
74 Haselden BM, Kay AB, Larché M: Immunoglobulin E-independent major histocompatibility complex-restricted T cell peptide epitope-induced late asthmatic reactions. J Exp Med 1999; 189:1885–1894.
75 Haselden BM, Larchè M, Meng Q, et al: Late asthmatic reactions provoked by intradermal injection of T-cell peptide epitopes are not associated with bronchial mucosal infiltration of eosinophils or T(h)2-type cells or with elevated concentrations of histamine or eicosanoids in bronchoalveolar fluid. J Allergy Clin Immunol 2001;108:394–401.

76 Piccinni M-P, Mecacci F, Sampognaro S, et al: Aeroallergen sensitization can occur during fetal life. Int Arch Allergy Immunol 1993;102:301–303.
77 Jones AC, Miles EA, Warner JO, et al: Fetal peripheral blood mononuclear cells proliferative responses to mitogenic and allergenic stimuli during gestation. Pediatr Allergy Immunol 1996;7:109–116.
78 Szepfalusi Z, Pichler J, Elsasser S, et al: Transplacental priming of the human immune system with environmental allergens can occur early in gestation. J Allergy Clin Immunol 2000;106: 441–443.
79 Piccinni M-P, Giudizi M-G, Biagiotti R, et al: Progesterone favors the development of human T helper cells producing Th2-type cytokines and promotes both IL-4 production and membrane CD30 expression in established Th1 cell clones. J Immunol 1995;155:128–133.
80 Piccinni MP, Beloni L, Livi C, et al: Role of type 2 T helper (Th2) cytokines and leukemia inhibitory factor (LIF) produced by decidual T cells in unexplained recurrent abortions. Nat Med 1998;4:1020–1024.
81 Michimata T, Tsuda H, Sadai M, et al: Accumulation of CRTH2-positive T-helper 2 and T-cytotoxic 2 cells at implantation sites in human deciduas in a prostaglandin D(2)-mediated manner. Mol Hum Reprod 2002;8:181–187.
82 Maggi E, Parronchi P, Manetti R, et al: Reciprocal regulatory role of IFN-γ and IL-4 on the in vitro development of human Th1 and Th2 cells. J Immunol 1992;148:2142–2147.
83 Parronchi P, De Carli M, Manetti R, et al: IL-4 and IFN(s) (alpha and gamma) exert opposite regulatory effects on the development of cytolytic potential by Th1 or Th2 human T cell clones. J Immunol 1992;149:2977–2982.
84 Manetti R, Parronchi P, Giudizi MG, et al: Natural killer cell stimulatory factor (interleukin-12) induces T helper type 1 (Th1)-specific immune responses and inhibits the development of IL-4-producing Th cells. J Exp Med 1993;177:1199–1204.
85 Romagnani S: Regulation of Th2 development in allergy. Curr Opin Immunol 1994;6:838–846.
86 Shirikawa T, Enomoto T, Shimazu SI, Hopkin J: The inverse association between tuberculin responses and atopic disorders. Science 1997;3:350–400.
87 Matricardi PM, Rosmini F, Ferrigno L, et al: Cross-sectional retrospective study of prevalence of atopy among Italian military students with antibodies against hepatitis A virus. BMJ 1997; 314:999–1003.
88 von Hertzen L, Klaukka T, Mattila H, Haahtela T: Mycobacterium tuberculosis infection and the subsequent development of asthma and allergic conditions. J Allergy Clin Immunol 1999; 104:1211–1214.
89 Alm JS, Swartz J, Lilja G, et al: Atopy in children of families with an anthroposophic lifestyle. Lancet 1999;353:1485–1488.
90 Kilpelainen M, Terho EO, Helenius H, Koskenvuo M: Farm environment in childhood prevents the development of allergies. Clin Exp Allergy 2000;30:201–208.
91 Riedler J, Eder W, Oberfeld G, Schreuer M: Austrian children living on a farm have less hay fever, asthma and allergic sensitization. Clin Exp Allergy 2000;30:194–200.
92 Von Ehrenstein OS, Von Mutius E, Illi S, et al: Reduced risk of hay fever and asthma among children of farmers. Clin Exp Allergy 2000;30:187–195.
93 Braun-Fahrlander C, Ridler J, Herz U, et al: Environmental exposure to endotoxin and its relation to asthma in school-age children. N Engl J Med 2002;347:869–877.
94 Lauener RP, Birchler T, Adamski J, et al: Expression of CD14 and Toll-like receptor 2 in farmers' and nonfarmers' children. Lancet 2002;360:465–466.
95 Baldini M, Lohman IC, Halonen M, et al: A polymorphism in the 5′-flanking region of the CD14 gene is associated with circulating soluble CD14 levels and with total serum IgE. Am J Respir Cell Mol Biol 1999;20:976–983.
96 Martinez FD: The coming-of-age of the hygiene hypothesis. Respir Res 2001;2:129–132.
97 Yazdanbakhah M, Kremsner PG, van Ree R: Allergy, parasites, and the hygiene hypothesis. Science 2002;296:490–494.
98 Umetsu DT, McIntire JJ, Macaubas C, DeKruyff RH: Asthma: An epidemic of dysregulated immunity. Nat Immunol 2002;3:715–720.
99 Wills-Karp M, Santeliz J, Karp CL: The germless theory of allergic disease: Revisiting the hygiene hypothesis. Nat Rev Immunol 2001;1:69–75.
100 Bach JF: The effect of infections on susceptibility to autoimmune and allergic diseases. N Engl J Med 2002;347:911–920.

101 Holt PG: Parasites, atopy, and the hygiene hypothesis: Resolution of a paradox? Lancet 2000;356:1699–1700.
102 Atkinson MA, Wilson SB: Fatal attraction: Chemokines and type 1 diabetes. J Clin Invest 2002;110:1611–1613.
103 Tang L, Benjaponpitak S, DeKruyff H, Umetsu DT: Reduced prevalence of allergic disease in patients with multiple sclerosis is associated with enhanced IL-12 production. J Allergy Clin Immunol 1998;102:428–435.
104 Tremlett HL, Evand J, Wiles CM, Luscombe DK: Asthma and multiple sclerosis: An inverse association in a case-control general practice population. QJM 2002;95:753–756.
105 van Roon JAG, Bijlsma JWJ: Th2 mediated regulation in RA and the spondyloarthropathies. Ann Rheum Dis 2002;61:951–954.
106 Parronchi P, Brugnolo F, Annunziato F, et al: Phosphorothioate oligodeoxynucleotides promote the in vitro development of human allergen-specific CD4+ T cells into Th1 effectors. J Immunol 1999;163:5946–5953.
107 Brugnolo F, Sampognaro S, Liotta F, et al: The novel synthetic immune response modifier R-848 (Resiquimod) shifts human allergen-specific CD4+ Th2 lymphocytes into IFN-gamma-producing cells. J Allergy Clin Immunol 2003;111:380–388.
108 Renz H, von Mutius E, Illi S, et al: Th1/Th2 immune response profiles differ between atopic children in eastern and western Germany. J Allergy Clin Immunol 2002;109:338–342.
109 Wierenga EA, Snoek M, Jansen HM, et al: Human atopen-specific types 1 and 2 T helper cell clones. J Immunol 1991;147:2942–2949.

Discussion

Dr. Lack: Thank you for a very clear talk. The evidence is very compelling that Th2 plays a role in allergy. In your early work, more than 10 years ago, you used a purified protein derivative (PPD) and tetanus as paradigms of Th1 and Th2 immunity. Tetanus reproducibly produces the Th2 response with measurable levels of IL-4 similar to children with peanut or egg allergy, and you see no IgE [1]. So is Th2 a sufficient condition or is it a necessary condition for the development of allergic responses?

Dr. Romagnani: This is a very important question. Indeed when we started in atopic donors to compare the profile of T-cell clones specific for allergens with that of clones specific for bacterial antigens using both PPD and tetanus toxoid as bacterial components, we surprisingly found that in these subjects the profile of PPD-specific T cells was different not only from that of allergen-specific T cells, but also from toxoid-specific T cells. The profile of PPD-specific T cells was indeed definitely Th1, whereas the profile of many tetanus toxoid-specific T-cell clones was more oriented toward the Th2 profile, like that of allergen-specific T cells [2]. The reason is probably that the T-cell memory to PPD is due to a previous infection with corpuscular antigens, such as mycobacteria or Calmette-Guérin bacillus, whereas the memory to tetanus toxoid is the consequence of an artificial immunization with a soluble antigen. Indeed, it is known that corpuscular antigens usually induce Th1 responses, whereas soluble antigens preferentially evoke complex responses characterized by the production of both Th1 and Th2 cytokines. My feeling is that if we continue to inject tetanus toxoid more than 2–3 times during the life time, high levels of specific IgE may be produced and even anaphylactic shock to tetanus toxoid may be provoked.

Dr. Lack: The second question is that you mentioned immunotherapy as evidence, suggesting that the shift from Th2 to Th1 may be in favor of the hypothesis. If allergic disease is a Th2 disease, with a deficiency in interferon-γ production, how would you explain the failure of high-dose interferon-γ in clinical trials for atopic dermatitis, asthma and allergic rhinitis?

Dr. Romagnani: First of all, at least in a small proportion of subjects, immunologic changes were observed following the administration of aerosolized interferon [3].

Moreover, the Th1-inducing activity of specific immunotherapy was also confirmed by the study of Hamid et al. [4] showing increased skin levels of IL-12 in treated subjects. Interferon injection probably does not induce a clear-cut shift because systemic injection does not enable sufficient concentrations of this cytokine to reach the microenvironment where allergen presentation occurs without inducing heavy side effects. With regard to the Th1-shifting effects of specific immunotherapy I would like to make an additional comment. They rarely occur because the adjuvant we are presently using favors Th2 responses. The same adjuvant is used in all types of vaccines currently used, such as diphtheria, tetanus toxoid, etc. I think that we should search for different adjuvants able to favor Th1-oriented responses. This probably might have some effect on reducing the risk of developing allergy.

Dr. Schiffrin: You have shown a lot of evidence for the bronchi and the lungs. Is there anything comparable in the intestine for allergy or, for example, if I can go a little bit further, Crohn's disease and ulcerative colitis? Can you show this paradigm?

Dr. Romagnani: We published one of the first studies showing that Crohn's disease is characterized by a prevalent Th1 phenotype of intestinal T cells and this is due to abnormal IL-12 production in the intestinal environment [5]. Now there is general agreement that Crohn's disease is a Th1-dominant disorder. By contrast, the profile of T cells in ulcerative colitis is probably different. In our study we could not demonstrate a clear-cut Th2 profile of T cells in this disease; however, it is know that eosinophils are frequent in the intestine of these subjects, thus suggesting that the production of IL-5 occurs.

Dr. Neijens: I noticed that the arguments you brought in were based on studies under standardized conditions: you challenge with allergens and then take out material and show a Th2 response including signal transduction proteins. However, clinical medicine is much more complicated, we have variable situations, variable doses, we have infections occurring. Under these conditions what do we know about the responses, in particular in combination with infections or different doses that might be quite different?

Dr. Romagnani: I agree with you. Biologic responses are always complex and we often tend to oversimplify them. The same has been done with the Th1/Th2 paradigm. In all my talks I try to recommend that the image of a clear-cut dichotomy be forgotten because the Th-cell response is not that rigid. We can have a prevalent Th1 or a prevalent Th2 response according to the conditions in which it takes place, but often a shift from one profile to another is seen because all these responses are highly regulated and counterregulated. This is because they result from interactions between infectious agents and the host which both tend to avoid dangerous effects from the immune response. However, in the last 15 years I have studied the profile of the T-cell response at the level of target organs in many diseases and I can assure you that allergy is one of the pathological conditions in which polarization of allergen-specific T cells toward the Th2 profile is really a consistent phenomenon.

Dr. von der Weid: We saw in the previous presentation that bacterial colonization delivers a strong switch signal to the mucosal immune system. Is there any study in the mouse or in humans showing that bacterial colonization modulates one of those genes that you were talking about, the T-bet, STAT4, STAT6?

Dr. Romagnani: I think so far there are no studies on T-bet in different infections because this transcription factor has only very recently been identified. But we know that usually bacterial infections stimulate Toll-like receptors present on dendritic cells and therefore they induce the production by these cells and NK cells of cytokines, such as IL-12 and interferons, that provide an optimal local microenvironment for the development of Th1 responses. In this case it is clear that STAT-4 and T-bet are prevalently activated and this results in the cascade of intracellular events that lead to the activation of interferon-γ promoter and therefore to the Th1-oriented response. I would also like to remind you that T-bet expression is antagonistic for the development of Th2 responses. Indeed, allergic asthmatics exhibit reduced T-bet expression at the bronchial level in comparison with normal subjects [6]. So it is reasonable clear that many infectious agents may antagonize Th2 responses. I think this point will be discussed later.

Dr. Holt: I don't really disagree with anything that you have said, but as you know the story that I put up was a variation on the same thing. In fact some of the work with GATA-3 that you described was done in my laboratory, so clearly we understand what is happening in the adult world. I am working in a pediatric environment and I am continuously being reminded by my pediatric colleagues that children are not small adults, and also that pediatric asthma, for example, is not adult asthma. I think what we are starting to learn is that allergen-specific T-cell memory in childhood is not allergen-specific T-cell memory in adulthood because we are comparing an immune response that might be 2, 3, 4, 5, 10 years old to one that is 20, 30, 40, 50 years old. We are starting to think that during childhood there are developmental changes in the immune response that we are just beginning to understand. A number of the phenotypes I was describing don't appear to exist in the adult world or else they are small phenotypes or else people have been ignoring them. In particular when you do bronchial biopsy studies and in situ hybridization, as we have done, usually you have to go through about 150 slides to find the one that you want and you have to be convinced that the picture is very clean because we have seen lots of interferon-γ also in adults. So the situation in adults is different from the way you describe it, but there are other situations.

Dr. Romagnani: I agree with your comments. We only looked at the response of adults, who are clearly immunologically different from children. However, our data on the Th2 profile of allergen-specific T cells were confirmed by other groups using different experimental approaches such as in situ hybridization or confocal microscopy on bronchial biopsy specimens [7, 8]. We have also looked at the T-cell clones generated from bronchial biopsy specimens following allergen challenge and found that high numbers of T cells (25–30%) were specific for the allergen used for the challenge and the great majority of them exhibited a clear-cut Th2 profile [9]. More recently the same Th2 predominance was found by measuring cytokines in exhaled breath concentrate [10]. So I think that allergy is really a Th2-mediated disorder. Doubt no more on that!

Dr. Lack: There have been a number of immune defects recently recognized in the IL-12 interferon-γ axis. For example in interferon-γ receptor deficiency, these children have repeated mycobacterial infections. What is peculiar is that they have deficient Th1 responses, but you don't see eczema, asthma, allergies or IgE production anymore than in normal children. Why do you think that is?

Dr. Romagnani: I think that the number of children with these defects is too small to draw any definite conclusions. Indeed, to get allergic disorders not only the environment but also the existence of several genetic abnormalities are required.

Dr. Sorensen: I have always been puzzled by the fact that if you attend an allergy meeting the Th2 cell is the bad cell, if you go to infectious disease meetings the Th2 cell is the good cell that is essential to produce protective IgG antibodies, and I would like to find the clear explanation as to why we have such different opinions about the same cell.

Dr. Romagnani: This is right. Even in this field oversimplification is very common. The equation Th1 cell/cell-mediated immunity and Th2 cell/antibody production is not correct. Indeed Th1 cells are responsible for the so-called cell-mediated immunity, but the production of soluble antibodies is favored by both Th1 and Th2 cells.

The difference rests in the prevalence of Ig classes. In mice, Th1 cells induce IgG2a while Th2 cells induce IgG1 and IgE; in humans, Th1 cells induce IgG1, IgG2 and IgG3 while Th2 cells induce IgE and IgG4. Now, the majority of vaccines we are using are based on the induction of IgG production because neutralization of toxins or extracellular bacteria can be easily achieved by soluble antibodies. So to prevent these infections Th2 responses are sufficiently active. However, I believe that to get immunity against infections such as malaria or HIV we should be able to promote prevalent Th1 and CD8 responses. However, it is clear that even Th2 responses can be protective and I have a bias towards the attempts to cure allergy by globally suppressing Th2 responses. The goal I would like to achieve for the therapy of allergy is to develop novel therapeutic strategies that suppress or shift only the allergen-specific Th2 responses.

Dr. Al-Malik: In children, most of the time, either asthma or cow's milk allergy or egg allergy or atopic dermatitis disappear by the age of 5–7 years. As we said, they outgrow their allergy. Is it in children that that there is an overproduction of IL-13 and IL-4 that enhances their allergy, or are we dealing with a maturation process for Th1 that has not been at this stage of growth activity?

Dr. Romagnani: At the beginning of life, the immune response is prevalently Th2-oriented, even for maternal reasons. As you know pregnancy needs a Th2 environment to avoid the rejection of fetal transplant from the immune system of the mother. Then the child starts to have infections in the first years of life and infectious agents usually induce the production of IL-12 and interferons by dendritic and NK cells that results in a progressive polarization of the response toward the Th1 phenotype. Accordingly we know that the development of allergy in late age is a rare phenomenon. The reduced microbial burden during childhood may be the reason why the prevalence of allergy has strongly increased in the last decades in developed countries.

Dr. Rijntjes: A lot of patients with immune deficiency have high IgE. They have atopic dermatitis but clinically the difference is the itching because most of the time dermatitis does not itch. So do you think because the itching is faulted, especially irritation of the nerves, that neuropeptides play a special role in the predominance of the Th2 cells?

Dr. Romagnani: My answer is no.

Dr. Rijntjes: Why?

Dr. Romagnani: Because at the beginning of the 1990s we did a lot of experiments designed to demonstrate the effects of several hormones and neuropeptides on Th cell polarization, but we found that only progesterone had some effect in favoring Th2 differentiation.

Dr. West: You have talked about Th1 and Th2 cells and their respective cytokine patterns. Would you like to comment on the Th3 and regulatory T cells in relation to allergy?

Dr. Romagnani: As you know Th3 cells were first described in a particular model: the oral administration of myelin basic protein to prevent experimental autoimmune encephalomyelitis in mice. Th3 cells are able to suppress the disease mainly by producing TGF-β. However, there is still no convincing experimental evidence to support the role of TGF-β in suppressing allergy. You know that there are different families of T-regulatory cells: those that act by contact such as CD4+ CD25+ T cells, and those that act by producing cytokines such as IL-10 and TGF-β. However, so far it is clear that CD4+ CD25+ T cells suppress Th1 responses, but it is possible that they have no activity on Th2 cells. The role of IL-10 in suppressing allergy is better documented. However, we also know that IL-10 gene-deficient mice have increased Th1 responses but decreased Th2 responses. This suggests that in some conditions IL-10 may even favor Th2 responses. So additional studies are required before drawing definite conclusions on this topic.

Dr. von der Weid: There will be a session tomorrow morning on oral tolerance and I am sure that we will come back to regulatory T cells then. I have a question that I think has been hanging around for a long time. What is the earliest source of IL-4 and how is a Th2 response actually initiated?

Dr. Romagnani: This is one of the few unsolved mysteries of the Th1/Th2 story. At least three different possibilities have been suggested. The first possibility is that early IL-4 production, required for Th2 differentiation, is due to a particular cell type, known as NK1.1+ T cells because they have markers shared by NK and T cells. However, these cells cannot be operative in the majority of pathophysiologic conditions because they are only activated by some particular antigens. The second possibility is that there is a cell working in the opposite way to dendritic cells (which produce the Th1-inducing cytokine IL-12) and this may be the mast cell. Mast cells are able to produce high amounts of IL-4 which are stored in the granules following nonspecific or specific stimulation. However, it is difficult to think that all allergens possess some structure able to induce nonspecific mast cell stimulation. Indeed, to have specific stimulation, the presence of specific IgE antibodies bound on the surface of mast cells is required and specific IgE antibodies can only be produced by B cells under cooperation of Th2 cells. So it is not possible to have IL-4 specifically produced by mast cells in the absence of Th2 cells. My personal feeling is that the source of early IL-4 required for Th2 polarization is the naïve Th cell itself. Probably this early IL-4 production is due to both environmental and genetic reasons. Once a given threshold in IL-4 production has been exceeded, this results in additional IL-4 production, stimulation of STAT-6, and then activation of GATA-3, resulting in Th2 differentiation.

References

1 Turnacu V, Lack G: Characterisation of lymphocyte responses to peanut in normal children, peanut-allergic children and allergic children who acquired tolerance to peanuts. J Clin Invest 2003;111:1065–1072.

2 Parronchi P, Macchia D, Piccinni M-P, et al: Allergen- and bacterial antigen-specific T-cell clones established from atopic donors show a different profile of cytokine production. Proc Natl Acad Sci USA 1991;59:3768–3773.

3 Boguniewicz M, Martin RJ, Martin D, et al: The effects of nebulized recombinant interferon-gamma in asthmatic airways. J Allergy Clin Immunol 1995;95:133–135.

4 Hamid QA, Schotman E, Jacobson MR, et al: Increase in IL-12 messenger RNA+ cells accompany inhibition of allergen-induced late skin responses after successful grass pollen immunotherapy. J Allergy Clin Immunol 1997;99:254–260.

5 Parronchi P, Romagnani P, Scaletti C, et al: Type 1 T-helper cell predominance and interleukin-12 expression in the intestine of patients with Crohn's disease. Am J Pathol 1997;150: 823–832.

6 Finotto S, Neurath MF, Glickman JN, et al: Development of spontaneous airway changes consistent with human asthma in mice lacking T-bet. Science 2002;295:336–338.

7 Robinson DS, Hamid QA, Ying S, et al: Predominant Th2-linked bronchoalveolar T-lymphocyte population in atopic asthma. N Engl J Med 1992;326:298–304.

8 Panina-Bordignon P, Papi A, Mariani M, et al: The C-C chemokine receptors CCR4 and CCR8 identify airway T cells on allergen-challenged atopic asthmatics. J Clin Invest 2001;107: 1357–1364.

9 Del Prete GF, De Carli M, D'Elios MM, et al: Allergen exposure induces the activation of allergen-specific Th2 cells in airway mucosa of patients with allergic disorders. Eur J Immunol 1993;23:1445–1449.

10 Shahid SK, Kharitonov SA, Wilson NM, et al: Increased interleukin-4 and decreased interferon-gamma in exhaled condensate of children with asthma. Am J Respir Crit Care Med 2002; 165:1390–1293.

Isolauri E, Walker WA (eds): Allergic Diseases and the Environment.
Nestlé Nutrition Workshop Series Pediatric Program, Vol. 53, pp. 97–116,
Nestec Ltd.; Vevey/S. Karger AG, Basel, © 2004.

The Induction of Immunoregulation Prevents the Development of Immunopathology in Chronic Helminth Infections and Allergy

Anita H.J. van den Biggelaar and Maria Yazdanbakhsh

Department of Parasitology, Leiden University Medical Center, Leiden, The Netherlands

Introduction

Humans are exposed to aeroallergens worldwide, but only some (in the West an estimated 40%) become sensitized, i.e. produce allergen-specific IgE antibodies. In the West about a quarter of the sensitized population develops allergic diseases, whereas in rural areas of developing countries the sensitized population rarely develops allergy [1–3]. Since genetic predisposition alone cannot explain the tremendous rise in allergies in the West or urban centers of developing countries, environmental risk factors that change with progressive urbanization are likely to play a role. One risk factor, the decrease in experiencing infectious diseases, has been held responsible for the rise in allergic diseases and has led to the so-called 'hygiene hypothesis' [4–7].

Allergic diseases have in common that immunopathology is mediated by allergen-specific type-2 T-helper (Th2) cell responses. For example, in asthma both the production of IgE antibodies, which after cross-linking induce degranulation of mast cells, and the recruitment of effector cells, which cause damage to the epithelial layer of the airways, are orchestrated by the production of Th2 cytokines [8–11]. Moreover, atopic dermatitis is associated with the recruitment of eosinophils and Th2 cells to the skin [12], and also for food allergy increased Th2 responses play a central role in the expression of disease [13, 14]. Therefore, the postulation that Th2 responses are central in the immunopathogenesis of allergic diseases seems beyond dispute.

The immunological interpretation of the 'hygiene hypothesis' has been as follows: the rise in allergies results from a shift in the Th1/Th2 balance towards Th2 due to the decrease in experiencing Th1-inducing infectious diseases [15, 16]. This suggests that the increase in allergy is predominantly due to an increase in Th2 responses. However, the Th1/Th2 paradigm fails to explain why, simultaneous with the rise in allergy, Th1-mediated autoimmune diseases have become more prevalent [17–21], nor can this paradigm substantiate the finding that the risk to develop allergy is reduced in people who are infected with Th2-inducing helminths [22–26]. We therefore argue against the postulate that the development of allergic diseases is primarily due to a shift towards Th2. Without refuting the hypothesis that infectious diseases may counterbalance the development of allergy, we believe that another immunological mechanism involving the immunoregulatory network of the human immune system underlies the 'hygiene hypothesis' [27].

Here we will first discuss the responsiveness of the human immune system against helminth infections, and schistosomes in particular. Schistosome infections are immunologically characterized by a Th2 response but also the activation of an immunoregulatory response. The latter becomes activated during chronic infections and controls parasite-specific immune responses resulting in benefit to both the parasite and the infected host. Next, the concept will be discussed that parasite-induced immunosuppression may, as a result of spillover suppression, downregulate allergen-specific responses. Since there is increasing evidence that parasites are directly involved in inducing immunosuppression, the absence of parasites, as in Western populations, will have implications for the activation of this immunoregulatory response and consequently the control of immune responses against allergens.

Immunity, Immunopathology and Immunosuppression in Schistosome Infections

Parasite-Specific Th2 Responses: Do They Protect or Harm the Host?

Schistosomiasis, a parasitic disease caused by infection with trematodes belonging to the genus *Schistosoma*, is generally characterized by a skewing of the specific immune response towards Th2. Although in an endemic area a minor group of individuals (the 'endemic normals') is able to resist infection [28], the majority of the exposed endemic population will become infected. Typically, the prevalence and intensity of schistosome infection rise during childhood, followed by a decline during adulthood. Since differences in exposure cannot explain this age-infection curve and the peak in the age-infection curve occurs earlier in areas with higher transmission levels [29, 30], it has been postulated that humans may acquire immunity against schistosomes with an increased exposure to parasite antigens. The first immunoepidemological studies searching for immunological associates showed that parasite-specific IgE antibodies increased with age coinciding with the rise in infections [31, 32]. Parasite-specific IgE antibodies were therefore assumed to be mediators of immunity and specific Th2 responses were considered protective. Accordingly, chemotherapy studies showed that individuals who remained uninfected ('resistant') after treatment-induced parasite clearance produced higher levels of parasite-specific IgE than reinfected ('susceptible') subjects [33–35]. However, the active role of parasite-specific IgE antibodies in schistosome immunity became disputable when in recently exposed communities (where the time of exposure is independent of age) adults were found to be less susceptible to infection than children, whereas the levels of parasite-specific IgE antibodies were similar [36, 37]. In fact, in these areas levels of parasite-specific IgE were found to be associated with infection intensity [38, 39].

Considering that a relative long period of time is needed to develop protective immunity, it has been hypothesized that dying – and not living – adult worms may be the source delivering the stimulus for Th2-mediated acquired immunity [40]. Indeed, treatment with anthelminthics (that damage the adult worms) results in profound immunological changes such as an increased production of specific IL-4 and IL-5 and elevated levels of parasite-specific IgE and IgG1 antibodies [34, 41–45]. These observations gave rise to the postulation that repeated anthelminthic treatment would result in an accelerated acquisition of immunity [40]. However, we recently showed Gabonese that repeated anthelminthic treatment (Praziquantel, every 3 months for 2 years) of schoolchildren infected with *S. haematobium* did not result in an increased resistance to reinfection, despite the significant amplification of parasite-specific Th2 cytokines and antibody levels [45]. On the contrary, we found that elevated levels of parasite-specific IL-5 were associated with an increased risk of developing pathology one year later. Clinical manifestations of *S. haematobium* infection mainly result from eggs trapped in bladder tissue provoking a granulomatous inflammatory response. Although in mice schistosome-specific Th2 responses have been shown to be associated with the development of pathology [46, 47] and granuloma formation [48], this is the first evidence that in humans schistosome-specific Th2 responses may be associated with tissue damage. Parasite-induced Th2 responses in infected hosts should therefore be considered potentially protective and harmful.

Immunosuppression in Chronic Schistosome Infections: A Role for IL-10

Adult schistosome worms can survive for many years (approximately 3–7 years) in the human host, despite the presence of sometimes vigorous (Th2) responses. Interestingly, with prolonged time and intensity of infection, the proliferation and cytokine production of parasite-specific Th1 and Th2 cells appears to become suppressed [49]. Apparently during the course of infection a negative feedback loop becomes activated. This may be induced by the parasite itself, since parasite clearance by chemotherapy may restore immunoresponsiveness [42, 50]. It has been suggested that the immunosuppressive cytokine IL-10, which is increasingly produced during prolonged infection, may be a key player in this suppression, at least with regard to parasite-specific Th1 responses [51–54]. Whether IL-10 can act directly on Th2 cells is not clear, but IL-10 may affect the functions of eosinophils and mast cells [55–57]. There is an increasing interest in the so-called regulatory T cells, which seem central in the induction of immunosuppression [58]. However, whether these regulatory T cells also orchestrate the induction of hyporesponsiveness in schistosome-infected hosts is not clear. Considering that parasite-specific immune responses may be associated with parasite clearance as well as immunopathology, immunosuppression may benefit both the parasite and the host. The extent to which the immunoregulatory network can be activated to control parasite-specific immune responses may therefore turn out to be crucial.

Chronic Helminth Infections Control Allergy via the Immunoregulatory Network

Helminth infections and allergic diseases are both characterized by a skewing of the immune response towards Th2. Since humans have likely become infected with parasites since early mankind, it is a commonly held view that Th2 responses evolved to combat helminths. Th2 responses against de facto harmless allergens may therefore well represent a negative exponent of the anti-parasitic Th2 response. Interestingly, in the past decades allergic diseases mainly emerged in areas of the world where helminth infections are hardly present (the Western world and urbanized centers of developing countries), whereas in areas where chronic helminth infections are still endemic (rural areas of developing countries) allergic diseases remain rare [1, 22–26].

Importantly, the intensity of helminth infections appears to determine the association between helminth infections and allergy. As shown by a Venezuelan study heavily helminth-infected individuals were protected from skin test reactivity to mite, whereas skin test reactivity to mite was increased in subjects with light helminth infections [59]. This indicates that in lightly infected individuals the stimulation of parasite-specific Th2 responses may potentiate allergen-specific Th2 responses [60], whereas in heavily infected subjects putatively different immunological mechanisms become activated that are responsible for allergy suppression. Interestingly, in heavily infected individuals the risk of becoming sensitized, i.e. the production of allergen-specific IgE antibodies, was not suppressed [60]. In accordance, in a study in Gabon we showed that the percentage of children producing functional

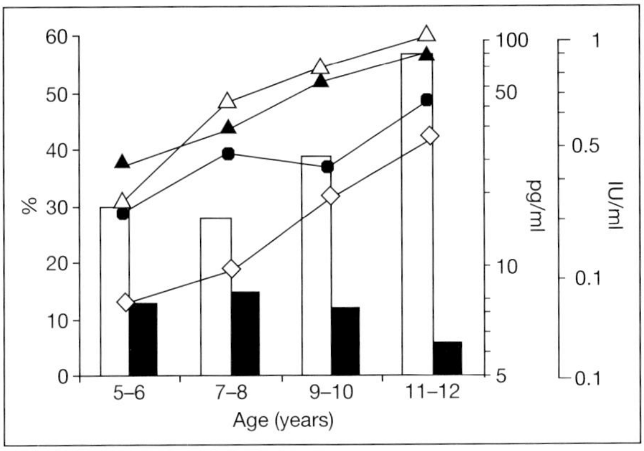

Fig. 1. Measurements of schistosome infection and atopy in Gabonese schoolchildren. Results of 520 Gabonese schoolchildren living in an area endemic for schistosome infections show that with increasing age the prevalence of schistosome infection increased (□). Accordingly, levels of parasite-specific IgE (▲; IU/ml) and the production of parasite-specific Th2 cytokines increased as shown by levels of parasite-specific IL-5 (●; pg/ml; the same pattern was found for IL-13; data not shown) and IL-10 (◇; pg/ml) that showed a marked increase (notably, immunological factors were assessed in a subgroup of 180 children). Interestingly, in the same group of children the prevalence of skin test reactivity to mite (■) decreased with age, whereas the production of mite-specific IgE antibodies increased (△). Schistosome infections were found to explain this inverse relationship between mite sensitization and skin test reactivity: in infected children the risk of a positive skin test result was reduced by 70% compared to uninfected children. Moreover, this suppressing effect of schistosome infections was found to be attributable to the increased production of the parasite-specific immunosuppressive cytokine IL-10 [61].

levels of mite-specific IgE (>1 IU/ml; 50%) outnumbered the percentage of children reacting positively to mite in skin-prick tests (11%). As illustrated in figure 1, in our study population levels of mite-specific IgE increased with age, whereas skin test reactivity to mite was decreasing. When we took into account the infection status of the children, we found that independent of mite-specific IgE the presence of schistosome infections reduced the risk of having a positive skin test result by 70% [61]. Accordingly, an Ethiopian study showed that the production of IgE antibodies against house dust mite was elevated in a rural compared to a urban setting, whereas the prevalence of asthma was higher in the city [2]. In a later nested case-control study this same research group reported that hookworm infections independently reduced the risk of wheeze by more than half and that the effect of sensitization to house dust mite on the risk of wheeze was greatly decreased with an increasing intensity of parasite infection [26]. The findings of these studies indicate that the mechanism that is responsible for suppressing allergic reactivity in chronically helminth-infected individuals interferes at a level that does not involve the production of allergen-specific IgE.

In order to put a finger on which part of the helminth-induced immune response is responsible for the suppression of allergic reactivity, we performed detailed cellular immunology in a subgroup of the Gabonese study population. As expected, schistosome-specific Th2 responses, such as the production of parasite-specific IL-5, IL-13 and IL-10, as well as levels of parasite-specific IgE and total IgE, were significantly elevated in the infected children. Next, using multiple logistic regression we studied which of the elevated schistosome-induced immunological factors could explain the reduced risk to respond to mite in skin tests in the schistosome-infected children. The one factor that was found to be independently and significantly associated with a reduced risk was the elevated production of parasite-specific IL-10 [61]. We therefore postulate that the suppression of allergic reactivity in chronically infected individuals can be explained by the activation of an immunoregulatory response. Indeed, it is known that hyporesponsiveness in chronic helminth infections may have a spillover effect on non-parasite antigens. For example, during chronic helminth infections the protective immune response induced by Calmette-Guérin bacillus vaccinations may be impaired [62, 63], and accordingly Th1 responses against tetanus toxoid have been shown to be weaker in helminth-infected individuals [64].

In order to prove that parasites themselves and no other cryptic factors mediate the suppression of allergic reactivity in chronically infected individuals, we performed a longitudinal study in which the effect of parasite clearance on skin test reactivity was studied. Gabonese schoolchildren who were skin test negative to mite at the onset of the study were followed for a period of 30 months during which they were treated every 3 months with anthelminthics or a placebo. Parasitological examinations as well as skin prick tests were performed every 6 months. Anthelminthic treatment was found to double the risk of children to convert to a positive skin prick test during these 30 months (Bigelaar, Journal of Infectious Diseases 2003, in press), by a mechanism that involved the treatment-induced clearance of helminth infections. This study confirms that parasites directly mediate the spillover suppression of skin test reactivity in chronic infected children.

Schistosomes and Immunoregulation: A Role for TLR-2?

Although the mechanism by which schistosomes may activate the immunoregulatory network is not known, in general antigen-presenting cells, which are part of the innate immune system, are known to be involved in the induction of tolerance. After antigen uptake dendritic cells (DCs) mature into a type-1 or type-2 DCs that after migration to the lymph nodes can polarize naïve Th cells into Th1 or Th2 [65, 66]. Interestingly, a third type of DC has been described which appears to tolerize instead of prime T cells and which may induce regulatory T cells [67, 68] by a mechanism that has not yet been clarified. Regulatory T cells produce high levels of anti-inflammatory cytokines such as IL-10 and are functionally characterized by their ability to suppress both Th1 and Th2 cells [66–68]. The polarization of DCs into immunogenic (type-1/type-2) or tolerogenic DCs is dependent on both the local microenvironment of the infected tissue as well as the pathogen encountered. DCs can recognize antigens by expression of pattern recognition receptors that bind antigen-associated evolutionarily well-conserved pathogen-associated molecular patterns (PAMPs) [72, 73]. Depending on the PAMP-Toll-like receptor (TLR) complex different immune responses may be induced [74, 75]. For example, lipopolysaccharide of gram-negative bacteria bound to TLR-4 [76, 77] is known to result in an increased transcription of the pro-inflammatory cytokine IL-12, which subsequently promotes the induction of Th1 cells. On the contrary the activation of TLR-2 has been associated with the induction of Th2 cells [78].

Molecular patterns present on schistosome stages that may bind to pattern recognition receptors expressed by cells of the innate immune response have not yet been characterized. However, de Jong et al. [79] provided the first evidence that schistosomes are able to interact with the innate immune system of the infected host by showing that culturing immature DCs in the presence of soluble schistosome egg antigens gave rise to type-2 DCs that polarize naïve T cells into Th2. More recently van der Kleij et al. [80] showed that DCs, matured in the presence of schistosome lipids, induced the development of naïve T cells into both Th2 cells and IL-10 inducing regulatory T cells, of which the latter could be inhibited by blocking TLR-2. This interesting finding indicates that schistosomes possess molecule patterns that can be recognized by the innate immune system and induce a tolerogenic response in vitro.

Interestingly, with respect to allergy, a recent study showed that in farmers' children, who have a reduced risk of developing atopic disease, the expression of CD14 and TLR-2 on isolated peripheral blood mononuclear cells was elevated compared to non-farmers' children [81]. This is an exciting observation since signaling through TLR-2 was shown to have a tolerogenic outcome in experiments with schistosome extracts. This may indicate that in the farmers' children allergic reactivity may be suppressed due to an elevated sensitivity to activate the tolerogenic pathway.

Pathogens in the West that May Induce (Spillover) Immunosuppression

Although the focus of this report has been chronic helminth infections, the same mechanisms may hold true for other chronic infectious diseases. For example, malaria infections [82], measles [83] and tuberculosis [84] have been

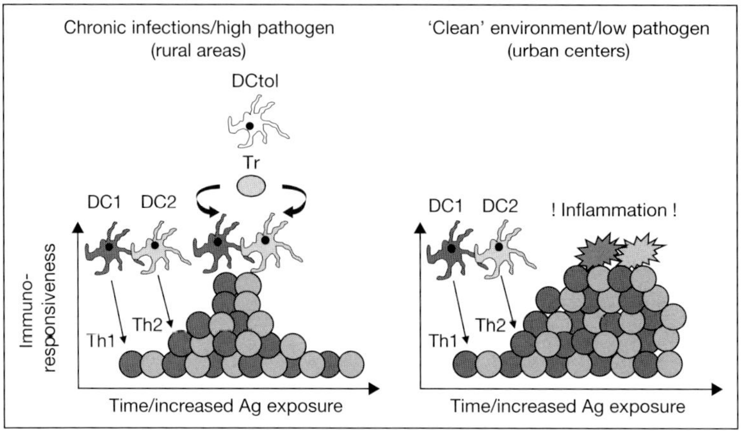

Fig. 2. Hypothetical concept of pathogen-induced (spillover) suppression. Depending on the microenvironment and pathogen encountered, DCs mature and develop into type-1 or type-2 DCs, which can polarize naïve T cells into Th1 and Th2 cells, respectively. By still unclarified mechanisms, with prolonged time and intensity of infection, pathogens may induce an immunoregulatory response, probably by inducing a tolerogenic DC that induces immunoregulatory T cells that may subsequently control specific Th1 and Th2 responses. As a spillover effect Th1 and Th2 responses against nonpathogenic antigens may be suppressed. In the situation that chronic pathogens are absent and the immune system is no longer repeatedly stimulated, the immunoregulatory response is no longer sufficiently activated and Th1 and Th2 responses will not be downregulated. The failure to induce an immunoregulatory response will result in a loss of control by spillover suppression and may result in increased risk to develop immunopathology, such as in allergic disorders and autoimmune diseases.

shown to result in immunosuppression and indeed a negative association with allergic reactivity has been shown [5, 86, 87].

In the Western world severe chronic infectious diseases such as helminth infections and malaria are largely controlled. Nevertheless, the immune system of Western individuals may be exposed to candidate pathogens (or their products) that putatively suppress allergic reactivity by activating the immunoregulatory network. For example, hepatitis A virus, *Toxoplasma gondii, Helicobacter pylori* and probiotics (products of lactobacilli in the gut flora) are pathogens that have been negatively associated with the development of atopy and asthma in the West [88, 89] and at least *T. gondii* and lactobacilli have been shown to stimulate the production of IL-10 [90, 94]. Moreover, simultaneously with the rise in allergy, the exposure to these food-borne and orofecal microbes has declined due to the increased consumption of sterilized food products [88]. Alternatively, endotoxins (lipopolysaccharides) of gram-negative bacteria are pathogens that are strong stimulators of the production of IL-10 [92–95] and the increased endotoxin exposure in the homes of farming families has been associated with a reduced risk of farmers' children to develop atopic disease compared to non-farmers' children [96–100].

Finally, a natural long-term exposure to high concentrations of cat allergens has been shown to result in a reduced risk of developing asthma, indicating that with prolonged exposure to cat allergens specific allergic immune responses become suppressed [101, 102]. Although it is yet to be proven that activation of the immunoregulatory network explains this 'cat desensitization', it indicates that immunotolerance to cat allergens is inducible, if the exposure to the allergens is high and continuous. However, for other allergens such an association has not been shown.

Conclusion

Although in both allergic diseases and helminth infections immunopathology appears to be associated with elevated Th2 responses, the mechanism underlying the development of immunopathology seems to be an inability to sufficiently activate the immunoregulatory network (fig. 2). Although there seems to be an increase in IgE responses to allergens in the West, we argue that the major cause of the rise in allergic disorders is the weak immunoregulatory network which is no longer capable of controlling immune responses against allergens in the West.

References

1 Beasley R, Keil U, Von Mutius E, Pearce N: Worldwide variation in prevalence of symptoms of asthma, allergic rhino-conjunctivitis, and atopic eczema: ISAAC. Lancet 1998;351:1225–1232.
2 Yemaneberhan H, Bekele Z, Venn A, et al: Prevalence of wheeze and asthma and relation to atopy in urban and rural Ethiopia. Lancet 1997;350:85–90.
3 Faniran AO, Peat JK, Woolcock AJ: Prevalence of atopy, asthma symptoms and diagnosis and the management of asthma: Comparison of an affluent and a non-affluent country. Thorax 1999;54:606–610.
4 Strachan DP: Hay fever, hygiene, and household size: BMJ 1989;299:1259–1260.
5 Shaheen SO, Aaby AJ, Barker DJP, et al: Measles and atopy in Guinea-Bissau. Lancet 1996;347:1792–1796.
6 Matricardi PM, Rosmini F, Ferrigno L, et al: Cross sectional retrospective study of prevalence of atopy among Italian military students with antibodies against hepatitis A virus. BMJ 1997;314:999–1003.
7 Kramer U, Heinrich J, Wjst M, Wichmann HE: Age of entry to day nursery and allergy in later childhood. Lancet 1999;353:450–454.
8 Hogg JC: Pathology of asthma. J Allergy Clin Immunol 1993;92:1–5.
9 Brightling CE, Bradding P, Syman FA, et al: Mast-cell infiltration of airway smooth muscle in asthma. N Engl J Med 2002;192:455–462.
10 Lee NA, Gelfand EW, Lee JJ: Pulmonary T cells and eosinophils: Coconspiritors or independent triggers of allergic respiratory pathology. J Allergy Clin Immunol 2001;107:945–957.
11 Walker C, Bode E, Boer L, et al: Allergic and non-allergic asthmatics have distinct patterns of T-cell activation and cytokine production in peripheral blood and bronchoalveolar lavage. Am Rev Respir Dis 1992;146:109–115.

12 Leung DYM: Atopic dermatitis: New insights and opportunities for therapeutic intervention. J Allergy Clin Immunol 2000;105:860–876.
13 Sampson HA, Ho DG: Relationship between food-specific IgE concentrations and the risk of positive food challenges in children and adolescents. J Allergy Clin Immunol 1997;100: 444–451.
14 Mishra A, Hogan SP, Brandt EB, Rothenberg ME: An etiological role for aeroallergens and eosinophils in experimental esophagitis. J Clin Invest 2001;107:83–90.
15 Cookson WO, Moffatt MF: Asthma: An epidemic in the absence of infection? Science 1997;275:41–42.
16 Matricardi PM, Bonini S: High microbial turnover rate preventing atopy: A solution to inconsistencies impinging on the hygiene hypothesis? Clin Exp Allergy 2000;30:1506–1510.
17 World Health Organization: The World Health Report 1998 – Life in the 21st Century: A Vision for All. Geneva, World Health Organization, 1998.
18 Karvonen M, Viik-Kajander M, Moltchanova E, et al: Incidence of childhood type 1 diabetes worldwide. Diabetes Mondiale (DiaMond) Project Group. Diabetes Care 2000;23: 1516–1526.
19 Stromberg LG, Ludvigsson GJ, Bjorksten B: Atopic allergy and delayed hypersensitivity in children with diabetes. J Allergy Clin Immunol 1995;96:188–192.
20 Stene LC, Nafstad P: Relation between occurrence of type 1 diabetes and asthma. Lancet 2001;357:607–608.
21 Kero J, Gissler M, Hemminki E, Isolauri E: Could TH1 and TH2 diseases coexist? Evaluation of asthma incidence in children with coeliac disease, type 1 diabetes, or rheumatoid arthritis: A register study. J Allergy Clin Immunol 2001;108:781–783.
22 Lynch NR, Hagel I, Perez M, et al: Effect of anthelmintic treatment on the allergic reactivity of children in a tropical slum. J Allergy Clin Immunol 1993;92:404–411.
23 Lynch NR, Hagel IA, Palenque ME, et al: Relationship between helminth infection and IgE response in atopic and nonatopic children in a tropical environment. J Allergy Clin Immunol 1998;101:217–221.
24 van den Biggelaar AHJ, Lopuhaa C, Van Ree R, et al: The prevalence of parasite infestation and house dust mite sensitization in Gabonese schoolchildren. Int Arch Allergy Immunol 2001;126:231–238.
25 Araujo MI, Lopes AA, Medeiros M, et al: Inverse association between skin response to aeroallergens and *Schistosoma mansoni* infection. Int Arch Allergy Immunol 2000;123: 145–148.
26 Scrivener S, Yemaneberhan H, Zebenigus M, et al: Independent effects of intestinal parasite infection and domestic allergen exposure on risk of wheeze in Ethiopia: A nested case-control study. Lancet 2001;358:1493–1499.
27 Yazdanbakhsh M, Kremsner PG, Van Ree R: Allergy, parasites and the hygiene hypothesis. Science 2002;296:490–494.
28 Viana IR, Sher A, Carvalho OS, et al: Interferon-gamma production by peripheral blood mononuclear cells from residents of an area endemic for *Schistosoma mansoni*. Trans R Soc Trop Med Hyg 1994;88:466–470.
29 Woolhouse ME, Taylor P, Matanhire D, Chanidwana SK: Acquired immunity and epidemiology of *Schistosoma haematobium*. Nature 1991;351:757–759.
30 Woolhouse MEJ: Patterns in parasite epidemiology. Parasitol Today 1998;14:428–434.
31 Hussain R, Hofstetter M, Goldstone A, et al: IgE responses in human schistosomiasis. I. Quantitation of specific IgE by radioimmunoassay and correlation of results with skin test and basophil histamine release. Am J Trop Med Hyg 1983;32:1347–1355.
32 Ndhlovu P, Cadman H, Vennervald BJ, et al: Age-related antibody profiles in *Schistosoma haematobium* infections in a rural community in Zimbabwe. Parasite Immunol 1996;18: 181–191.
33 Hagan P, Blumenthal UJ, Dunn D, et al: Human IgE, IgG4 and resistance to reinfection with *Schistosoma haematobium*. Nature 1991;349:243–245.
34 Dunne DW, Butterworth AE, Fulford AJ, et al: Immunity after treatment of human schistosomiasis: Association between IgE antibodies to adult worm antigens and resistance to reinfection. Eur J Immunol 1992;22:1483–1494.
35 Dunne DW, Hagan P, Abath FG: Prospects for immunological control of schistosomiasis. Lancet 1995;345:1488–1491.

36 Stelma FF, Talla I, Polman K, et al: Epidemiology of *Schistosoma mansoni* infection in a recently exposed community in northern Senegal. Am J Trop Med Hyg 1993;49: 701–706.
37 Ouma JH, Fulford AJ, Kariuki HC, et al: The development of schistosomiasis mansoni in an immunologically naive immigrant population in Masongaleni, Kenya. Parasitology 1998; 117:123–132.
38 Van Dam GJ, Stelma FF, Gryseels B, et al: Antibody response patterns against *Schistosoma mansoni* in a recently exposed community in Senegal. J Infect Dis 1996;173:1232–1241.
39 Naus CW, Kimani G, Ouma JH, et al: Development of antibody isotype responses to *Schistosoma mansoni* in an immunologically naïve immigrant population: Influence of infection duration, infection intensity, and host age. Infect Immun 1999;67:3444–3451.
40 Woolhouse ME, Hagan P: Seeking the ghost of worms past. Nat Med 1999;5:1225–1227.
41 Grogan JL, Kremsner PG, van Dam GJ, et al: Antischistosome IgG4 and IgE responses are affected differentially by chemotherapy in children versus adults. J Infect Dis 1996;173: 1242–1247.
42 Grogan JL, Kremsner PG, Deelder AM, Yazdanbakhsh M: Elevated proliferation and interleukin-4 release from CD4+ cells after chemotherapy in human *Schistosoma haematobium* infection. Eur J Immunol 1996;26:1365–1370.
43 Mutapi F, Ndhlovu PD, Hagan P, Woolhouse ME: Changes in specific anti-egg antibody levels following treatment with praziquantel for *Schistosoma haematobium* infection in children. Parasite Immunol 1998;20:595–600.
44 Mutapi F, Ndhlovu PD, Hagan P, et al: Chemotherapy accelerates the development of acquired immune responses to *Schistosoma haematobium* infection. J Infect Dis 1998;178: 289–293.
45 van den Biggelaar AHJ, Borrmann S, Kremsner P, Yazdanbakhsh M: Immune responses induced by repeated treatment do not result in protective immunity to *Schistosoma haematobium:* Interleukin (IL)-5 and IL-10 responses. J Infect Dis 2002;186:1474–1482.
46 Cheever AW, Williams ME, Wynn TA, et al: Anti-IL-4 treatment of *Schistosoma mansoni*-infected mice inhibits development of T cells and non-B, non-T cells expressing Th2 cytokines while decreasing egg-induced hepatic fibrosis. J Immunol 1994;153:753–759.
47 Kaplan MH, Whitfield JR, Boros DL, Grusby MJ: Th2 cells are required for the *Schistosoma mansoni* egg-induced granulomatous response. J Immunol 1998;160:1850–1856.
48 Hesse M, Modolell M, La Flamme AC, et al: Differential regulation of nitric oxide synthase-2 and arginase-1 by type 1/type 2 cytokines in vivo: Granulomatous pathology is shaped by the pattern of *L*-arginine metabolism. J Immunol 2001;167:6533–6544.
49 De Jesus AM, Almeida RP, Bacellar O, et al: Correlation between cell-mediated immunity and degree of infection in subjects living in an endemic area of schistosomiasis. Eur J Immunol 1993;23:152–158.
50 Grogan JL, Kremsner PG, Deelder AM, Yazdanbakhsh M: Antigen-specific proliferation and interferon-gamma and interleukin-5 production are down-regulated during *Schistosoma haematobium* infection. J Infect Dis. 1998;177:1433–1437.
51 Grogan JL, Kremsner PG, Deelder AM, Yazdanbakhsh M: The effect of anti-IL-10 on proliferation and cytokine production in human schistosomiasis: Fresh versus cryopreserved cells. Parasite Immunol 1998;20:345–349.
52 Sher A, Fiorentino D, Caspar P, et al: Production of IL-10 by CD4+ T lymphocytes correlates with down-regulation of Th1 cytokine synthesis in helminth infection. J Immunol 1991;147:2713–2716.
53 King CL, Mahanty S, Kumaraswami V, et al: Cytokine control of parasite-specific anergy in human lymphatic filariasis. Preferential induction of a regulatory T helper type 2 lymphocyte subset. J Clin Invest 1993;92:1667–1673.
54 King CL, Medhat A, Malhotra I, et al: Cytokine control of parasite-specific anergy in human urinary schistosomiasis. IL-10 modulates lymphocyte reactivity. J Immunol 1996;156: 4715–4721.
55 Takanaski S, Nonaka R, Xing Z, et al: Interleukin 10 inhibits lipopolysaccharide-induced survival and cytokine production by human peripheral blood eosinophils. J Exp Med 1994; 180:711–715.
56 Ohkawara Y, Lim KG, Xing Z, et al: CD40 expression by human peripheral blood eosinophils. J Clin Invest 1996;97:1761–1766.

57 Royer B, Varadaradjalou S, Saas P, et al: Inhibition of IgE-induced activation of human mast cells by IL-10. Clin Exp Allergy 2001;31:694–704.
58 Groux H, O'Garra A, Bigler M, et al: A CD4+ T-cell subset inhibits antigen-specific T-cell responses and prevents colitis. Nature 1997;389:737–742.
59 Lynch NR, Lopez RI, Di Prisco-Fuenmayor MC, et al: Allergic reactivity and socio-economic level in a tropical environment. Clin Allergy 1987;17:199–207.
60 Lynch NR, Palenque M, Hagel I, DiPrisco MC: Clinical improvement of asthma after anthelminthic treatment in a tropical situation. Am J Respir Crit Care Med 1997;156: 50–54.
61 van den Biggelaar AHJ, van Ree R, Rodrigues LC, et al: Decreased atopy in children infected with *Schistosoma haematobium*: A role for parasite-induced interleukin-10. Lancet 2000; 356:1723–1727.
62 Malhotra I, Mungai P, Wamachi A, et al: Helminth- and bacillus Calmette-Guérin-induced immunity in children sensitized in utero to filariasis and schistosomiasis. J Immunol 1999;162:6843–6848.
63 Elias D, Wolday D, Akuffo H, et al: Effect of deworming on human T cell responses to mycobacterial antigens in helminth-exposed individuals before and after bacillé Calmette-Guérin (BCG) vaccination. Clin Exp Immunol 2001;123:219–225.
64 Sabin EA, Araujo MI, Carvalho EM, Pearce EJ: Impairment of tetanus toxoid-specific Th1-like immune responses in humans infected with *Schistosoma mansoni*. J Infect Dis 1996;173:269–272.
65 Kapsenberg ML, Hilkens CM, Wierenga EA, Kalinski P: The paradigm of type 1 and type 2 antigen-presenting cells. Implications for atopic allergy. Clin Exp Allergy 1999;29: 33–36.
66 Kalinski P, Hilkens CM, Wierenga EA, Kapsenberg ML: T-cell priming by type-1 and type-2 polarized dendritic cells: The concept of a third signal. Immunol Today 1999;20:561–567.
67 Jonuleit H, Schmitt E, Schuler G, et al: Induction of interleukin 10-producing, nonproliferating CD4(+) T cells with regulatory properties by repetitive stimulation with allogeneic immature human dendritic cells. J Exp Med 2000;192:1213–1222.
68 McGuirk P, McCann C, Mills KH: Pathogen-specific T regulatory 1 cells induced in the respiratory tract by a bacterial molecule that stimulates interleukin 10 production by dendritic cells: A novel strategy for evasion of protective T helper type 1 responsive by *Bordetella pertussis*. J Exp Med 2002;195:221–231.
69 Doetze A, Satoguina J, Burchard G, et al: Antigen-specific cellular hyporesponsiveness in a chronic human helminth infection is mediated by Th3/Tr1-type cytokines IL-10 and transforming growth factor-β but not by a T(h)1 to T(h)2 shift. Int Immunol 2000;12: 623–630.
70 Cavani A, Nasorri F, Prezzi C, et al: Human CD4+ T lymphocytes with remarkable regulatory functions on dendritic cells and nickel-specific Th1 immune responses. J Invest Dermatol 2000;114:295–302.
71 Levings MK, Sangregorio R, Galbiati F, et al: IFN-γ and IL-10 induce the differentiation of human type 1 T regulatory cells. J Immunol 2001;166:5530–5539.
72 Cottrez F, Hurst SD, Coffman RL, Groux H: T regulatory cells 1 inhibit a Th2-specific response in vivo. J Immunol 2000;165:4848–4853.
73 Reis e Sousa C: Dendritic cells as sensors of infection. Immunity 2001;14:495–498.
74 Underhill D, Ozinsky A: Toll-like receptors: Key mediators of microbe detection. Curr Opin Immunol 2002;14:103–110.
75 Huang Q: The plasticity of dendritic cell responses to pathogens and their components. Science 2001;294:870–875.
76 Hirschfeld M: Signalling by toll-like receptor 2 and 4 agonists results in differential gene expression in murine macrophages. Infect Immun 2001;69:1477–1482.
77 Chow JC, Young DW, Golenbock DT, et al: Toll-like receptor-4 mediates lipopolysaccharide-induced signal transduction. J Biol Chem 1999;274:10689–10692.
78 O'Neill LAJ: Toll-like receptor signal transduction and the tailoring of innate immunity: A role for Mal? Trends Immunol 2002;23:296–300.
79 De Jong EC, Vieira PL, Kalinski P, et al: Microbial compounds selectively induce Th1 cell-promoting or Th2 cell-promoting dendritic cells in vitro with diverse Th cell-polarizing signals. J Immunol 2002;168:1704–1709.

80 Van der Kleij D, Latz E, Brouwers JFHM, et al: A novel host-parasite cross talk: Schistosomal lyso-phosphahtidylserine activates Toll-like receptor 2 and affects immune polerization. J Biol Chem 2002;277:48122–48129.
81 Lauener RP, Birchler T, Adamski J, et al: Expression of CD14 and Toll-like receptor 2 in farmers' and non-farmers' children. Lancet 2002;360:465–466.
82 Greenwood BM, Bradley-Moore AM, Bryceson AD, Palit A: Immunosuppression in children with malaria. Lancet 1972;i:169–172.
83 Redpath S, Ghazal P, Gascoigne NR: Hijacking and exploitation of IL-10 by intracellular pathogens. Trends Microbiol 2001;9:86–92.
84 Hirsch CS, Hussain R, Toossi Z, et al: Cross-modulation by transforming growth factor beta in human tuberculosis: Suppression of antigen-driven blastogenesis and interferon gamma production. Proc Natl Acad Sci USA 1996;93:3193–3198.
85 Lell B, Borrmann S, Yazdanbakhsh M, Kremsner PG: Atopy and malaria. Wien Klin Wochenschr 2001;113:927–929.
86 Shirakawa T, Enomoto T, Shimazu S, Hopkin JM: The inverse association between tuberculin responses and atopic disorder. Science 1997;275:77–79.
87 Matricardi PM, Rosmini F, Riondino S, et al: Exposure to foodborne and orofecal microbes versus airborne viruses in relation to atopy and allergic asthma: Epidemiological study. BMJ 2000;320:412–417.
88 Kosunen TU, Hook-Nikanne J, Salomaa A, et al: Increase of allergen-specific immunoglobulin E antibodies from 1973 to 1994 in a Finnish population and a possible relationship to *Helicobacter pylori* infections. Clin Exp Allergy 2002;32:373–378.
89 Kaliomäki M, Salminen S, Arvilommi H, et al: Probiotics in primary prevention of atopic disease: A randomised placebo-controlled trial. Lancet 2001;357:1076–1079.
90 Lee YH, Channon JY, Matsuura T, et al: Functional and quantitative analysis of splenic T cell immune responses following oral *Toxoplasma gondii* infection in mice. Exp Parasitol 1999; 91:212–221.
91 Pessi T, Sutas Y, Hurme M, Isolauri E: Interleukin-10 generation in atopic children following oral *Lactobacillus rhamnosus* GG. Clin Exp Allergy 2000;30:1804–1808.
92 Rietschel ET, Schade U, Jensen M, et al: Bacterial endotoxins: Chemical structure, biological activity and role in septicaemia. Scand J Infect Dis 1982;31:8–21.
93 Frankenberger M, Pechumer H, Ziegler-Heitbrock HW: Interleukin-10 is upregulated in LPS tolerance. J Inflamm 1995;45:56–63.
94 Randow F, Syrbe U, Meisel C, et al: Mechanism of endotoxin desensitization: Involvement of interleukin 10 and transforming growth factor beta. J Exp Med 1995;181:1887–1892.
95 Junger WG, Hoyt DB, Liu FC, et al: Immunosuppression after endotoxin shock: the result of multiple anti-inflammatory factors. J Trauma 1996;40:702–709.
96 Braun-Fahrlander C, Gassner M, Grize L, et al: Prevalence of hay fever and allergic sensitization in farmer's children and their peers living in the same rural community. SCARPOL team. Swiss Study on Childhood Allergy and Respiratory Symptoms with Respect to Air Pollution. Clin Exp Allergy 1999;29:28–34.
97 Von Ehrenstein OS, Von Mutius E, Illi S, et al: Reduced risk of hay fever and asthma among children of farmers. Clin Exp Allergy 2000;30:187–193.
98 Riedler J, Eder W, Oberfeld G, Schreuer M: Austrian children living on a farm have less hay fever, asthma and allergic sensitization. Clin Exp Allergy 2000;30:194–200.
99 Von Mutius E, Braun-Fahrlander C, Schierl R, et al: Exposure to endotoxin or other bacterial components might protect against the development of atopy. Clin Exp Allergy 2000;30:1230–1234.
100 Gehring U, Bolte G, Borte M, et al, LISA Study Group: Lifestyle-related factors on the immune system and the development of allergies in childhood. Exposure to endotoxin decreases the risk of atopic eczema in infancy: A cohort study. J Allergy Clin Immunol 2001; 108:847–854.
101 Platts-Mills T, Vaughan J, Squillace S, et al: Sensitisation, asthma, and a modified Th2 response in children exposed to cat allergen: A population-based cross-sectional study. Lancet 2001;357:752–756.
102 Perzanowski M, Rönmark E, Platts-Mills TAE, Lundbäck B: Effect of cat and dog ownership on sensitisation and development of asthma among preteenage children. Am J Respir Crit Care Med 2002;166:696–702.

Discussion

Dr. Romagnani: I think that your talk demonstrates that there is no disagreement on the prevalent Th2 nature of allergic disorders, nor on the hygiene hypothesis as an explanation for the increased prevalence of allergy in developed countries. The true disagreement between us is on the immune mechanisms by which the reduced burden of infectious agents during childhood is capable of inducing 'allergic epidemics'. You say that immune deviation from a prevalent Th1 to a prevalent Th2 profile in the response is not important and that the increased prevalence of allergy is only due to the decreased immune suppression. In other words, while I believe that the reduced production of IL-12 and interferons (Th1-inducing, but Th2-antagonizing cytokines) is the main mechanism involved, you believe that the increased prevalence of Th2 responses to common environmental allergens is due to reduced activity of T regulatory cells and to decreased production of suppressive cytokines, such as IL-10 and TGF-β. However, I would like to object that while the role of missing immune deviation rests on solid experimental evidence, the possible role of reduced immune suppression is mainly based on epidemiological findings. The first epidemiological evidence comes from your studies on helminthic infections. However, I believe that the interpretation of your data represents a wrong checkpoint. First, the situation of Africa and South America cannot be used to explain the increased prevalence of allergy in Westernized countries because helminthic infections disappeared from Europe and the United States many decades ago, and for example, certainly at present there are no helminths in Estonia where the prevalence of allergy is as low as in Africa and South America. Secondly, you say that people infested by helminths have negative prick tests to allergens, but they have specific IgE in their serum. In my view this means that Th2 responses to allergens are not suppressed by helminthic infestations, rather some other event is suppressed in the effector phase of the Th2-mediated response that impairs the production of chemical mediators by mast cells. I believe that the old hypothesis of specific IgE dilution due to helminth-induced IgE hyperproduction that impairs the allergen to find two specific IgE antibody molecules so close on the surface of the mast cell to cross-link IgE receptors allowing mast cell degranulation is a more likely explanation for this phenomenon. The second epidemiological observation is that the prevalence of Th1-mediated disorders is also increased. This is also, at least in my view, a wrong checkpoint. Indeed, insulin-dependent diabetes mellitus (IDDM) is a short-lasting inflammatory disorder, limited to pancreatic β cells, which ends their destruction. So, it is not possible to compare allergy, which is a systemic disorder lasting for several years, with IDDM, which is a relatively rare, very limited and short-lasting inflammation which then rapidly becomes a pure metabolic disorder. Moreover, the Th1 nature of the immune response in IDDM is still controversial. With regard to Crohn's disease this is indeed a long-lasting, Th1-mediated disease, but that until some years ago the differential diagnosis between Crohn's disease and ulcerative colitis was virtually impossible and the two diseases were classified together as inflammatory bowel disorders. However, ulcerative colitis is probably not a Th1-dominated disorder. So I am not sure that the prevalence of Crohn's disease is really augmented. The same is for multiple sclerosis. Indeed, we can presently diagnose multiple sclerosis simply by performing magnetic resonance of the brain, which was not possible 10 years ago. Therefore it is clear that the prevalence of multiple sclerosis has increased but this may simply be due to the improved diagnostic tools. Moreover, you have to explain why allergy is very rare in patients with multiple sclerosis and has a low prevalence in rheumatoid arthritis, another systemic and long-lasting Th1-mediated inflammatory disorder.

Dr. van den Biggelaar: If I want to answer all these points, it would be better to repeat my presentation. The main point I tried to make in this presentation is that immunoregulation, thus immunosuppression, is the mechanism underlying the development of immunopathology: when you don't have this control within your immune system you may develop Th2-mediated disease as well as Th1-mediated disease. Regarding the paradigm on Th1 and Th2: yes, in experiments adding very high levels of Th1 cytokines has been shown to counteract Th2 [1, 2]. However, from immunotherapy studies it is not clear that Th1 responses are induced that counteract the Th2 response. Studies, like the one I mentioned on mice treated with *Mycobacterium vaccae* suspension [3] and also those with CpG oligodeoxynucleotides (CpG-ODN) [4], which are thought to activate Th1 responses, indicate that Th2 responses are counteracted by the induction of IL-10 producing regulatory T cells and not Th1. CpG-ODN studies in IL-12 and interferon-γ knockout mice show an effect in the absence of these Th1 cytokines, indicating it is not Th1 that controls allergic responses [5].

With respect to your comment on diabetes, I am not comparing the mechanisms by which diabetes and allergic reactivity are expressed, but I am discussing the origin of these two diseases; the mechanism that underlies the onset of these diseases. How the diseases are expressed is something different, and not what I am discussing. Whether diabetes is rising or not is perhaps an interesting question to ask our participants from Indonesia, because these are countries where things are changing very rapidly at the moment. I wonder whether they can confirm a high increase in allergic and autoimmune diseases in their countries. I expect that it is these parts of the world where things are rapidly changing, where infectious diseases are becoming controlled, we should worry about a rise in allergy and autoimmune diseases.

Dr. Walker: First of all your work was very well presented. As in many situations in medicine and biology, things are not as clear-cut as they appear to be, and that is probably true with the 'hygiene hypothesis'. As I understand it, it is not so straightforward that specific microbes can cause just a Th1 or just a Th2 response. Probably the issue is not so much either or, as it is the microbial burden that is brought to bear whether as a parasite or microorganism. I have one additional comment. There was an article in the *New England Journal of Medicine* [6], a study in Germany, showing that endotoxin seems to be a factor in decreasing the expression of allergic disease, but in that same journal there was a commentary by Bach [7] in which he addressed the issue of both increasing autoimmune disease and increasing allergy, again underscoring the fact that things are not as clear-cut as they are thought to be.

Dr. Guesry: I find your study in Lambaréné very interesting. However, it is a very special situation in which the babies are loaded with helminth and also with bacterial infection. It would be very interesting to know of any studies done in industrialized countries in which parasitic infestation still exists. In pediatrics we see a lot of children with ascaridiasis, for example, who do not get this huge load of bacterial infection. There are a lot of situations, particularly also in allergy, where a certain effect is obtained with a moderate load of allergens, and when you really push to the extreme with a huge load you get almost the reverse reaction. Do you know of any other study done in industrialized countries with parasitic infestation and less bacterial infection?

Dr. van den Biggelaar: In industrialized countries helminth infections are not chronic. The point is that the infection load is probably not high enough to stimulate the immunoregulatory network. In studies performed in Holland, infections with ascaris (personal commun.) and *Toxocara canis* [8] were found to stimulate allergic responses. Whether this relates to an increased or a decreased infection with bacteria, I do not know.

Dr. Guesry: So you say that in Holland with *T. canis* or ascaridiasis, there was an increase in allergy and Th2 deviation. So that partly answers my question.

Dr. van den Biggelaar: Yes, and that is also exactly what I tried to explain before.

Dr. Holt: I would like to go back to the issue of IL-10 which, for a number of reasons, I still think is interesting. But I don't think we know really how it operates. We have data from our group that say if your forget parasites and look in a Western country like Australia and simply collect a large number of children who are skin prick test positive to house dust mite and then stimulate their T cells in vitro and get a full cytokine profile, and put all the data in the computer and ask what associates with the size of the skin prick wheal, then all of the Th2 cytokines are positively associated and IL-10 is negatively associated, even to the extent that you can have some children that make massive IL-4, IL-5 and IL-13 responses, but if it is balanced by a conjoint high IL-10 response then the skin prick wheal instead of being 10 or higher is ≤2. So that is something rather special about what that can do in that microenvironment. But also I am struck by early work comparing East and West Germany and comparing Sweden and Estonia, in which skin prick test reactivity was also tested. Both carefully controlled studies came out with the finding that the size of the histamine wheal was actually lower in eastern European populations. Now I remember from a conversation with you a while back that you did not find this in your study population and yet the finding was very consistent in terms of the east–west gradient in Europe. So maybe what this is telling us is that the mechanism responsible for the east–west gradient in allergy in Europe might not be the same as the one responsible for the Europe–Third World gradient. After all we are talking about logarithm difference in terms of the level of antigenic stimulation.

Dr. van den Biggelaar: You are right that in our study we only see a negative association of parasite-specific IL-10 with mite-specific skin test responses and not with the histamine control. The way we interpret our data is that IL-10 indicates the involvement of an immunoregulatory mechanism with suppression at the level of the mast cells that are responsible for the response to the mite in skin prick testing. And what the difference might be regarding the setting in Estonia and Germany is a good question. Are these different mechanisms?

Dr. Marini: I will make a point concerning juvenile type-1 diabetes. Now in Europe and in Western countries many babies are born in the second trimester which suggests that something wrong is happening in the fetus in the first trimester and may be related to some kind of viral infection. Another point, juvenile diabetes is now being diagnosed earlier than it was years ago. It is a fact that juvenile type-1 diabetes is 3 times higher in babies born from diabetic fathers than from diabetic mothers. Some say that the diabetic milieu in fetal life can protect the fetus. This is important because we have shown that if you do very strict metabolic control of diabetes in the mothers you have an increase in diabetes type-1 in the babies [9]. I have another question for people who work in allergy: what is the relationship between obesity in adolescents and allergy?

Dr. van den Biggelaar: There may be a link with obesity and leptin, since leptin is known to be associated with immunosuppression. However, this is still a very much unknown field. Regarding the onset of diabetes, there is possibly a lot to be achieved by studying the innate immune response. We may learn more from studying the polymorphism of Toll-like receptors, whether there is a genetic link. For example premature birth was mentioned this morning, and it has been shown to be associated with a polymorphism of one of the Toll-like receptors because women are more susceptible to infections during pregnancy. I wish I could answer all these questions because then we would have achieved a lot, but I think this is really the field that we should try to explore in more detail.

Dr. Bindslev-Jensen: I was a little puzzled 2 years ago when I saw a Danish study published on the possible relationship or the opposite between diabetes and atopic dermatitis. I think it was published in the *British Medical Journal* and, based on data from a central computer which was functioning in Denmark, it demonstrated very clearly that if you had diabetes type-1 as a child then the risk of later developing atopic dermatitis was dramatically decreased, and the opposite way around was in fact also the case with more than 7,000 children or something like that. You showed data in which it sometimes goes up, sometimes down and sometimes nothing happens. One of the answers might lie in the fact that these patients only reportedly had asthma, but what kind of asthma did they have, did they have allergic asthma or things like that. So what we need in that respect is to also clarify this in a prospectively conducted study and see what is going to happen if we really try to figure out what the phenotypes are and the association between them. I call them fingerprints and my colleague from Holland calls them phenotypes.

Dr. Rijntjes: You call this *Schistosoma haematobium*, and I was wondering, is there a difference between whether the helminth is invasive or not because the schistosome goes to the bladder, the haematobium and the ascaris go to the lungs and cause pneumonia? Is there a difference in the possibility to induce immunomodulation?

Dr. van den Biggelaar: Regarding schistosomes and also filarial worms, which are both tissue- and blood-dwelling helminths, there have been a lot of studies on these parasites and the human immune system. Since these are chronic infections, meaning they can survive for many years in the infected host, it is a perfect model to study immunoregulation. With respect to ascaris and other intestinal helminths, much less is known, or the results are contradictory. For example, it is not yet quite clear whether ascaris induces Th2 responses such as schistosomes and filarial worms do, nor whether they induce immunoregulatory responses such as an increased production of IL-10 and TGF-β or other markers of immunoregulation. In a longitudinal study we showed that when the infection with intestinal helminths was cleared, this was associated with an increased risk of responding to skin testing for mites. Although we cannot show that this acts via immunoregulation, we do show that interrupting a chronic infection in the school-age children results in a conversion to atopic reactivity. Your second point on the route of infestation, schistosomes indeed enter via the skin, indicating that there may be reactions taking place in the skin by antigen-presenting cells that immediately react with the entering parasites. Regarding ascaris, parasite stages are known to pass the lungs, which may induce bronchial responsiveness to ascaris antigens.

Dr. Lack: I have a question for both protagonists. If you desensitize with immunotherapy in established allergy, the effect is antigen-specific. So your skin prick test with specific IgE will only change to the allergen you have desensitized with. Lymphocyte function will only change in an antigen-specific way. But there are now 3 studies in immunotherapy in children showing that, if you desensitize at an early age to one allergen, you prevent neo-sensitization to other allergens; so you cross allergen specificity. I ask both of you how do you account for this suppression of further sensitization either using the Th1, Th2 paradigm or an alternative immunoregulatory paradigm? How do you explain this protective effect?

Dr. van den Biggelaar: For immunotherapy it has been shown that cross-regulation in desensitization may occur according to the existence of cross-sensitization in allergic people who are often sensitized to more than one allergen which might also change during life. For helminths cross-suppression of responses to other antigens is known to exist. From the helminth point of view, our immune system likely got shaped in the presence of helminths. Therefore immunoregulation likely developed to control harmful responses against parasites, but it was likely not shaped to control responses against allergens because there is no direct danger. However, I don't dare to claim that the same mechanism by which cross-suppression between helminths and other antigen-specific cells acts also underlies the cross-suppression of allergen-specific responses.

Dr. Romagnani: My view is that both immunological mechanisms, i.e. missing immune deviation from Th2 to Th1 and reduced immune suppression, may cooperate in inducing the increased prevalence of allergy. Due to the lower microbial burden in infancy, the reduced production of IL-10 and TGF-β may result in the increased response of the immune system to all allergens including common environmental allergens. At the same time, the reduced production of IL-12 and interferons results in reduced antagonization of Th2 development and polarization. I would like to say, however, that so far there is solid experimental evidence in favor of the possibility of inducing a Th1 shift of allergen-specific Th2 responses by using cytokines, such as IL-12 and interferons, or microbial products, such as CpG motif-containing oligodeoxynucleotides and double-stranded RNA, whereas there is no convincing experimental evidence available so far on the role of regulatory T cells on the Th2 response. As I mentioned before, IL-10 gene-deficient mice exhibit increased Th1 responses, which means that IL-10 suppresses the activity of Th1 cells, whereas Th2 responses are reduced, suggesting that IL-10 can even favor this type of response.

Dr. van den Biggelaar: As I emphasized we do not claim that IL-10 is doing the whole job; IL-10 is a measure of regulatory responsiveness. What I am trying to say is that we should first increase our knowledge on the immunoregulatory system, since this is still a very newly developing area of research, before we start giving IL-10 to people.

Dr. Romagnani: IL-10 has been administered to people suffering from Crohn's disease with therapeutic effects not much different from those of a placebo. So IL-10 seems to be unable to cure even Th1 disorders, although its suppressive effect on Th1 cells has been clearly demonstrated.

Dr. van den Biggelaar: I can give a similar reply that giving interferon-γ may also be very dangerous. You argue for inducing a Th1 response, however so far there is no clear evidence that Th1 is the mechanism. In IL-12 knockout mice as well as interferon-γ knockouts, the effect is still there.

Dr. Neijens: In this respect, where you observe that the parasites induce IL-10, it is important to make observations to what extend this effect is age-related in children or depending on the genetic information. Oberle et al. [10] were able to show that the effect is expressed most if they are exposed in pregnancy and in early life. In a large cohort recently Matricardi et al. [11] observed that the effects of hepatitis A are most pronounced if it was increased early in life. In your observations, could you find an effect of the age of the children? Is it most pronounced early or does it work later on in chronic infections, and is it dependent on risk factors, genetic risk factors?

Dr. van den Biggelaar: In this study we did not include any genetic risk factors. The children were included at school age, they were between 5 and 13 years old when we started the study. Our longitudinal study was for 2.5 years, and yes, it is true that most of the children who converted to a positive skin test result to mites were relatively younger children. Thus in children who were about between 13 and 15 years at the end of the study the effect was less clear. However, in migrant studies [12, 13] it has been shown that people who at an adult age move out of a highly endemic area to a cleaner area, depending on their genetic background, they are still at risk of developing allergic reactivity, indicating that it is not solely based on the young age.

Dr. Sorensen: Just very briefly going back to the preceding question on the number of allergens to which you are sensitized. Martinez (personal commun.) studied clearly segregated families, some who are sensitized to one allergen while others are sensitized to multiple allergens. I wonder how long you follow these subjects who tend to get sensitized to a lot of allergens? So before accepting that immunotherapy is the cause of it, you have to make sure that you are not just scaring the population. In the United States, and particularly in my state of Louisiana, we are facing a real epidemic of type-2 diabetes linked to obesity, and obesity is clearly now being considered an inflammatory disease with the evidence that there are a number of inflammatory processes going on. So I wonder if you came across any study regarding asthma, type-2 diabetes and allergy?

Dr. van den Biggelaar: A few years ago Castro-Rodriguez et al. [14] showed an increase in asthma symptoms in obese teenage girls who matured very young. I am not sure where this research was headed: whether these girls suffered from the same phenotype of asthma as mostly seen in other asthmatics, or whether it was a different type of asthma? Since obesity is also a risk factor for type-2 diabetes, it may be possible that an alternative mechanism underlies these two diseases.

Dr. Holt: A comment and perhaps a question addressed back to an issue that Dr. Lack just raised which I think is going to turn out to be of major importance in some of the intervention strategies, and that is the emerging evidence that if you desensitize children to one of the major inhalant allergens, it seems to have a spreading effect, as it were, in relation to the prevention of new sensitizations. I don't think it matters mechanistically whether Dr. Romagnani or Dr. van den Biggelaar is right. The key probably is simply that if one can reduce the totality of the Th2 drive at the level of the airway mucosa, which is the port of entry for the new allergens responsible for sensitization, then this might 'short circuit' the progression of allergic sensitization. It is very clear from animal models that Th2 responses at the airway mucosa drive other (bystander) Th2 responses. They do this primarily by altering the functional phenotype of the local antigen-presenting cells, in particular by bombardment of the airway dendritic cell population with Th2 cytokines, which primes them so that the response to new allergens will continue to default to Th2 phenotype. If we can cut down that drive through desensitization then we have quite a reasonable chance of stopping this progressive expression of new sensitizations which occurs in atopics.

References

1 Parronchi P, De Carli M, Manetti R, et al: IL-4 and IFN (alpha and gamma) exert opposite regulatory effects on the development of cytolytic potential by Th1 or Th2 human T cell clones. J Immunol 1992;149:2977–2988.
2 Manetti R, Gerosa F, Giudizi MG, et al: Interleukin 12 induces stable priming for interferon gamma (IFN-gamma) production during differentiation of human T-helper (Th) cells and transient IFN-gamma production in established Th2 cell clones. J Exp Med 1994;179:1273–1283.
3 Zuany-Amorim C, Sawicka E, ManliusC, et al: Suppression of airway eosinophilia by killed *Mycobacterium vaccae*-induced allergen-specific regulatory T-cells. Nat Med 2002;8:625–629.
4 Kitagaki K, Jain VV, Businga TR, et al: Immunomodulatory effects of CpG oligodeoxynucleotides on established Th2 responses. Clin Diagn Lab Immunol 2002;9:1260–1269.
5 Kline JN, Krieg AM, Waldschmidt TJ, et al: CpG oligodeoxynucleotides do not require Th1 cytokines to prevent eosinophilic airway inflammation in a murine model of asthma. J Allergy Clin Immunol 1999;104:1258–1264.
6 Braun-Fahrlander C, Riedler J, Herz U, et al, Allergy and Endotoxin Study Team: Environmental exposure to endotoxin and its relation to asthma in school-age children. N Engl J Med 2002;347:869–877.
7 Bach F: Commentary. N Engl J Med 2002;347:965–970.
8 Buijs J, Borsboom G, Renting M, et al: Relationship between allergic manifestations and Toxocara seropositivity: A cross-sectional study among elementary school children. Eur Respir J 1997;10:1467–1475.
9 Marini A, Li Destri M, Cattaneo F, Dozio N: Short- and Long-term results on offspring of diabetic mothers kept under a very tight metabolic control during pregnancy. V. Incidence of juvenile type 1 diabetes. Pediatr Res 2001;50:20A.
10 Oberle D, Mutius E, Kries R: Childhood asthma and continuous exposure to cats since the first year of life with cats allowed in the child's bedroom. Allergy 2003;58:1033–1036.
11 Matricardi PM, Rosmini F, Riondino S, et al: Exposure to foodborne and orofecal microbes versus airborne viruses in relation to atopy and allergic asthma: Epidemiological study. BMJ. 2000;320:412–417.

12 Ballin A, Somekh E, Geva D, Meytes D: High rate of asthma among immigrants. Med Hypothese 1998;51:281–284.
13 Rosenberg R, Vinker S, Zakut H, et al: An unusually high prevalence of asthma in Ethiopian immigrants to Israel. Fam Med 1999;31:276–279.
14 Castro-Rodriguez JA, Holberg CJ, Morgan WJ, et al: Increased incidence of asthmalike symptoms in girls who become overweight or obese during the school years. Am J Respir Crit Care Med 2001;163:1344–1349.

Isolauri E, Walker WA (eds): Allergic Diseases and the Environment.
Nestlé Nutrition Workshop Series Pediatric Program, Vol. 53, pp. 117–132,
Nestec Ltd.; Vevey/S. Karger AG, Basel, © 2004.

Mechanisms Governing Non-Responsiveness to Food Proteins

Cathryn Nagler-Anderson and W. Allan Walker

Massachusetts General Hospital and Harvard Medical School,
Charlestown, Mass., USA

Introduction

Dietary antigens and the luminal bacterial load are the major sources of chronic antigenic stimulation in gut-associated lymphoid tissue (GALT). Experimentally, oral administration of soluble protein antigens induces systemic non-responsiveness ('oral tolerance') to peripheral antigen challenge [for review see, 1]. Clinically, the induction of non-responsiveness to food antigens is essential for avoiding hypersensitivity reactions to food while tolerance of the commensal flora prevents chronic intestinal inflammation [for review see, 2]. In this review we will examine the mechanisms by which this non-responsiveness is induced and how their breakdown can contribute to the induction of food allergy.

Maintenance of the Intestinal Epithelial Barrier

Most infectious microbes enter the body via the respiratory or gastrointestinal tracts. In the intestine, the barrier formed by the single-cell-layered epithelium is protected by both specialized adaptations (table 1) and the innate and adaptive immune systems [for review see, 3]. The primary function of enterocytes, i.e. terminal digestion and absorption of dietary nutrients, is accomplished by the densely packed absorptive microvilli that coat its apical surface. At the tips of the microvilli a layer of membrane-anchored glycoproteins forms the filamentous brush border glycocalyx and prevents microbes and macromolecules from crossing the epithelial barrier [4]. In some portions of the epithelium, however, specialized enterocytes, known

Table 1. Adaptations that support intestinal epithelial barrier function

Tight junctions	Ring of proteins that seals apical epithelium; includes the integral membrane proteins occludin and claudin in association with cytoplasmic zonula occludins proteins [43]
Secretory IgA	Predominant form of Ig found at mucosal surface; secreted as a dimer joined by a J chain. Typically neutralizing, secretory IgA binds complement very weakly [44]
Mucins	Secreted glycoproteins that form a viscoelastic gel at apical surface [45]
Trefoil peptides	Three small proteins, secreted by goblet cells, which function in epithelial protection and repair [45]
Defensins (cryptidins)	Anti-microbial peptides secreted by Paneth cells in the villus crypt [46]
Filamentous brush border glycocalyx	Thick (400–500 nm) layer of membrane anchored glycoproteins at tips of microvilli [4]

as M cells, lack this glycocalyx and facilitate the uptake and transport of both microbes and soluble antigens.

As schematized in figure 1, the mucosal immune system of the small intestine is comprised of both organized lymphoid structures such as the Peyer's patch (PP) and populations of effector cells scattered throughout the lamina propria (LP) of the intestinal villi. The GALT can also be divided functionally into inductive (PP) and effector (LP) sites. Microbes bind to M cells ① and are transported into the PPs where they are taken up by antigen-presenting cells (APCs, particularly dendritic cells, DCs) ② in the subepithelial dome. Recent studies have suggested that DCs that extend their processes through the intercellular tight junctions of the villus epithelium ③ provide another mechanism for transport across this barrier [5]. Secretory IgA responses are initiated in B-cell follicles in the PP ④ and play an important role in protecting the epithelium against microbial invasion. IgA-secreting plasma cells and memory T-effector cells migrate into the intestinal LP ⑤ via high endothelial venules where they are poised to mount a rapid and efficient response to any breach of the epithelial barrier.

Antigenic components of both dietary proteins and the luminal commensal bacteria also gain access to the mucosal immune system and induce systemic non-responsiveness rather than immunity. Although it is not yet clear how they are taken up, the distinction between innocuous antigens and pathogens is likely to occur at the level of antigen presentation. Some evidence suggests that, in the absence of the inflammatory response induced by infection, soluble antigens from food or commensal bacteria are taken up by immature DCs (see discussion below). Unique patterns of cytokine production by mucosally derived DCs are likely to be important to the generation of

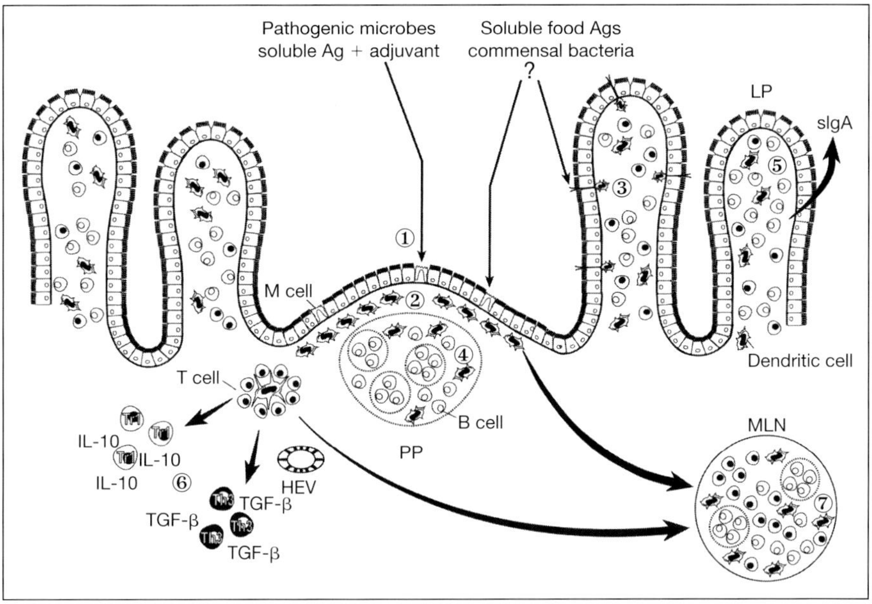

Fig. 1. Antigen sampling and the induction of tolerance and immunity in the gut associated lymphoid tissue. HEV = High endothelial venules; MLN = mesenteric lymph node. See description in text.

regulatory cells secreting anti-inflammatory cytokines like interleukin (IL)-10 and transforming growth factor-β. (TGF-β) ⑥ Antigen-bearing DCs also migrate from the mucosal surface and carry antigen to the draining (mesenteric) lymph node ⑦ for presentation to naïve T cells and the induction of systemic non-responsiveness.

Activation of the Innate Immune System Regulates Tolerance and Immunity

Microbial recognition by the innate immune system represents a rapidly deployed, first line of defense. The initial response to microorganisms involves the detection of broadly conserved microbial structural elements by pattern recognition molecules such as Toll-like receptors (TLRs) [6, 7]. The pattern recognition receptors of the innate immune system are relatively non-specific and are encoded in the germline. Some of the pathogen-associated molecular patterns recognized include: the lipopeptides and peptidoglycans of gram-positive bacteria (TLR-2), lipopolysaccharide (LPS) of gram-negative bacteria (TLR-4), bacterial flagellin (TLR-5), double-stranded viral RNA (TLR-3) and hypomethylated bacterial CpG DNA (TLR-9). Each encounter of

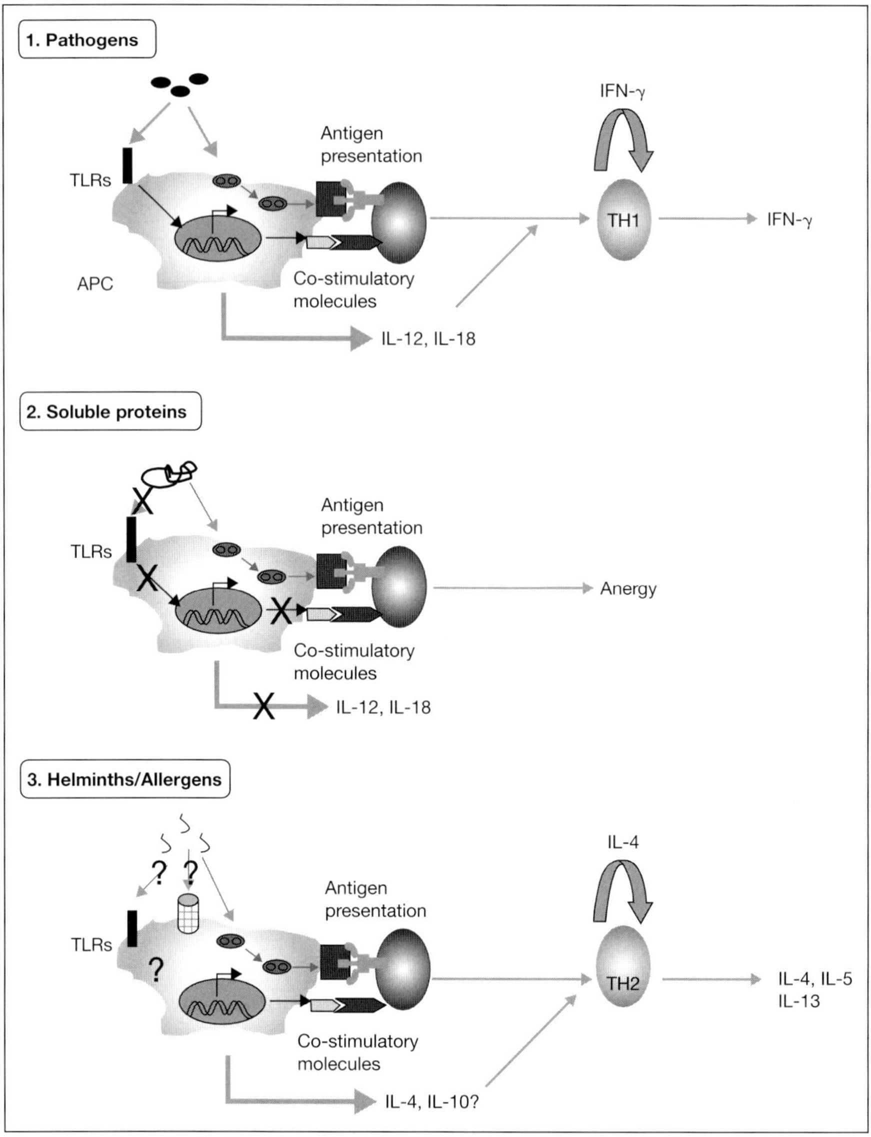

Fig. 2. Signaling via the innate immune system sets the stage for the adaptive immune response. Antigen-presenting cells (APC) process microbial antigens to generate peptide fragments for presentation to naïve T cells in the context of MHC class-I and class-II proteins. 1: Most Th1-polarizing microbial pathogens bear pathogen-associated molecular patterns (PAMPs) that signal via a family of pattern recognition molecules called Toll-like receptors (TLRs). TLR signaling activates genes that upregulate the co-stimulatory molecules that provide the 'second signal' for a productive immune response and induce the secretion of the cytokines (IL-12 and IL-18) required for the initiation of a Th1 response. IFN-γ is the prototypic Th1 cytokine and is both secreted

the innate immune system with an antigen occurs without recall of past antigen encounters.

Recognition by the innate immune system sets the stage for the adaptive immune response. Following the initial identification of foreign microbial antigens, the adaptive immune system generates lymphocytes with receptors with unique antigenic specificities. DNA rearrangement creates the T-cell and B-cell receptors required for the recognition of the universe of potential antigens. Whereas B-cell receptors (Ig) recognize intact proteins folded in their native configuration, T-cell receptors recognize antigenic fragments (peptides) presented in the context of class-I or class-II major histocompatibility complex (MHC) proteins. However, this recognition event is not sufficient to generate a productive immune response. A second or 'co-stimulatory' signal is required for T-cell activation. Members of the best-characterized co-stimulatory family B7.1 and B7.2 (CD80/86) bind the T-cell ligands CD28 and CTLA-4. The high affinity T-cell ligand CTLA-4 preferentially binds to APC expressing low levels of CD80/86; binding to CD28 is favored in the context of high CD80/86 expression. TLR signaling facilitates the adaptive immune response by inducing the upregulation of the MHC proteins and co-stimulatory molecules required for T-cell activation and optimization of antigen presentation (fig. 2).

By contrast, soluble proteins (including those in the diet) that do not trigger the innate immune system by signaling via TLRs are presented in the presence of low levels of co-stimulatory signals and typically induce non-responsiveness (anergy; fig. 2). Several reports have shown that transient T-cell activation and proliferation is the initial response to both soluble dietary antigens and pathogenic microbes and is observed primarily in the GALT [8–10]. Work in our laboratory has shown that, upon subsequent peripheral exposure to antigen, the proliferative capacity of antigen-specific cells from mice fed soluble protein antigens is reduced when compared to mice that have received antigen in an immunogenic form [10]. The reduction in proliferative capacity induced by the recognition of a tolerogenic form of antigen is due to the preferential binding of the B7 co-stimulatory molecules to their T-cell ligand CTLA-4 [11]. Tolerance to an intravenous administration of soluble antigen cannot be induced in mice bearing antigen-specific, T-cell receptor, transgenic T cells lacking CTLA-4

by these cells and required for their clonal expansion. 2: Soluble proteins do not signal via TLRs. Co-stimulatory molecules are not upregulated. Low levels of co-stimulation favor binding to the inhibitory T-cell ligand CTLA-4 and functional anergy ensues (see text for discussion). 3: Helminths and allergens uniquely induce a polarized Th2 response. It is not yet clear whether they signal via TLRs or an alternative pathway for pattern recognition. Signaling via these stimuli generate Th2-inducing cytokines (IL-4) and immunoregulatory mediators like IL-10. Co-stimulatory molecules are also induced. IL-4 both induces and drives a polarized Th2 response, characterized by the secretion of IL-4, IL-5 and IL-13.

because the mutant T cells cannot downregulate cell cycle progression via CTLA-4 signaling [11]. A recent study has shown that signaling via CTLA-4 is also required for the induction of tolerance to orally administered antigen [12]. When soluble antigen is administered either orally or, in the periphery, antigen-specific clones fail to expand and either become anergic or die. Immunogenic forms of antigen activate the innate immune system and prime for the clonal expansion of antigen-specific cells.

Antigen Uptake in the GALT

While the failure to engage TLRs and activate of the innate immune system provides an explanation for orally induced non-responsiveness at a molecular level, where and by what subset of APCs, antigen is presented to naïve T cells also plays a critical role in determining the ultimate outcome. The immature DCs that are found in abundance below the dome of the PP are highly phagocytic cells optimized for antigen uptake. As mentioned above, signaling via the innate immune system induces the 'maturation' of DCs to a form that functions primarily to present antigen to T cells. MHC and co-stimulatory molecules are upregulated and phagocytic capacity is greatly reduced. The migration of DCs has also been linked to this maturation process. In the gut, however, perhaps due to the constant exposure to potentially inflammatory stimuli, immature DCs can continuously pick up antigens at the epithelial surface and transport them to the T-cell areas of the mesenteric lymph node [13]. The cargo of these DCs includes fragments of epithelial cells shed from the villus tips as the epithelium regenerates [13]. The identification of this constitutive migratory pathway has opened up the possibility that DCs may also pick up other types of antigen from the intestinal lumen, including those derived from food or commensal bacteria, without inducing their own maturation. The observation that DCs can extend their dendrites between enterocytes to sample the luminal contents suggests a mechanism by which this could occur [5]. The constitutive migration of antigen-laden DCs from the epithelial surface also suggests a mechanism by which immature DCs could present mucosa-derived antigens to naïve T cells and induce tolerance in peripheral sites. Alternatively, these migratory DCs might tolerize naïve peripheral T cells by transferring their antigenic cargo to a specialized subset of tolerance-inducing DC, resident in T-cell areas of the lymph node [14]. A great deal of effort has been devoted to the identification of functionally specialized subsets of DCs and has resulted in their classification into two major groups based largely on their cell surface markers [15, 16]. The DCs that are localized prominently in the subepithelial dome of the PP belong to the myeloid (CD11c+CD11b+) subset and are also found in the marginal zone of the spleen and in the subcapsular sinus of the lymph node [17]. The activation, and subsequent migration, of myeloid DCs to the T-cell areas of secondary lymphoid organs has been associated with the induction of a type-2 T-helper (Th2) type of response. By contrast, the lymphoid (CD11c+CD8α+) DCs found in the T-cell areas of lymphoid organs have been associated with the induction of a Th1 (inflammatory) type of response. However, newer studies have emphasized the functional plasticity of these DC subsets and suggest that T-cell priming and polarization is also strongly influenced by antigen dose, immunoregulatory mediators and tissue microenvironment [18]. Indeed, in the PP high level production of the Th2-type cytokines IL-4 and IL-10 by DCs appears to slant the mucosal immune response in an anti-inflammatory direction [17, 19]. The IL-10 produced has been attributed to the myeloid CD11b+ DCs located in the subepithelial dome of the PP [19]. Moreover, only PP DCs constitutively express mRNA for TGF-β. DCs in the gut therefore constitutively (and uniquely?) produce the growth factors required for maintenance and expansion of two major subsets of immunoregulatory T cells, IL-10-secreting T-regulatory 1 (Tr1) cells [20–22] and TGF-β secreting Th3 cells [23, 24].

Regulatory T Cells

Active suppression, clonal deletion and clonal anergy are typically cited as the primary mechanisms through which peripheral tolerance to oral (or intravenous) administration of antigens is induced. The active suppression of immune responses by the secretion of immunoregulatory cytokines and the induction of non-responsiveness (clonal anergy) in the presence of low levels of co-stimulation may represent two independent mechanistic pathways for the induction of tolerance. Alternatively, the 'functionally non-responsive' T cells may themselves act as regulatory cells through the secretion of immunoregulatory cytokines. Subsets of regulatory/suppressor T cells secreting TGF-β have long been implicated in oral tolerance [for review see, 25]. Regulatory T cells (Treg) dependent on both TGF-β and signaling via CTLA-4 have been described [26, 27] and, as mentioned above, signaling via CTLA-4 is required for the induction of tolerance to orally administered antigen [12]. Other work indicates that apoptotic T cells release TGF-β, again suggesting overlap between the secretion of immunoregulatory cytokines and a mechanism for the induction of tolerance [28].

Tolerance to self requires deletion and/or suppression of T cells with potentially self-reactive specificities. In recent years data have rapidly accumulated suggesting that self-reactivity is controlled by a specialized subset of naturally occurring Treg in both mice and humans [29, 30]. These Treg are CD4+ and constitutively express CD25, the IL-2 receptor α chain. At least some of the cells in this subset exit the thymus in a functionally mature form. In addition to their role in controlling organ-specific autoimmunity, CD4+CD25+ Treg regulate responses to environmental antigens at mucosal surfaces in models of both intestinal inflammation and allergy and can be induced by both oral and intravenous administration of soluble antigen [31]. In a well-characterized model of colitis induced by the transfer of 'pathogenic' CD4+CD45RB^{hi} T cells, pathology is ameliorated by the transfer of CD4+CD25+ CD45RB^{lo} Treg which appear to function in a cytokine (IL-10 and TGF-β)-dependent fashion [32]. However, other evidence suggests that the cytokine secretion profiles that define Th3 and Tr1 cells do not represent functional subsets within the broader CD4+CD25+ regulatory cell category but are distinct cell lineages [33]. Interestingly, similarities between the multiorgan autoimmune diseases which develop in patients with the X-linked recessive diseases XLAAD (X-linked autoimmunity-allergic dysregulation syndrome) or IPEX (immune dysregulation, polyendocrinopathy, enteropathy X-linked syndrome) and those seen in a mutant mouse strain (Scurfy) have led to the identification of the genetic defect responsible for these disorders. The gene, *Foxp3*, encodes a transcription factor that controls the development of CD4+CD25+ T cells, emphasizing the critical role of these cells in maintaining immune homeostasis and in preventing hyperreactivity to both self antigens and potential allergens [34]. The identification of this genetic marker should help to clarify the mechanisms by which CD4+CD25+ Treg suppress immune responsiveness and their relationship to other subsets of Treg.

Dysregulated Immune Responsiveness to Intestinal Microbes and the Development of Food Allergy

As mentioned above, activation of the innate immune system is required for the induction of a productive immune response. Experimentally, various microbial products can act as adjuvants and induce systemic and mucosal immune responses to co-administered soluble protein antigens [3]. Our laboratory has shown that infection with an enteric helminth can also act as an adjuvant to prime for an antigen-specific Th2 response to a model dietary antigen [10]. Helminthic parasites and allergens are unique in their ability to induce a polarized Th2 response and the production of IgE. Using a well-characterized murine model of food allergy [35], we examined whether chronic gastrointestinal helminthiasis could also induce an allergic response to a dietary antigen [36]. We found that an IgE response to an orally administered antigen was not induced in helminth-infected mice, despite the ability of this Th2-polarized environment to prime for a Th2 response to this typically tolerogenic stimulus. Although they do not generate the Th1-biased inflammatory response associated with other pathogenic microbes, helminths (and allergens) activate the innate immune system and induce the upregulation of co-stimulatory molecules. Whether this occurs via as yet unidentified pathogen-associated molecular patterns and signaling through TLRs or is mediated by a novel, TLR-independent pathway is not yet known (fig. 2). Why is an allergic (IgE) response induced when a dietary antigen is administered with the Th2 inducing mucosal adjuvant cholera toxin but not when the GALT is Th2 polarized by helminth infection? When antigen plus cholera toxin is administered to helminth-infected mice, the antigen-specific, IgE-mediated, anaphylactic response is greatly reduced. The downregulation of antigen-specific IgE observed in helminth-infected mice is accompanied by a reduction in antigen-specific T cells secreting IL-13. A reduced incidence of allergic disease in patients from areas in which chronic infection with helminthic parasites is endemic has been reported in clinical studies and attributed to parasite-induced immunoregulatory cytokines, particularly IL-10 [37, 38]. When we treated infected mice with neutralizing antibody to IL-10 the infection-mediated protection against allergic symptoms was abrogated, suggesting that helminth-dependent protection against allergic disease involves immunoregulatory mechanisms that block production of allergen-specific IgE [36].

Another interesting interrelationship between microbes and the induction of allergy involves the commensal bacteria that colonize the gastrointestinal tract. The Th2/T-regulatory cell dominant tone of the GALT is shaped, in part, by antigenic stimulation by these luminal bacteria and protects against the development of intestinal inflammation [for review see, 3]. Microbial stimulation seems to provide counter-regulatory signals necessary to overcome the inherent Th2 bias of the mucosa-associated lymphoid tissue to prevent allergic disease. As mentioned above, TLR-4 has been identified as the receptor for bacterial LPS. Mice of the C3H/HeJ strain have a point mutation in the intracellular domain of TLR-4 that blocks LPS signaling, and are therefore hypo-responsive to LPS [39, 40]. We have examined whether the inability to signal via TLR-4 is linked to susceptibility to an allergic response to food [41]. We have found that administration of a food allergen (peanut) with a mucosal adjuvant induces allergen-specific IgE, elevated plasma histamine levels and anaphylactic symptoms in strains of mice lacking a functional receptor for bacterial LPS (TLR-4) but not in MHC-matched controls. The link between the allergic phenotype and mutant TLR-4 observed in 3 separate strains of mice strongly suggests that bacterial components act via TLR-4 to negatively regulate the development of allergy. Decontamination of the gut with antibiotics renders wild-type mice susceptible to food allergy, demonstrating that the commensal flora of the intestine is the source of these bacterial signals. The induction of allergic disease is associated with an apparently dysregulated antigen-specific IL-13 response. The recent description of Treg that express TLR-4 and are activated by LPS suggests the intriguing possibility that the absence of a functional subset of these cells in the TLR-4 mutant mice may play a role in their susceptibility to allergic responses to food in our model [42].

The GALT exists in a dynamic equilibrium with antigenic stimulation from the luminal contents. As we have discussed above, in the healthy individual, multiple immunoregulatory mechanisms are in place to maintain intestinal homeostasis. However, stimuli from both infectious microbes (helminths) and the luminal flora can perturb this balance and dramatically alter the mucosal microenvironment. Detailed examination of the mechanisms by which non-responsiveness to food/commensal antigens is normally maintained, and their alteration by microbial stimuli, are challenging and exciting areas for future study.

Acknowledgments

We thank Drs. Bobby Cherayil and Mohamed Bashir for their critical review of the manuscript. This work was supported by RO-1 DK 55678 and by the Center for the Study of Inflammatory Bowel Disease at the Massachusetts General Hospital and the Clinical Nutrition Research Center at Harvard.

References

1 Nagler-Anderson C, Shi HN: Peripheral nonresponsiveness to orally administered soluble protein antigens. Crit Rev Immunol 2001;21:121–131.
2 Spiekermann G, Walker WA: Oral tolerance and its role in clinical disease. J Pediatr Gastroenterol Nutr 2001;32:237–255.
3 Nagler-Anderson C: Man the barrier! Strategic defenses in the intestinal mucosa. Nat Rev Immunol 2001;1:59–67.
4 Kraehenbuhl J-P, Neutra MR: Epithelial M cells: Differentiation and function. Annu Rev Cell Dev Biol 2000;16:301–332.
5 Rescigno M, Urbano M, Valzasina B, et al: Dendritic cells express tight junction proteins and penetrate gut epithelial monolayers to sample bacteria. Nat Immunol 2001;2:361–367.
6 Akira S, Takeda K, Kaisho T: Toll-like receptors: Critical proteins linking innate and acquired immunity. Nat Immunol 2001;2:675–680.
7 Medzhitov R: Toll-like receptors and innate immunity. Nat Rev Immunol 2001;1:135–145.
8 Sun J, Dirden-Kramer B, Ito K, et al: Antigen-specific T cell activation and proliferation during oral tolerance induction. J Immunol 1999;162:5868–5875.
9 Blanas E, Davey GM, Carbone FR, Heath WR: A bone marrow-derived APC in the gut-associated lymphoid tissue captures oral antigens and presents them to both CD4+ and CD8+ T cells. J Immunol 2000;164:2890–2896.
10 Shi HN, Liu HY, Nagler-Anderson C: Enteric infection acts as an adjuvant for the response to a model food antigen. J Immunol 2000;165:6174–6182.
11 Greenwald RJ, Boussiotis VA, Lorsbach RB, et al: CTLA-4 regulates induction of anergy in vivo. Immunity 2001;14:145–155.
12 Fowler S, Powrie F: CTLA-4 expression on antigen-specific cells but not IL-10 secretion is required for oral tolerance. Eur J Immunol 2002;32:2997–3006.
13 Huang FP, Platt N, Wykes M, et al: A discrete subpopulation of dendritic cells transports apoptotic intestinal epithelial cells to T cell areas of mesenteric lymph nodes. J Exp Med 2000;191:435–443.
14 Sallusto F, Lanzavecchia A: Mobilizing dendritic cells for tolerance, priming and chronic inflammation. J Exp Med 1999;189:611–614.
15 Pulendran B, Maraskovsky E, Banchereau J, Maliszewski C: Modulating the immune response with dendritic cells and their growth factors. Trends Immunol 2001;22:41–47.

16 Henri S, Vremec D, Kamath A, et al: The dendritic cell populations of mouse lymph nodes. J Immunol 2001;167:741–748.
17 Iwasaki A, Kelsall BL: Freshly isolated Peyer's patch, but not spleen, dendritic cells produce interleukin 10 and induce the differentiation of T helper type 2 cells. J Exp Med 1999;190: 229–239.
18 Kelsall BL, Biron CA, Sharma O, Kaye PM: Dendritic cells at the host-pathogen interface. Nat Immunol 2002;3:699–702.
19 Iwasaki A, Kelsall BL: Unique functions of CD11b+, CD8α+, and double-negative Peyer's patch dendritic cells. J Immunol 2001;166:4884–4890.
20 Groux H, O'Garra A, Bigler M, et al: A CD4+ T cell subset inhibits antigen-specific T cell responses and prevents colitis. Nature 1997;389:737–742.
21 Cottrez F, Hurst SD, Coffman RL, Groux H: T regulatory cells 1 inhibit a Th2-specific response in vivo. J Immunol 2000;165:4848–4853.
22 Roncarolo MG, Levings MK, Traversari C: Differentiation of T regulatory cells by immature dendritic cells. J Exp Med 2001;193:F5–F9.
23 Chen Y, Inobe J, Marks R, et al: Peripheral deletion of antigen-reactive T cells in oral tolerance. Nature 1995;376:177–180.
24 Weiner HL: Oral tolerance: Immune mechanisms and treatment of autoimmune diseases. Immunol Today 1997;19:335–339.
25 Mowat AM, Weiner HL: Oral tolerance. Physiological basis and clinical applications; in Ogra PL, Mestecky J, Lamm ME, et al (eds): Mucosal Immunology. New York, Academic Press, 1999, pp 587–618.
26 Chen W, Jin W, Wahl SM: Engagement of cytotoxic T lymphocyte-associated antigen 4 (CTLA-4) induces transforming growth factor β (TGF-β) production by murine CD4+ T cells. J Exp Med 1998;188:1849–1857.
27 Read S, Malmstrom V, Powrie F: Cytotoxic T lymphocyte-associated antigen 4 plays an essential role in the function of CD25+CD4+ regulatory cells that control intestinal inflammation. J Exp Med 2000;192:295–302.
28 Chen WJ, Frank ME, Jin W, Wahl SM: TGF-β released by apoptotic T cells contributes to an immunosuppressive milieu. Immunity 2001;14:715–725.
29 Shevach EM: Certified professionals: CD4+CD25+ suppressor T cells. J Exp Med 2001;193: F41–F45.
30 Shevach EM: CD4+CD25+ suppressor T cells: More questions than answers. Nat Rev Immunol 2002;2:389–400.
31 Thorstenson KM, Khoruts A: Generation of anergic and potentially immunoregulatory CD25+CD4+ T cells in vivo after induction of peripheral tolerance with intravenous or oral antigen. J Immunol 2001;167:188–195.
32 Maloy KJ, Salaun L, Cahill R, et al: CD4+CD25+ Tr cells suppress innate immune pathology through cytokine-dependent mechanisms. J Exp Med 2003;197:111–119.
33 Levings MK, Sangregorio R, Sartirana C, et al: Human CD25+CD4+ T suppressor cell clones produce transforming growth factor β, but not interleukin 10, and are distinct from type 1 regulatory T cells. J Exp Med 2002;196:1335–1346.
34 Hori S, Nomura T, Sakaguchi S: Control of regulatory T cell development by the transcription factor Foxp3. Science 2003;299:1057–1061.
35 Li XM, Zhang TF, Huang CK, et al: A murine model of peanut anaphylaxis: T- and B-cell responses to a major peanut allergen mimic human responses. J Allergy Clin Immunol 2000; 106:150–158.
36 Bashir MEH, Andersen P, Fuss IJ, et al: An enteric helminth infection protects against an allergic response to dietary antigen. J Immunol 2002;169:3284–3292.
37 van den Biggelaar AHJ, van Ree R, Rodrigues LC, et al: Decreased atopy in children infected with *Schistosoma haematobium:* A role for parasite-induced interleukin-10. Lancet 2000; 356:1723–1727.
38 Yazdanbakhsh M, Kremsner PG, Van Ree R: Allergy, parasites and the hygiene hypothesis. Science 2002;296:490–494.
39 Poltorak A, Merlin T, Nielsen PJ, et al: A point mutation in the IL-12Rβ2 gene underlies the IL-12 unresponsiveness of LPS-defective C57Bl/10ScCr mice. J Immunol 2001;167:2106–2111.
40 Qureshi ST, Lariviere L, Leveque G, et al: Endotoxin-tolerant mice have mutations in Toll-like receptor 4 (TLR4). J Exp Med 1999;189:615–625.

41 Bashir MEH, Shi HN, Nagler-Anderson C: TLR-4 signaling by intestinal microbes determines susceptibility to food allergy in a murine model. Submitted for publication, 2003.
42 Caramalho I, Lopes-Carvalho T, Ostler D, et al: Regulatory T cells selectively express Toll-like receptors and are activated by lipopolysaccharide. J Exp Med 2003;197:403–411.
43 Madara JL: Regulation of movement of solutes across tight junctions. Annu Rev Physiol 1998;60:143–159.
44 Robinson JK, Blanchard TG, Levine AD, et al: A mucosal IgA mediated excretory immune system in vivo. J Immunol 2001;166:3688–3692.
45 Podolsky DK: Mucosal immunity and inflammation. V. Innate mechanisms of mucosal defense and repair: The best offense is a good defense. Am J Physiol 1999;277:G495–G499.
46 Ayabe T, Satchell DP, Wilson CL, et al: Secretion of microbial α-defensins by intestinal Paneth cells in response to bacteria. Nat Immunol 2000;1:113–118.

Discussion

As the author of this paper was unable to join the workshop, the presentation and the discussion were conducted by W. Allan Walker, USA.

Dr. Sorensen: This was a challenging talk because it is hard to really know where this is going to lead now and perhaps you will to tell us more later on today. How are we going to know when a bacteria is a pathogen and does bad things, and when it is a good bacteria that will shift immunity in the right direction?

Dr. Walker: Actually I plan to address this in my second talk. Let me try to comment however. I personally think this is one of the most interesting and exciting areas of investigation right now. What was presented is a basic observation made in a mouse model and I don't mean to imply that you can directly apply this to patients. We have to approach this in multiple steps but we are getting some clues as to how the process from basic research works. One of the bases for preventing allergy is understanding better how the initial colonization of the gut occurs and how, through its commensal bacteria, it stimulates an appropriate immune responsiveness, e.g., downregulation of response to food antigens and at the same time an appropriate response to pathogens and tolerating commensal bacteria. The next step is investigations to explain what are the best organisms to accomplish this effect. When Dr. Isolauri presents some of the work she is doing, we will hear more about how we are going to be able to effect these observations made in an animal model and apply them to patient care.

Dr. Murch: In the interpretation of regulatory cells there seem to be a lot of shared pathway Th1 responses, it is mediated by Toll receptors, NF-κB. In the early stages of generating TGF-β responses you have a transient interferon-γ response so presumably there is some kind of trip switch along the Th1 pathway which then deviates towards the regulatory cells. IL-10 is in the frame for that. Do you think that at some point we are going to have small molecules which will deviate responses from Th1 to a regulatory one without necessarily going towards the Th2?

Dr. Walker: Again I am trying to present Dr. Nagler-Anderson's work, so it is not really my area. But what I think is going on is that there might be a differential innate immune response that may be developmentally regulated, which is something I know you are very interested in. There may be a circumstance where other signal transduction pathways in addition to the classic TLR4, IL-1 signal transduction molecules affect NF-κB and then activation. Alternatively there could be another response at a certain point in development that actually turns off inflammation. I am going to talk a little bit about this in some work we are showing with commensal bacteria in the immature gut. So it is a very fascinating area, we have to know more about it at the cellular level before we can begin to deal with it at the clinical level.

Dr. Neijens: It would be very interesting to learn how these observations might work in practice and in clinical medicine. We did this type of investigation with regard to respiratory pathogens, both in a mouse model and in children, looking at the development of atopic diseases and also the interaction with the respiratory pathogen, respiratory syncytial virus, rhino virus and influenza. We noticed in both the animal model and in humans that it is highly dependent on the genetic background, the degree of sensitization and also the time and the intensity of the microorganism which is available. I wonder if in your experiments the background is also important, the genetic background, and the degree of sensitization, and also the time and the dose because you induce either a high or a low dose, and also the activation of the dendritic cells and the T cells is highly dependent on the dose?

Dr. Walker: You are absolutely right. What I showed you is a manipulated system. We used an inbred strain of mouse that respond to peanut antigen with allergy. Perhaps the same thing pertains in humans, although we don't understand quite as well as to whether it may be a genetic predisposition. Although the environment is important it only affects those individuals who have a subtle genetic predisposition to an allergic response. There are probably human models like the mouse model but I would say we can't study these patients in the same way. My point is that it is very important for us to understand as best we can what is going on in animals and cells lines, but we can't then assume that the same thing is going on in humans because the human is a much more complex organism and there could be multiple steps we are missing that we just need to get sorted out. The problem is you can't go to the human and start trying to make observations that allow you to understand the actual mechanism. You can see whether it is stimulated or suppressed but you don't know the basis for the responses. You need both approaches in parallel to answer the mechanism question.

Dr. Neijens: But this is so complicated in practice that the effect of the microorganism is so dependent on the time, the age and the time of development.

Dr. Walker: You are absolutely right. The dose, the nature of the antigen, the time when the antigen is administered, etc., are critical questions. Let me just underscore what you are suggesting. Yesterday there were comments made about why an interferon-γ trial does not work in a Th1-mediated process such as Crohn's disease, and then another question why IL-10 does not work in another process. These discrepancies underscore how complex the human immune system is, so you can't really say what works in the inbred mouse also works in humans. Therefore we have to address this at both levels. Your point is very well taken.

Dr. Hill: Can I just push that a little more. You have shown very elegantly that you can switch a Th2 to a Th1 response. My question is how far do you pursue and demonstrate true tolerance to the antigen? If you go beyond the time point, is there evidence that you are inducing tolerance or maybe just switching one mechanism to another?

Dr. Walker: If I understood you correctly, you are asking how you turn on tolerance but what about the long-term effect and its process? That is also a very good question. Tolerance has been studied very carefully for a long time and we still don't know much about its mechanism. What is exciting about Dr. Nagler-Anderson's work is the fact that there are other subsets of T-helper cells that can release factors able to modulate both anti-inflammation and tolerance, and whether or not these persistently have the same effect periodically. Therefore whether or not there is a waxing and waning, or whether or not it is a long-term process I don't know. What Dr. Murch will probably discuss is the fact that one can prime to produce tolerance at a certain stage but you can't do it in a very young immature animal or human. There is something about maturation of the immune response and how antigens are handled that is going to determine this response.

Dr. Papageorgiou: I was wondering about the mouse model you just described. Are there any experiments in which dietary proteins are fed versus gavaging them? Is there any difference in the tolerance induction?

Dr. Walker: Did you say the whole protein versus the hydrolysate?

Dr. Papageorgiou: No, giving it by mouth versus gavaging them directly into the stomach.

Dr. Walker: There isn't much difference whether you infuse by gavage or you give it orally because it is crossing the mucosa surface, so in both circumstances it is probably going to be the same type of response. Did I answer your question?

Dr. Papageorgiou: I was just interested to know if the process starts in the mouth.

Dr. Walker: I don't know.

Dr. Lack: I was just surprised that in this model the regulatory response actually seems to affect humoral immunity as far as IgE is concerned and the question I had for you is what happens to IgG1, IgG2 and other isotypes. Does chronic helminthic infection downregulate antigen-specific humeral responses in general or is it specific to IgE?

Dr. Walker: The data I showed you imply that a helminth infection specifically turns off the IgE response. I don't know what it does to other humoral responses, but what Dr. Nagler-Anderson demonstrated is because of its effect on upregulating IL-10, not downregulating IL-13, you don't get a switch to IgE being produced. That is what she is implying. It is possible that she studied that, and that it could have turned off other components of the humeral immune response. Your point is extremely well taken. This is just a specific step in turning off a specific response to an antigen. This is what she is trying to show.

Dr. Al-Malik: In the last slide you showed that the suppression of TGF-β was being produced by Th3, and that nitric oxide synthetase has an inhibitory effect on the mechanism for tolerance. Would you comment on these two please?

Dr. Walker: I am just presenting Dr. Nagler-Anderson's work and I don't know if she has studied that more. Her last slide was more of a general nature. Her work has necessarily examined TGF-β, which is an extremely important molecule. Beyond that statement, I have no information.

Dr. Hourihane: With Dr. Strobel in London we developed a model of oral tolerance with peanut in which tolerance was induce without cholera toxin or any other toxin. In the model you describe, do you know whether they tried doing it with peanut with or without adjuvants or toxins?

Dr. Walker: They haven't. Again this is an area that we have to study more carefully. It could be that it is the toxin itself that has a different response. The last two slides are from an article just published in the *Journal of Immunology* [1], and there are plans to do additional observations but they haven't been done yet.

Dr. Hourihane: About the switch of the other antibody levels: we got a conventional tolerance switch of G1 and 2A. My second question is, is the peanut chow a purified protein, or is it a crude protein mixture?

Dr. Walker: I guess it is a purified protein. Actually you would probably know more about that, but the model system was adapted from a model that Sampson has used and they are using the same antigen.

Dr. von der Weid: I have one comment and one question. Probably 2 or 3 years ago, Cottrez et al. [2], the inventor of T-regulatory cells, already published quite a nice paper showing that transfer of TR1 cells specific to ovalbumin could suppress Th2 responses in vivo. I think this is very direct evidence that regulatory-type cells that produce high levels of IL-10 can suppress allergy. You showed that Toll-like receptor-4 (TLR4) is probably important for suppressing allergy, therefore microorganisms containing lipopolysaccharide (LPS) would be protective. So how do you reconcile this with some epidemiological studies [3, 4] showing that coliforms seem to be increased in allergic infants?

Dr. Walker: What you are referring to is that there might be different intestinal flora that exist in allergic compared to nonallergic patients. The problem is you are dealing with more cells in the gut that are probiotic, but just defining the intestinal flora doesn't answer the question. There are enough commensal organisms in the gut that have gram-negative LPS that they can stimulate TLR4. Therefore we have to be more specific in implicating specific bacterial flora.

Dr. Schiffrin: You show the relevance of TLR4 in this model. Do you know if Dr. Nagler-Anderson has also looked into the importance of intracellular pattern recognition receptors like Nod1 or Nod2 since the Nod2 variant seems to be related to inflammatory bowel disease for example?

Dr. Walker: What you are suggesting is that there are intracellular receptors that interact with LPS that can actually modulate inflammation. To my knowledge she hasn't studied that yet. Her next step is to determine if TLR2 knockout and other surface molecules may affect the process.

Dr. Isolauri: I have one comment and one question concerning the differences in intestinal flora between allergic infants and healthy infants. Does this not mean that these differences, for instance observed for coliforms, existed before and are causal to the development of allergy? We know that allergic inflammation in allergic individuals leads to changes in gut flora secondary to inflammation and the net result might be decreasing bifidobacteria. Different changes have been seen at the stage when allergic disease develops as compared to fully established allergic disease. So we cannot extrapolate from one stage to another. For instance the number of bifidobacteria is very low and coliforms are not the key issue in that. But one question. You showed that Toll-like receptor CD14 transmit the message from microbes; can you explain what the role of soluble receptors in that situation could be? We have measured CD14 soluble receptors.

Dr. Walker: The study of the LPS–TLR4 interaction is a very complex one. As you know it requires LPS-binding protein to form a complex and then binds to CD14. CD14 then facilitates the interaction to TLR4 which will cause a surface protein to be expressed, and then a series of steps happens after that. It is a very complex problem. I would suspect that in the absence of CD14 or LPS-binding protein that there would be a similar non-response to LPS as seen with a point mutation in TLR4.

Dr. van den Biggelaar: Do you know whether Dr. Nagler-Anderson has looked at all Toll-like receptors because yesterday I mentioned that the production of IL-10 upon stimulation with schistosome antigens can be blocked by anti-TLR2, indicating the helminth signals via TLR2. Did she look at TLR2 or other Toll-like receptors?

Dr. Walker: The next step is to work on TLR2, this is just the initial step. It just happens that the TLR4 knockouts or modulated point mutations are more readily available. However, the next step is to study TLR2. It is very likely that there could be a similar process mediated through TLR2.

Dr. Fritsche: Yesterday we talked about IL-10 in clinical studies. Could you say a little bit more on this topic?

Dr. Walker: About IL-10 in the human?

Dr. Fritsche: Because in this model IL-10 is very important. Have approaches been made?

Dr. Walker: Again this was in a mouse model, we are not dealing with human studies. But she demonstrated two observations clearly. One that IL-10 was involved in downregulating the allergic response in the infected animals and that it seems to be mediated through a downregulation of IL-13 as opposed to IL-5. IL-13 is also necessary for the switch to IgE production. That is what she has demonstrated, but again I am not sure that is exactly what is happening in the human.

References

1 Bashir ME, Andersen P, Fuss IJ, et al: An enteric helminth infection protects against an allergic response to dietary antigen. J Immunol 2002;169:3284–3292.
2 Cottrez F, Hurst SD, Coffman RL, Groux H: T regulatory cells 1 inhibit a Th2-specific response in vivo. J Immunol 2000;165:4848–4853.
3 Bjorksten B, Naaber P, Sepp E, Mikelsaar M: Intestinal microflora in allergic Estonian and Swedish 2-year-old children. Clin Exp Allergy 1999;29:342–346.
4 Kirjavainen PV, Arvola T, Salminen SJ, Isolauri E: Aberrant composition of gut microbiota of allergic infants: A target of bifidobacterial therapy at weaning? Gut 2002;51:51–55.

Isolauri E, Walker WA (eds): Allergic Diseases and the Environment.
Nestlé Nutrition Workshop Series Pediatric Program, Vol. 53, pp. 133–151,
Nestec Ltd.; Vevey/S. Karger AG, Basel, © 2004.

Oral Tolerance and Gut Maturation

Simon Murch

Paediatric Gastroenterology, Centre for Paediatric Gastroenterology,
Royal Free and University College School of Medicine, London, UK

Introduction

The maturation of intestinal function varies greatly between species. Clear maturational changes are seen in both enterocyte function and immune responses. The normal intestinal flora plays a much greater role in both processes than previously recognized, and has a profound impact on mucosal and systemic immune tolerance. While much conceptual advance has followed from study of genetically immunodeficient mouse strains, the major challenge in the unraveling of allergic and immunopathological disease is to extrapolate meaningfully from these data, to understand why changing infectious exposures appear to impact so greatly on the mechanisms of immune tolerance in apparently immunocompetent children in the developed world.

The evolutionarily ancient innate immune system is particularly important in intestinal immune responses. The increasing evidence for a central role of innate immunity in the mechanisms of oral tolerance show that normal gut homeostasis requires an actively maintained immunological response. Study of the integration between the innate and adaptive systems has developed in the last decade into an area of great conceptual interest, which may have important practical implications in reducing the incidence of allergic disease and autoimmunity [1, 2]. There is increasing evidence that the proinflammatory responses that are made to microorganisms by cells of innate immune origin, particularly dendritic cells (DCs), may determine the polarization of subsequent adaptive immune responses. In particular, in the development of oral tolerance there appears to be a requirement for specific input from the normal intestinal flora to innate immune cells such as macrophages and DCs, which allows generation of regulatory lymphocyte populations.

The Effects of Innate Immunity on T-Cell Responses

Early studies of macrophage subpopulations within the intestine identified distinct phenotypes dependent on location, with evidence of functional differences in terms of phagocytosis and antigen presentation [3]. The interactions between innate and adaptive immunity are complex and extensive, but the control of antigen presentation by innate immune cells is critical for determining subsequent T-cell reactivity (table 1). Recent work on professional antigen-presenting cells has demonstrated the importance of distinct DC lineages in determining the polarized response of T cells following antigen presentation [4]. Thus either type-1 T-helper (Th1) or type-2 T-helper (Th2) reactions are promoted by different populations of DCs. DCs of myeloid origin (DC1 cells) usually skew T-cell responses towards Th1 through release of IL-12, while, by contrast, those of plasmacytoid origin (DC2 cells) promote Th2 responses through IL-10 production [4]. However this dichotomy is not absolute, and the bacterial exposures of these cell types appear functionally important in determining final polarity. Protein derived from helminths caused myeloid DCs to develop into DC2 cells, inducing a Th2 response through upregulation of the OX-40 ligand, while bacterial or viral exposures induced a stable DC1 phenotype [5]. Plasmacytoid cells can also develop a Th1 phenotype on exposure to CpG DNA with appropriate cell surface contact [6]. As DC lineage and function can be modulated at the precursor stage by the exposure to bacterial or viral components, resulting in a phenotype that may be stably fixed through multiple division cycles, the early infectious exposures of the nascent immune system are clearly of unusual importance and may have very long-term relevance.

The discovery of the conserved family of Toll-like receptors (TLRs), each recognizing a distinct bacterial, fungal or viral component and inducing a proinflammatory response via the nuclear factor-κB (NFκB) pathway (table 1), has allowed fundamental advance in understanding the contribution of innate immunity to adaptive responses [7]. On the basis of TLR expression, there is evidence to suggest different evolutionary lineage and pathogen response of human DC types, with expression of TLRs 1, 2, 4, 5 and 8 in monocytes (pre-DC1 cells), TLRs 7 and 9 in plasmacytoid DC precursors (pre-DC2 cells) and TLRs 1, 2 and 3 in immature DCs [8]. Thus bacteria with cell surface peptidoglycans (recognized by TLR-2) are able to activate pre-DC-1 and immature DCs, but not pre-DC2 cells. By contrast, those expressing lipopolysaccharide (LPS; recognized by TLR-4) could activate only pre-DC1 cells, while pre-DC2 cells only responded to oligodeoxynucleotides from bacterial DNA, containing unmethylated CpG motifs. Immature DCs responded either to peptidoglycan or the viral RNA analogue poly I:C [8].

Plasmacytoid DCs show remarkable plasticity in functional response, and their production of type-1 interferons (IFNs)may represent a central link between innate and adaptive responses [6]. After initial IFN production, they

Table 1. Some potential interactions between innate immune cells and the intestinal flora which may affect adaptive immune responses [79]

Recognition element	Distribution	Microbial component recognized	Effect transduced
Mannose receptor	Dendritic cells, macrophages,	High-mannose carbohydrates	Increased efficiency of antigen presentation
Natural antibody	Secreted by peritoneal and intestinal B-1 cells	Surface glycans	Modulation of T-cell activation
Complement	Synergy with natural antibody	O- and N-linked glycans	Opsonization. Also regulates T-cell activation and B-cell tolerance
Toll-like receptors	Dendritic cells, macrophages, T cells, enterocytes Variable expression of TLRs on different lineages	TLR1: Mycobacterial lipoprotein (+TLR2), May Inhibit TLR4 TLR2: Peptoglycans TLR3: Viral ds-RNA TLR4: LPS TLR5: Flagellin TLR6: Diacylated lipopeptide (+TLR2) TLR7, 8: Antiviral synthetic peptide TLR9: Bacterial DNA (unmethylated CpG repeats) TLR10: Unknown	MyD88-dependent NFκB activation MyD88-independent upregulation of surface class-II MHC and co-stimulatory ligand expression
Mannan-binding lectin	Serum-derived, binds to macrophages, monocytes and B cells	Carbohydrates on gram-negative and gram-positive bacteria	Activates complement directly via serine proteases MASP-1 MASP-2
Nod receptors	Intracellular recognition molecules in innate immune	Nod1: LPS Nod2: Muramyl dipeptide	NFκB signaling pathway
Vα24 NK T cells, Vδ1 γδ T cells	Epithelial lymphocyte subsets Invariant T cell receptor chains	Conserved glycolipid sequences presented by nonclassical MHC (CD1d)	Modulate enterocyte responses, polarize towards Th1 and mucosal IgA production

may develop a DC1 phenotype after exposure to CpG DNA with surface contact from CD40-ligand, a DC2 phenotype in the presence of IL-3 and an indeterminate phenotype on viral exposure [6]. Studies of mature DC populations have shown less evidence of a potential for phenotype conversion, but the relative numbers of DC1 and DC2 cells in a mixed population may be altered by infectious exposures. Both dose of antigen and bacterial exposures induced a skewed response from a mixed population of differentiated DCs, suggesting the possibility of later shifts in functional polarization by appropriate immunotherapy [9].

The ability of DCs to produce IL-12 is an important regulator of protective Th1 responses. IL-12 production capacity is reduced in young infants and children, and recent evidence suggests that this deficiency lies in impaired function of circulating plasmacytoid DCs, rather than those of monocyte origin [10]. Indeed, the response to enteric bacteria of cord blood mononuclear cells, including IL-12 production, is as strong as that elicited from adult cells [11]. Thus an understanding of the molecular basis of maturation of plasmacytoid DCs may be important in developing strategies to overcome childhood allergic diseases.

Adaptive Immunity within the Intestine

Intestinal T and B lymphocytes show evidence of compartmentalized functions and developmental change in infancy. There is anatomical division into either organized lymphoid structures, such as Peyer's patches (cryptopatches and lymphocyte-filled villi are more recently recognized organized structures thought important in extrathymic lymphocyte maturation [12, 13]), or diffuse tissue infiltration in both the lamina propria and intraepithelial compartments. The mucosal immune system differs from the circulating immune system in several important ways, including the presence of high numbers of IgA-producing plasma cells, and T cells which have matured outside the thymus, with a notable over-representation of evolutionarily ancient lineages such as $\gamma\delta$ and Vα24 T cells, which recognize antigen in a manner distinct from 'conventional' circulating cells [14, 15]. Much of the functional data of these cell types comes from murine studies, with little known about the function of individual cell types in mucosal tolerance and even less about their role in early infancy. There is some evidence that $\gamma\delta$ cells may stimulate mucosal IgA responses [14, 15].

Peyer's patches are the principal sites of initiation of gut immune responses. Their precursors are found in human fetal intestine by 16 weeks of gestation, with organization into distinct T- and B-cell areas by 19 weeks [16]. They are well developed by 5 months gestation, and develop further after birth. In addition to Peyer's patches, isolated lymphoid follicles are commonly seen on small intestinal biopsies in young childhood, and hypertrophy of these follicles has been linked to allergic sensitization [17]. The milieu within the Peyer's patches differs from regional lymph nodes, and favors generation of regulatory lymphocytes (TR). The cytokines TGF-β and IL-10 may be particularly important in the generation and function of suppressor-type lymphocytes [18, 19].

The lamina propria of human intestine at birth contains few lymphoid cells, and these appear later in development than Peyer's patches or intraepithelial lymphocytes (IEL) [20]. Recent murine studies show that IELs may derive from cryptopatches situated just beneath the epithelial basement membrane [12], and that isolated lymphoid follicles are also detectable [21]. Analysis of T-cell variable region expression within fetal intestine shows traces of oligoclonal responses, although the stimulus for local expansion is unlikely to be of bacterial origin [22]. The human equivalents of cryptopatches have yet to be clarified, although lymphocyte-filled villi have been reported in a study of surgically resected specimens [13]. Early life exposures may be important in determining whether sensitization or tolerance occurs, and neonatal excision of organized mucosal lymphoid tissue by appendectomy prevented the much later development of colitis in transgenic mice [23]. Regression of Peyer's patches due to apoptosis also predated the onset of colitis in Gαi2 mice by many weeks [24] (the equivalent of years in human terms) further demonstrating that aberrant early life responses within organized mucosal lymphoid tissue may remain clinically silent for extended periods before subsequent immunopathology manifests. This may be analogous to the phenomenon of early life sensitization to inhaled antigens, with overt expression of allergy only becoming apparent much later [25]. While much adult disease is now thought to have a fetal origin, the basis for immunopathological disorders may lie in the first days and months of life.

Oral Tolerance

Oral tolerance is characterized by immunological tolerance to ingested foreign substances that would induce an inflammatory response if administered systemically [26, 27]. Whether oral tolerance is fundamentally different from other forms of peripheral immune tolerance remains controversial. Tolerance to the enteric flora may be mediated similarly to that of dietary antigen [26, 27]. Several factors may be important in generating tolerance, including the dose of antigen, as high-dose antigen induces T-cell anergy while low doses of antigen induce the production of transforming growth factor-β (TGF-β) by T-cell clones within Peyer's patches [27, 28]. Experimental studies demonstrate that T-cell apoptosis may be induced in Peyer's patches by ingestion of extremely large doses of antigen [29], although data in humans are lacking. It remains unclear whether these regulatory responses are directly analogous to those seen in more recent studies of circulating regulatory T-cell populations, and what may be the relative roles of cell–cell contact and secreted cytokines. However, it was notable from murine studies that low-dose oral tolerance was particularly difficult to establish in neonatal animals, and that paradoxical sensitization could occur which was not seen in older animals [30]. Whether dosage of dietary antigen is a factor determining sensitization or tolerance in infancy is an important question.

Control of T-Cell Reactivity within the Normal Intestine

There is potential for reciprocal inhibition of cell activation between Th1 and Th2 cells, with IFN-γ from Th1 cells inhibiting Th2 cytokine production and IL-10 and IL-4 from Th2 cells in turn inhibiting Th1 responses [14]. This was thought to be of central importance after the first reports of spontaneous inflammatory bowel disease in mice with targeted deletion of either the Th2 cytokine IL-10 [31] or the Th1 cytokine IL-2 [32]. The disease occurred only after intestinal colonization, showing that the continuous proinflammatory drive of the luminal flora requires a balanced immune response.

This view of simple cross-inhibition between Th1 and Th2 T-cell effector responses (TE) responses has been supplanted by a growing body of evidence that regulatory T cell (TR) populations determine whether or not T cells activate in response to antigen [18, 33]. There is still some confusion in nomenclature, and substantially more murine than human evidence. The cytokines TGF-β and IL-10 are clearly important in these regulatory reactions, and act to suppress activation of surrounding cells by a process of 'bystander tolerance' [18, 26, 27]. Reported TR T-cell populations include Th3 cells, which produce TGF-β, and TR1 cells, which produce IL-10 [14, 18], although either or both may be overlap populations with the important regulatory population of CD4+CD25+ cells, initially recognized by their low surface expression of CD45RB in murine adoptive transfer studies [18, 33]. Cell surface contact has also been shown to be important in inducing systemic immune tolerance, and the CD4+CD25+ TR-cell population clearly has an important regulatory role [33]. The transcription factor *Foxp3* is a master regulator of regulatory lymphocyte production [34], and mutation of *Foxp3* induces a severe multifocal inflammatory phenotype including an autoimmune enterocolitis, in both mice and humans, by preventing the development of regulatory lymphocytes [35]. There is also evidence that CD8 as well as CD4 cells may mediate systemic tolerance [36], and a regulatory CD8+CD28– population has been generated by cell–cell contact with enterocytes [37]. The clinical significance of these populations remains to be determined.

It is notable that the CD4+CD25+ TR population is dominated in adults by old cells which have undergone repeated antigen-specific division, as evidenced by their short telomere length [38]. While these cells suppress responses to dietary antigen, it may be difficult to invoke such multiply exposed cells as major mediators of mucosal T-cell suppression in early life, as the great majority of T cells in early infancy are of naïve phenotype. It is possible that these cells represent a distinct long-lived lineage. However recent murine evidence suggests that CD8 cells may play a central role in the induction of immune tolerance in neonates [39], which appears distinct from the situation in older animals, where CD4 cells make up the dominant suppressor populations. Further studies of putative suppressor cell populations in childhood will be necessary to clarify the role of candidate suppressor lineages in neonatal oral tolerance. Certainly there is evidence of an abnormally low percentage of TGF-β producing mucosal lymphocytes in children who are sensitized to dietary antigen [40–42].

It is evident that such a tolerogenic response within the intestine would be inappropriate when confronted by pathogens. Recent data show that the suppressive effect of the murine CD4+CD25+ cell population can be abrogated by a Toll pathway-dependent response amongst DCs, which is partly based on IL-6 production [33]. While allowing an effective T-cell response to pathogens, as evidenced by the Th1 skewing of astrovirus-reactive HLA-DR-restricted mucosal T cells in adult small intestine [43], this may also explain why tolerance to dietary antigen may be broken in infants by enteropathogens.

Antigen Entry

The maintenance of tolerance is critically dependent on epithelial integrity. Induced leakiness of crypt epithelium in transgenic mice with a dominant negative n-cadherin [44] led to severe transmural inflammation. Paracellular permeability is particularly high during acute gastroenteritis in children [45], emphasizing that this may be a time when enteric inflammation is initiated. As peptides of only up to 11 amino acids can cross the epithelial barrier by the paracellular pathway, even during glucose absorption [46], antigen exclusion is probably important in preventing sensitization. The bulk of the antigen is taken up directly by the enterocytes, processed within endosomal compartments and presented to the immune system in an inherently non-sensitizing manner [47]. Increased permeability bypasses these mechanisms and favors immunological response [48]. Maturation of the intestinal epithelium is modulated by many factors, including breast milk components [49], which may act directly or through induced changes in the flora [50].

Unlike other species, there is no evidence in human infants of excessive gut hyperpermeability at birth followed by 'gut closure' [51], and thus initial immune responses are unlikely to be mediated by bypassing of the epithelial barrier. However, repeated pathogen challenge may undermine the integrity of the epithelial barrier, as induced IFN-γ production increases epithelial leakiness [52], although the regulatory cytokines TGF-β and IL-10 limit this change [53, 54]. It is thus notable that the growth of developing world infants mirrors that of those in privileged countries while exclusively breast-feeding, before falling away sharply at weaning, with mean weight of Gambian infants at 1 year equivalent to the 2nd percentile by UK standards. It is striking that progression to malnutrition in Gambian infants is highly associated with increased paracellular permeability [55]. There is evidence of a sharp decline in TGF-β+ mucosal lymphocyte density during progression to marasmus in this population [56]. Disruption of oral tolerance mechanisms may thus have a more widespread implication than allergic sensitization alone. Randomization of marasmic Zambian infants to an elemental formula, compared to isocaloric quantities of fermented cow's milk, was associated with significant additional improvements in weight gain [57].

The Gut Flora and Allergic Sensitization

Socioeconomic conditions are important in childhood allergies, and rapid progression to a Western world economic status is followed by a rise in allergic sensitization [58, 59]. Exposure to gastroenterological pathogens reduced the risk of allergic sensitization amongst young European adults [60]. Rural upbringing and exposure to bacterial endotoxin offers protection against later allergy [61, 62]. There may thus be an important role for early environmental exposures, particularly via the gastrointestinal tract, in the determination of immune tolerance, modulating the effects of genetic predisposition. There is increasing evidence of an obligatory role for the normal gut flora, and possibly an additional effect of pathogens in the establishment of immune tolerance [1, 63, 64]. One distinct component of the 'clean child' hypothesis [63] may thus be intestinal infectious exposures, and in particular the effects of these exposures on the generation of regulatory lymphocytes [65]. Exposure to mycobacterial components, usually acquired by ingestion from soil, induced generation of regulatory lymphocytes which attenuated pulmonary eosinophilia in a murine model of asthma [66].

The final pathway in the generation of regulatory lymphocytes appears to be shared with Th1 reactions, with NFκB responses by innate immune cells potentially important to both pathways [1, 7, 67]. For both dietary antigen and the intestinal flora, prevention of a normal initial response to the commensal flora impairs the establishment and maintenance of immune tolerance. In transgenic mice with a single T-cell population specific for hen egg lysozyme, and thus able to respond to the gut flora only through innate immune cells, tolerance to dietary hen egg lysozyme was maintained under normal conditions [67]. However, when production of prostaglandin E2 (PgE2) was prevented by cyclooxygenase-2 antagonists, tolerance was abrogated and enteropathy developed [67]. One explanation for this result is that DCs produce high levels of IL-10 on exposure to LPS, and that this is prevented by blockade of PgE2 production [68]. In LPS-resistant mice, who are genetically deficient in TLR-4, spontaneous colitis develops [69]. Mutation of several other components of the NFκB pathway, in both mice and humans, also induces a paradoxically inflammatory phenotype, although the relative roles of immune regulation, immunodeficiency and control of apoptosis remain to be elucidated [70]. However, the concept that an inadequate NFκB response to bacterial products may lead to sensitization is demonstrated by the genetic association of Crohn's disease with a loss-of-function mutation in Nod2, an intracellular pathogen-associated molecular pattern sensor which induces an NFκB response to bacterial muramyl dipeptide [71, 72]. Thus the consensus finding is that a suboptimal initial NFκB response to normal gut bacterial challenges is a sensitizing event, leading to a potential for later loss of immune tolerance. Genetic adaptation to a heavy enteric pathogen exposure in infancy, the lot of all mankind until the last century, may have contributed to the limitation of pro-inflammatory responses by the immune system of young children, and current reduced early life exposures in the Western world may be inadequate to trigger the development of regulatory lymphocyte populations in those who have the lowest responses [64, 65].

Initial Colonization May Determine Later Immunological Responses

Initial colonization of the intestine is one of the major immunological challenges faced during the lifetime of the organism. While animals maintained strictly germ-free may not show overt abnormality, they require approximately 30% more calories than colonized animals, and show clear abnormalities of crypt architecture, epithelial turnover and IEL numbers [73]. In addition, induction of oral tolerance does not occur normally without gut bacteria, in xenobiotic mice [74].

When commensal bacteria are introduced, they induce clear immunological responses, including expansion of IEL populations with increased crypt cell proliferation [63]. However, quite fundamental additional responses occur [75], with induction of multiple genes within enterocytes and even stimulation of angiogenesis within the villi [76]. It is notable that different bacteria stimulate expression of different genes. One important change is the induction of fucosyl transferases, leading to alterations in glycosylation of the glycocalyx [77]. While the microheterogeneity of these changes in the glycocalyx remains understudied, it is likely that this provides selective advantage for the initial colonizing bacteria. It is notable that probiotic administration to young infants leads to stable and permanent colonization whereas administration after 1 year gives only transient expression [78]. Changes in initial colonization patterns may thus have long-term consequences.

It is important to recognize that the changes in initial gut colonization during the last century have been quite dramatic in evolutionary terms. This has clear potential to affect the induction of mucosal tolerance [79, 80]. There is now reduced early colonization by previously dominant species such as bifidobacteria, together with frequent discordance between the flora of the mother and her child [81–83]. Improvement of neonatal practices is often overlooked as a target for effective immunotherapy. As cesarean-born infants show permanent alterations in the gut flora and a higher incidence of allergies [84], the high rate of operative delivery in some centers appears very short-sighted. Breast-feeding provides important advantages for the infant, including important input to the immune system and the gastrointestinal flora [85]. Inappropriate use of broad-spectrum antibiotics in the neonatal period is now unfortunately commonplace [86], and almost nothing is known about the long-term immunological consequences of this.

These changes in colonization patterns have not been seen in developing world populations to anything like the same extent, and it is likely that this contributes to the low incidence of allergic disease in underprivileged countries [82]. It is notable that colostral and breast milk lymphocytes are dominated by gut-derived populations, such as $\gamma\delta$ and $\beta 7+$ T cells [87] and that these lymphocytes transfer immunological input to the infant's immune system [88]. It remains to be seen whether mismatching of maternal immune input from breast milk lymphocytes specific for her own flora, with that from a non-maternal colonizing flora based on hospital-derived strains has any immunological consequence for the nascent mucosal immune system. Study of initial infant handling in the 1970 UK national birth cohort showed significant excess of later atopic disease in infants nursed away from their mothers on the first night of life [89]. Further support that early-life colonization is a determinant of later sensitization has been provided by studies of gut flora in Estonian and Swedish children, and allergic children from either country showed reduced lactobacilli and anaerobes but higher numbers of coliforms and *Staphylococcus aureus* [90, 91]. These changes are detectable very early in life, before the development of clinical allergies.

Evidence that early colonization may affect the development of mucosal tolerance was demonstrated by the perinatal administration of probiotics to infants at risk of later allergies, which induced a remarkable reduction in later eczema [92]. However it was notable that systemic IgE responses were unaffected in the treated infants, arguing for compartmentalization of mucosal and cutaneous responses [79]. It looks increasingly likely that previous focus on IgE responses as the determinant of allergic sensitization may need to be replaced by primary consideration of tolerance induction at mucosal surfaces. Interaction between bacterial exposures in early infancy and genetically determined responses in innate immune cells may determine whether an adequate tolerogenic response occurs.

References

1 Fearon DT, Locksley RM: The instructive role of innate immunity in the acquired immune response. Science 1996;272:50–54.
2 Medzhitov R, Janeway CA Jr: Innate immunity: Impact on the adaptive immune response. Curr Opin Immunol 1997;9:4–9.

3 Selby WS, Poulter LW, Hobbs S, et al: Heterogeneity of HLA-DR-positive histiocytes in human intestinal lamina propria: A combined histochemical and immunohistological analysis. J Clin Pathol 1983;36:379–384.
4 Liu YJ, Kadowaki N, Rissoan MC, Soumelis V: T cell activation and polarization by DC1 and DC2. Curr Top Microbiol Immunol 2000;251:149–59.
5 de Jong EC, Vieira PL, Kalinski P, et al: Microbial compounds selectively induce Th1 cell-promoting or Th2 cell-promoting dendritic cells in vitro with diverse Th cell-polarizing signals. J Immunol 2002;168:1704–1709.
6 Kadowaki N, Liu YJ: Natural type I interferon-producing cells as a link between innate and adaptive immunity. Hum Immunol 2002;63:1126–1132.
7 Barton GM, Medzhitov R: Toll-like receptors and their ligands. Curr Top Microbiol Immunol 2002;270:81–92.
8 Kadowaki N, Ho S, Antonenko S, et al: Subsets of human dendritic cell precursors express different toll-like receptors and respond to different microbial antigens. J Exp Med 2001; 194:863–869.
9 Manickasingham SP, Edwards AD, Schulz O, Sousa CR: The ability of murine dendritic cell subsets to direct T helper cell differentiation is dependent on microbial signals. Eur J Immunol 2003;33:101–107.
10 Upham JW, Lee PT, Holt BJ, et al: Development of interleukin-12-producing capacity throughout childhood. Infect Immun 2002;70:6583–6588.
11 Karlsson H, Hessle C, Rudin A: Innate immune responses of human neonatal cells to bacteria from the normal gastrointestinal flora. Infect Immun 2002;70:6688–6696.
12 Suzuki K, Oida T, Hamada H, et al: Gut cryptopatches: Direct evidence of extrathymic anatomical sites for intestinal T lymphopoiesis. Immunity 2000;13:691–702.
13 Moghaddami M, Cummins A, Mayrhofer G: Lymphocyte-filled villi: Comparison with other lymphoid aggregations in the mucosa of the human small intestine. Gastroenterology 1998; 115:1414–1425.
14 Walker-Smith JA, Murch SH: The immune system of the small intestine; in Walker-Smith JA (ed): Diseases of the Small Intestine in Childhood, ed 4. Oxford, Isis Medical Media, 1999, pp 45–61.
15 Benlagha K, Bendelac A: CD1d-restricted mouse Vα14 and human Vα24 T cells: Lymphocytes of innate immunity. Semin Immunol 2000;12:537–542.
16 Spencer J, MacDonald TT, Finn T, Isaacson PG: The development of gut associated lymphoid tissue in the terminal ileum of fetal human intestine. Clin Exp Immunol 1986;64:536–543.
17 Kokkonen J, Karttunen TJ: Lymphonodular hyperplasia on the mucosa of the lower gastrointestinal tract in children: An indication of enhanced immune response? J Pediatr Gastroenterol Nutr 2002;34:42–46.
18 Groux H, Powrie F: Regulatory T cells and inflammatory bowel disease. Immunol Today 1999; 20:442–446.
19 Oida T, Zhang X, Goto M, et al: CD4(+)CD25(–) T cells that express latency-associated peptide on the surface suppress CD4(+)CD45RB(high)-induced colitis by a TGF-β-dependent mechanism. J Immunol 2003;170:2516–2522.
20 Spencer J, Dillon SB, Isaacson PG, MacDonald TT: T cell subclasses in fetal human ileum. Clin Exp Immunol 1986;65:553–558.
21 Hamada H, Hiroi T, Nishiyama Y, et al: Identification of multiple isolated lymphoid follicles on the antimesenteric wall of the mouse small intestine. J Immunol 2002;168:57–64.
22 Thomas R, Schurmann G, Lionetti P, et al: T cell receptor Vβ expression in human intestine: Regional variation in postnatal intestine and biased usage in fetal gut. Gut 1996;38:190–195.
23 Mizoguchi A, Mizoguchi E, Chiba C, Bhan AK: Role of appendix in the development of inflammatory bowel disease in TCR-α mutant mice. J Exp Med 1996;184:707–715.
24 Öhman L, Franzén L, Rudolph U, et al: Regression of Peyer's patches in Gαi2 deficient mice prior to colitis is associated with reduced expression of Bcl-2 and increased apoptosis. Gut 2002;51:392–397.
25 Holt PG, Macaubas C, Stumbles PA, Sly PD: The role of allergy in the development of asthma. Nature 1999;402(suppl):B12–B17.
26 Strobel S, Mowat AM: Immune responses to dietary antigens: Oral tolerance. Immunol Today 1998;19:173–181.
27 Weiner HL: Oral tolerance: Immune mechanisms and treatment of autoimmune diseases. Immunol Today 1997;18:335–343.

28 Friedman A, Weiner HL: Induction of anergy or active suppression following oral tolerance is determined by antigen dosage. Proc Natl Acad Sci USA 1994;91:6688–6692.
29 Chen Y, Inobe J, Marks R, et al: Peripheral deletion of antigen-reactive T cells in oral tolerance. Nature 1995;376:177–180.
30 Miller A, Lider O, Abramsky O, Weiner HL: Orally administered myelin basic protein in neonates primes for immune responses and enhances experimental autoimmune encephalomyelitis in adult animals. Eur J Immunol 1994;24:1026–1032.
31 Kühn R, Löhler J, Rennick D, et al: Interleukin-10 deficient mice develop chronic enterocolitis. Cell 1993;75:263–274.
32 Sadlack B, Merz H, Schorle H, et al: Ulcerative colitis in mice with a disrupted interleukin-2 gene. Cell 1993;75:253–261.
33 Pasare C, Medzhitov R: Toll pathway-dependent blockade of CD+CD25+ T cell-mediated suppression by dendritic cells. Science 2003;299:1033–1036.
34 Hori S, Nomura T, Sakaguchi S: Control of regulatory T cell development by the transcription factor Foxp3. Science 2003;299:1057–1061.
35 Wildin RS, Smyk-Pearson S, Filipovich AH: Clinical and molecular features of the immunodysregulation, polyendocrinopathy, enteropathy, X linked (IPEX) syndrome. J Med Genet 2002;39:537–545.
36 Filaci G, Bacilieri S, Fravega M, et al: Impairment of CD8+ T suppressor cell function in patients with active systemic lupus erythematosus. J Immunol 2001;166:6452–6457.
37 Allez M, Brimnes J, Dotan I, Mayer L: Expansion of CD8+ T cells with regulatory function after interaction with intestinal epithelial cells. Gastroenterology 2002;123:1516–1526.
38 Taams LS, Vukmanovic-Stejic M, Smith J, et al: Antigen-specific T cell suppression by human CD4+CD25+ regulatory T cells. Eur J Immunol 2002;32:1621–1630.
39 Field AC, Caccavelli L, Bloch MF, Bellon B: Regulatory CD8(+) T cells control neonatal tolerance to a Th2-mediated autoimmunity. J Immunol 2003;170:2508–2815.
40 Chung HL, Hwang JB, Park JJ, Kim SG: Expression of transforming growth factor β1, transforming growth factor type I and II receptors, and TNF-α in the mucosa of the small intestine in infants with food-protein induced enterocolitis syndrome. J Allergy Clin Immunol 2002;109: 150–154.
41 Beyer K, Castro R, Birnbaum A, et al: Human milk-specific mucosal lymphocytes of the gastrointestinal tract display a TH2 cytokine profile. J Allergy Clin Immunol 2002;109: 707–713.
42 Pérez-Machado M, Ashwood P, Sim R, et al: Evidence at protein and mRNA level of reduced TH3 lymphocytes in multiple food allergy. J Pediatr Gastroenterol Nutr 2000;31:S127–S128.
43 Molberg Ø, Nilsen EM, Sollid LM, et al: CD4+ T cells with specific reactivity against astrovirus isolated from normal human small intestine. Gastroenterology 1998;114:115–122.
44 Hermiston ML, Gordon JI: Inflammatory bowel disease and adenomas in mice expressing a dominant negative N-cadherin. Science 1995;270:1203–1207.
45 Ford RPK, Menzies IS, Phillips AD, et al: Intestinal sugar permeability: Relationship to diarrhoeal disease and small bowel morphology. J Pediatr Gastroenterol Nutr 1985;4:568–574.
46 Atisook K, Madara JL: An oligopeptide permeates intestinal tight junctions at glucose-elicited dilatations. Implications for oligopeptide absorption. Gastroenterology 1991;100:719–724.
47 Mayer L: Mucosal immunity and gastrointestinal antigen processing. J Pediatr Gastroenterol Nutr 2000;30:S4–S12.
48 Sanderson IR, Walker WA: Uptake and transport of macromolecules by the intestine: Possible role in clinical disorders (an update). Gastroenterology 1993;104:622–639.
49 Cummins AG, Thompson FM: Effect of breast milk and weaning on epithelial growth of the small intestine in humans. Gut 2002;51:748–754.
50 Sanderson IR: Nutritional factors and immune functions of gut epithelium. Proc Nutr Soc 2001;60:443–447.
51 Keller KM, Knobel R, Ewe K: Fecal α1-antitrypsin in newborn infants. J Pediatr Gastroenterol Nutr 1997;24:271–275.
52 Adams RB, Planchon SM, Roche JK: IFN-γ modulation of epithelial barrier function. Time course, reversibility, and site of cytokine binding. J Immunol 1993;150:2356–2363.
53 Planchon SM, Martins CA, Guerrant RL, Roche JK: Regulation of intestinal epithelial barrier function by TGF-β1. Evidence for its role in abrogating the effect of a T cell cytokine. J Immunol 1994;153:5370–5379.

54 Madsen KL, Lewis SA, Tavernini MM, et al: Interleukin 10 prevents cytokine-induced disruption of T84 monolayer barrier integrity and limits chloride secretion. Gastroenterology 1997; 113:151–159.
55 Lunn PG, Northrop-Clewes CA, Downes RM: Intestinal permeability, mucosal injury, and growth faltering in Gambian infants. Lancet 1991 338:907–910.
56 Campbell DI, Murch SH, Sullivan PB, et al: Chronic T cell-mediated enteropathy in rural West African children: Relationship with nutritional status and small bowel function. Pediatr Res 2003;54:306–311.
57 Amadi B: Role of food antigen elimination in treating children with persistent diarrhea and malnutrition in Zambia. J Pediatr Gastroenterol Nutr 2002;34(suppl 1):S54–S56.
58 von Mutius E, Weiland SK, Fritzsch C, et al: Increasing prevalence of hay fever and atopy among children in Leipzig, East Germany. Lancet 1998;351:862–866.
59 Goh DY, Chew FT, Quek SC, Lee BW: Prevalence and severity of asthma, rhinitis, and eczema in Singapore schoolchildren. Arch Dis Child 1996;74:131–135.
60 Matricardi PM, Rosmini F, Riondino S, et al: Exposure to foodborne and orofecal microbes versus airborne viruses in relation to atopy and allergic asthma. BMJ 2000;320:412–417.
61 Braun-Fahrländer C, Riedler J, Herz U, et al: Environmental exposure to endotoxin and its relation to asthma in school-age children. N Engl J Med 2002;347:869–877.
62 Lewis SA: Animals and allergy. Clin Exp Allergy 2000;30:153–157.
63 Sebra JJ: Influences of microbiota on intestinal immune system development. Am J Clin Nutr 1999;69(suppl):1046S–1051S.
64 Rook GAW, Stanford JL: Give us this day our daily germs. Immunol Today 1998;19:113–116.
65 Yazdanbakhsh M, Kremsner PG, van Ree R: Allergy, parasites, and the hygiene hypothesis. Science 2002;296:490–494.
66 Zuany-Amorim C, Sawicka E, Manlius C, et al: Suppression of airway eosinophilia by killed *Mycobacterium vaccae*-induced allergen-specific regulatory T-cells. Nat Med 2002;8:625–629.
67 Newberry RD, Stenson WF, Lorenz RG: Cycloxygenase-2-dependent arachidonic acid metabolites are essential modulators of the immune response to dietary antigen. Nat Med 1999;5: 900–906.
68 Harizi H, Juzan M, Pitard V, et al: Cyclooxygenase-2-issued prostaglandin E2 enhances the production of endogenous IL-10, which down-regulates dendritic cell functions. J Immunol 2002;168:2255–2263.
69 Poltorak A, He X, Smirnova I, et al: Defective LPS signalling in C3H/HeJ and C57BL/10ScCr mice: Mutations in Tlr4 gene. Science 1998;282:2085–2088.
70 Smahi A, Courtois G, Rabia SH, et al: The NF-κB signalling pathway in human diseases: From incontinentia pigmenti to ectodermal dysplasias and immune-deficiency syndromes. Hum Mol Genet 2002;11:2371–2375.
71 Ogura Y, Bonen DK, Inohara N, et al: A frameshift mutation in Nod2 associated with susceptibility to Crohn's disease. Nature 2001;411:603–606.
72 Girardin SE, Boneca IG, Viala J, et al: Nod2 is a general sensor of peptidoglycan through muramyl dipeptide (MDP) detection. J Biol Chem 2003;278:8869–8872.
73 Hooper LV, Gordon JI: Commensal host-bacterial relationships in the gut. Science 2001;292: 1115–1118.
74 Sudo N, Sawamura S, Tanaka K, et al: The requirement of intestinal bacterial flora for the development of an IgE production system susceptible to oral tolerance induction. J Immunol 1997;159:1739–1745.
75 Hooper LV, Wong MH, Thelin A, et al: Molecular analysis of commensal host-microbial relationships in the intestine. Science 2001;291:881–884.
76 Stappenbeck TS, Hooper LV, Gordon JI: Developmental regulation of intestinal angiogenesis by indigenous microbes via Paneth cells. Proc Natl Acad Sci USA 2002;99:15451–15455.
77 Lu L, Walker WA: Pathologic and physiologic interactions of bacteria with the gastrointestinal epithelium. Am J Clin Nutr 2001;73(suppl):1124S–1130S.
78 Heilig HG, Zoetendal EG, Vaughan EE, et al: Molecular diversity of *Lactobacillus* spp. and other lactic acid bacteria in the human intestine as determined by specific amplification of 16S ribosomal DNA. Appl Environ Microbiol 2002;68:114–123.
79 Murch SH: Toll of allergy reduced by probiotics. Lancet 2001;357:1057–1059.
80 Murch SH: The immunologic basis for intestinal food allergy. Curr Opin Gastroenterol 2000;16:552–557.

81 Grutte FK, Muller-Beuthow W: Wandlung der normalen Darmflora des menschlichen Säuglings innerhalb der letzen 20 Jahre. Nahrung 1979;23:455–465.
82 Simhon A, Douglas JR, Drasar BS, Soothill JF: Effect of feeding on infants' faecal flora. Arch Dis Child 1982;57:54–58.
83 Bettelheim KA, Breadon A, Faiers MC, et al: The origin of O serotypes of Escherischia coli in babies after normal delivery. J Hyg (Camb) 1974;72:67–70.
84 Gronlund MM, Lehtonen OP, Eerola E, Kero P: Fecal microflora in healthy infants born by different methods of delivery: Permanent changes in intestinal flora after cesarean section. J Pediatr Gastroenterol Nutr 1999;28:19–25.
85 Hanson LA, Korotkova M, Haversen L, et al: Breast-feeding, a complex support system for the offspring. Pediatr Int 2002;44:347–352.
86 Tan S, Holliman R, Bedford Russell AR: Hazards of widespread use of erythromycin for preterm prelabour rupture of membranes. Lancet 2003;361:437.
87 Gibson CE, Eglington BA, Penttila IA, Cummins AG: Phenotype and activation of milk-derived and peripheral blood lymphocytes from normal and coeliac subjects. Immunol Cell Biol 1991; 69:387–393.
88 Hanson LA: The mother-offspring dyad and the immune system. Acta Paediatr 2000;89: 252–258.
89 Montgomery SM, Wakefield AJ, Morris DL, et al: The initial care of newborn infants and subsequent hayfever. Allergy 2000;55:916–922.
90 Björksten B, Naaber P, Sepp E, Mikelsaar M: The intestinal microflora in allergic Estonian and Swedish 2-year old children. Clin Exp Allergy 1999;29:342–346.
91 Björksten B, Sepp E, Julge K, et al: Allergy development and the intestinal microflora during the first year of life. J Allergy Clin Immunol 2001;108:516–520.
92 Kalliomaki M, Salminen S, Arvillomi H, et al: Probiotics in primary prevention of atopic disease: A randomised placebo-controlled trial. Lancet 2001;357:1076–1079.

Discussion

Dr. Walker: In the studies in the Gambia on malnutrition, it could be that you are dealing with micronutrient deficiency and that could be an important factor in the lack of immune responsiveness.

Dr. Murch: A point completely well taken. Clearly we know that vitamin A, for example, is critically important. In many of our children who become micronutrient deficient with total parenteral nutrition, we see that it does dreadful things to their immune response. I completely agree with that.

Dr. Walker: Can I make one additional comment? This is for the clinicians in the audience. A lot can be learned about clinical medicine from some of the observations we made, and here are two examples. There is an article that Walker-Smith [1] published in *Archives of Disease in Childhood* many years ago suggesting that after a viral gastroenteritis, when you continue to feed milk you are very likely going to produce an allergic reaction. At that time we all thought this is because of the increased intestinal permeability of antigens. However, what happens is that there is a balance which is disrupted by an infection which then triggers a change from a tolerogenic response to an immunogenic, inflammatory response [2]. This may be an explanation for why that happens. Patients with inflammatory bowel disease (IBD) are different in response. When we saw these children, invariably or many times they would present what appeared to be a bacterial or viral enteritis, and when it persisted we realized that they have the chronic disease IBD. Again we are dealing with a genetic defect that is superposed upon an excessive inflammatory stimulation which then triggers the disease. We can learn a lot from this basic observation.

Dr. Murch: Again I completely agree with both these points. The one study that has been done on viral reactive T cells in adult life was from Molberg et al. [3] who extracted T cells from adult patients, which they pulsed with astrovirus and then pulled out the reactive T cells, all of which were Th1-skewed. So at the time of childhood astrovirus infections there was a clear Th1-dominated response. In terms of the IBD, the other point that I think is relevant is that in some models the progression down that path is initiated in the very first days of life. I think Bhan et al. [4] showed that taking out mucosal lymphoid tissue at birth, neonatal appendectomy, prevented the development of IBD later on in animals that otherwise normally always got this. The point about that model is that there was a silent period where clearly the cells had initially been sensitized and were polarized or maintained silent. Here the question is whether the role of intercurrent infections does actually provide the response allowing this very small and silent clone of flora-reactive Th1 cells to then expand and cause disease [5]. Very frequently the first episode of IBD occurs around the time of gastroenteritis. It has also been shown that relapse of IBD is associated with a whole variety of intercurrent viral infections. I think virus has remained rather understudied in most of the mouse models.

Dr. Schiffrin: I think you are proposing that dendritic cells are polarized very early in life and they remain so for most of the life time. This is kind of a pessimistic view because do we have some room for intervention once this has happened or is there a turnover of dendritic cells, of immature dendritic cells, that we can still direct to a better response?

Dr. Murch: You may have cells which are just inevitably committed, but they are part of an overresponding group and there is some evidence that you can then get a selective expansion of cells that go the other way. Just because one dendritic cell in its lineage is polarized does not mean that the overall effect to response is there and the animal is Th1-polarized. I don't think we have human data and I have mixed murine and human data in this talk. I know that they may not be exactly analogous, but I think the conceptual background is to interpret the fragments of human data that we do have. In man we don't know if dendritic cell A is going to remain that way for ever, we don't know what causes dendritic cells to survive or not, and whether there is a replenishment from the marrow. So it is not a pessimistic scenario, but I would suggest that there is very good evidence that you can have a silent immune deviation that requires a second hit later in life to unmask. This is really a plea just to consider the very early changes and the use of antibiotics at birth or, as we said yesterday, the obstetrician who does a cesarean section may have a long-term impact on the immune development of a person, and we need to do more of these basic human studies.

Dr. Sorensen: I would like to ask you if there could be other alternatives to the results of the low expression of NF-κB, because recently there have been several descriptions of immune deficiencies due to Nemo mutations, the essential modulator of NF-κB. Actually I got into that because we recently had a patient ourselves. This mutation leads to a combined immune deficiency and one of the very striking observations is that they develop very high IgA concentrations. They start with no immunoglobulins and then the IgA goes into the hundreds and thousands. So having a problem in that pathway sometimes predisposes or leads to an overproduction of IgA. I don't know if the IgA is functional but they do not produce IgE but huge amounts of IgA. I wonder if you can try to help me understand what is going on there?

Dr. Murch: I think the Nemo is a very difficult model to interpret. It does have an effect on systemic tolerance. In general the patients get anhidrotic ectodermal dysplasia, plus or minus immunodeficiency depending on the size of the mutation. It is very high in the NF-κB induction pathway. The Nemo pathway is quite near the tumor necrosis factor receptor and the induction of the apoptosis pathway, so you could quite easily argue that Nemo is a mutation that simply prevents normal apoptosis and you therefore get autoimmunity because of that. The IgA response in Nemo is interesting. Walker-Smith [1] again reported that many children with intractable ulcerating enterocolitis in infancy with time have gone on to develop lymphomas. We looked after some – all of them had sky-high IgA as well but we don't know the functionality of their IgA. There is certainly a group of children in whom IgA responses are maintained, and you might suggest IL-4 and transforming growth factor-β (TGF-β) may be preserved. It might also be that there is some other cell-to-cell contact that is affected because of Nemo mutation. I think that the whole question of the fine regulation of NF-κB simply remains to be determined. That is probably the single most important task in the field of allergy and immunology.

Dr. Neijens: I have more experience with immunology of the respiratory system and it is an interesting comparison. You made observations and depicted NF-κB as the critical variable. That might be true at least for part of the microorganism, depending on what kind of receptors are activated. But the critical thing is what is the important cell. You touched on γδ cells or α cells. It might be very important to compare the respiratory and the gut systems because gastrointestinal tract immunology is much more keen to induce tolerance than the respiratory system. I think in the future respiratory allergy should be treated via the gut. Then we have to know how to become tolerant, what kind of cells are critical there? Do you have information to what extent γδ cells and α cells are critical or take the lead?

Dr. Murch: This is a very good and important point. Within the microenvironment the phenotype of macrophages is quite different and they coexpress molecules, RFD7 and RFD1, which would have a suppressive function. It is quite difficult to induce sensitization in the lung in comparison to the gut. I don't know anything about γδ populations within the lung and whether they are thought to be involved in tolerance, but I think that when you have quite clear differences in major mesodermal lineages such as macrophages then they are there for a reason and there may be quite different rules of engagement. In terms of the data that γδ cells are an important it has been shown that γδ knockout mice, although phenotypically quite normal, had an inhibited inflammatory response to infection of the gut with a pathogen so that there is going to be redundancy within different functions. You can knockout various components of the cellular immune response and still get a reasonable phenotype unless found by pathogens.

Coming back to the clinical situation, again I am struck by the fact that my food allergy clinic has an under-representation of children with asthma because we get the later responders. A lot of children with asthma have peanut allergy, and very clearly there are children with eczema who go on to hay fever without asthma, and others who make immediate responses go on to asthma without hay fever. For me the biggest challenge remains how do we extrapolate from these very fine murine details into the human system? I think what we must do is pay attention to what good clinicians are pointing out, you cannot ignore clinical practice. I know this is anecdotal and we haven't got a double-blind controlled trial, but give me an hour with somebody who really knows the phenotype of asthmatic children or food allergic children.

Dr. Zakiudin Munasir: Indirect helminth infection can protect against allergy through IL-10 that can block IgE-specific production. My question is, what role does IgE play in the elimination of the parasite in this case?

Dr. Murch: I think parasite elimination requires several things. In Canada it has been shown very clearly that T-cell responses change motility. So one of the most important things that happens with parasite infection is a change in the motility response so that the migrating motility becomes faster and more intense, there is stimulation of production of mucus. In the UK we haven't really got anything like the parasites that you have in Malaysia. But when our UK children get worm infestation in the rectum they also get mucus that is an important part of the response. I think that having an exaggerated IgE response is probably helpful, it is part of the coordinated worm expulsion response. My prejudice in the allergic child is not that it causes allergy but that it makes sensitization that has occurred go in a certain direction and in a clinically obvious direction.

Dr. Papageorgiou: Regarding the immunological abnormalities that you found in food-allergic children, do you think this is a maturation process or is it permanent? How old were the children you studied?

Dr. Murch: In the 1970s Soothill identified this as a maturational problem. At the population level in Iceland, an IgA level that was in the low quartile of the normal range was much more strongly predictive of allergy than was IgE. But what Soothill found was that by the age of 4 or 5 it returned to normal, and that is exactly what we are seeing with the IgG subclass deficiency responses. The big question is whether probiotics actually stimulate that response toward normal and these are studies that need to be done. Following these children up again, a lot of our children who predominantly have delayed responses only go on to get big adenoids, and have adenoidectomies. They then end up at the age of 5 or 6 with quite normal IgA and IgG subclasses. The question is then not whether this is a life-long immunodeficiency but whether that period of relative immunodeficiency was associated with abnormal sensitization. I am really worried about this population because of the high instance of autoimmunity in their mothers, 25% of the mothers have autoimmunity and only 10% of the grandparents. So I think we need to lift our eyes beyond getting this child through peanut allergy. If we follow these young people through adult life, we are looking at a cohort of children in whom immune regulation is not being instituted normally right in the start. This is the population to study, the children who are presenting with immune dysregulation.

Dr. Schiffrin: You have given a large role to TGF-β in the preservation of gut homeostasis, and you have shown that TGF-β can be produced in the epithelial layer and in the lamina propria lymphocytes. I wonder whether you have some ideas or speculations on what the main source for homeostasis preservation is, and also if you think that with a lack of TGF-β, exogenous administration of TGF-β could restore this homeostasis?

Dr. Murch: Flow cytometry source is not in the lymphocyte population. The one thing that we learned with cytology of mucosal lymphoid tissue is when we gate on IL-10 or TGF-β, the dominant population, are outside the lymphocyte gates, and we know so little about the importance of that, both IL-10 and TGF-β are in the epithelium and the inducted pathways of that remain uncertain. TGF-β may be important. In an excellent article, Sampson recently reported how they derived milk-reactive T-cell clones from allergic and nonallergic children, and found that the dominant feature was a failure of the milk-reactive allergic clones that produce TGF-β.

Dr. Nousia Arvanitaki: Do you think that children receiving antibiotics during the first 2–3 days of life or even children repeatedly receiving antibiotics later in life are more prone to allergic reactions?

Dr. Murch: This is a question that I think nobody has really looked at very systematically. There are lots of anecdotal links that children with allergies often have a history in the first year of life of needing antibiotics. You could view it the other way around: if the child who is becoming allergic has low natural killer cells and low CD8 cells and low immunoglobulins it makes him get more colds, and the baby is then taken to the general practitioner who gives him antibiotics. It is an area that we intend to study, the whole area of neonatal antibiotics. There was an article in the *Lancet* a couple of weeks ago about the wide-spread use of broad-spectrum antibiotics for various reasons in London-born infants, and that is another major question.

Dr. Walker: Let me try to respond to the question because I will be discussing this topic next. The use of broad-spectrum antibiotics disrupts the colonizing process in the gut, and a disruption of the colonizing process in the gut results in mucosal immunologic responses. Therefore I do think this is a factor.

Dr. Al-Malik: How would you explain an adult who has been eating fish for quite a long time and then develops multiple fish allergy, meaning that he had a mature gut, T cells are matured, both the Th1 and Th2?

Dr. Murch: It is hard to explain. The disposition towards allergic reactions is probably not just antibody mediated. I was referring today to patterns of sensitization in South-East Asia, major differences from country to country despite largely similar dietary intakes. In order to become sensitized to fish you may well have to have a specific major histocompatibility complex type in the first place. You have got to then have an unmasking event. I don't know why I developed hay fever for the first time when I was 30. It is quite a common pattern that an adult may manifest sensitization for the first time later on. We don't know why a person who was completely tolerant to fish before not only has reactions, but can have anaphylaxis and repeated anaphylaxis. Something clearly is occurring in the T-cell clones to prime them or something is occurring to engender very highly reactive antibody. It may be that in the past the immune system was quite balanced and then pathogens may change that in a global way. In quite a lot of our children with immunodeficiencies, we have seen that they are never the same again after getting Epstein-Barr Virus (EBV) the enveloped form of virus. So you may have a very complex scenario with a genetic predisposition.

Dr. Bindslev-Jensen: How sure are we that sensitization takes place in the intestine of adults? I mean could it be via the skin, it could be via the nose, via the eye, via the lungs? What do we basically know about that?

Dr. Murch: We don't. Lack et al. [6] wrote an article in the *New England Journal of Medicine* which is a brilliant example that sensitization can occur by the skin. There are different rules of engagement in regional lymph nodes that drain inflamed skin to those within the intestine. The generation of tolerogenic lymphocytes clearly takes place as a default within Peyer's patches, within the lymph node draining inflamed skin, then you get out of the Th2- or Th1-dominated pathway. I don't think there is any good evidence that you get tolerogenic exposures in that way. Another recent important article showed the role of *Staphylococcus aureus* in determining whether eczema persists. We have got defensin in expression at many mucosal surfaces and you are going to get different patterns of sensitization, that is absolutely clear. There are anecdotes on exposure and sensitization in all kinds of ways: you can sensitize rectally, you can tolerize rectally, and the same will occur within the lung. The gut is central, and I think the gut has come from being an organ that was considered completely irrelevant to one which plays an important role in someway in many cases. You might argue that skin sensitization occurs because of your gut flora.

Dr. Guesry: The title of your talk is 'Oral Tolerance and Gut Maturation' and I was expecting, hoping, to hear about what we were discussing a lot 20 years ago. There was the work of Ferguson and Strobel [7], putting a lot of emphasis on the timing of the first contact with the allergen. Also in clinics, in the first study we did with Dr. Vandenplas, we showed that 2 months of hypoallergenic infant formula was insufficient. There are a lot of papers, mostly from Scandinavia, showing that even breastfeeding for 2 months is not efficient again. So definitely it seems that the gut maturation part of your talk, which is really passing a threshold, passing a critical period, is important, but I did not see new indications of this important phenomenon in your talk.

Dr. Murch: I think it is because the studies have not been revisited. I think the interpretation of those former studies has to be reviewed in the light of the basic mechanisms involved in tolerance. Studies performed 20–30 years ago were using different feeds for example; maternal diet was very different 20 years ago. We have a radically different maternal diet. London used to be viewed as the desert of cooking, you could not get any kind of interesting tasting food whatsoever. I don't think you can extrapolate directly from the work that was done then. 25 years ago in the UK the standard infant formula, in the early 1970s, was much more sensitizing than the formula we have now. I think that these studies have simply not been repeated in a way that we can interpret, and I think they are difficult to interpret. I would have thought that timing clearly does matter. If you suggested 20 years ago that infants could become sensitized to multiple antigens eaten by their mothers then I think this would have been viewed as very unorthodox indeed. My background is in terms of mucosal responses and therefore there are people in the audience who would better than I be able to argue for the role of timing inclusion.

Dr. Manjra: You know that sublingual immunotherapy works for respiratory allergy. Do you know the reason why it doesn't work very well for food allergy?

Dr. Murch: Again we don't know if we have got the dosage right. I just think that the whole thing about desensitization is getting the dose and the timing right, and we may not have done that yet.

Dr. Lack: I just wanted to make a comment about sublingual immunotherapy related to food allergy. One of the reasons you can't do it with food allergens but you can do it with respiratory allergens is that it is too dangerous to do with food allergens. What characterizes a food allergen is stability to change in pH, temperature and resistance to enzymatic digestion. Respiratory allergens are modified almost immediately in the oral mucosa and retain very little allergenicity; so you can presumably take in the relevant peptides and tolerize to respiratory allergens, but you just could not take in enough of a food allergen because it would cause anaphylaxis. That is the problem, for example, with subcutaneous desensitization to peanut, which has been attempted, treatment is relatively unsuccessful and dangerous because of type-1 reactions.

References

1 Walker-Smith J: Rotavirus gastroenteritis. Arch Dis Child 1978;53:355–362.
2 Shah U, Walker WA: Pathophysiology of intestinal food allergy. Adv Pediatr 2002;49:299–316.
3 Molberg O, Nilsen EM, Sollid LM, et al: CD4+ T cells with specific reactivity against astrovirus isolated from normal human small intestine. Gastroenterology 1998;114:115–122.
4 Bhan AK, Miziguchi E, Smith RN, Mizoguchi A: Spontaneous chronic colitis in TCR alpha-mutant mice: An experimental model of human ulcerative colitis. Int Rev Immunol 2000;19:123–138.
5 Russel MG, Stockbrugger RW: Is appendectomy a causative factor in ulcerative colitis? Eur J Gastroenterol Hepatol 1998;10:455-457.
6 Lack G, Fox D Northstone K, Golding J: Factors associated with the development of peanut allergy in childhood. N Engl J Med 2003;348:977–985.
7 Strobel S, Ferguson A: Immune response to fed antigen in mice. Systemic tolerance of priming is related to age at which antigen is first encountered. Pediatr Res 1984;18:588–594.

Isolauri E, Walker WA (eds): Allergic Diseases and the Environment.
Nestlé Nutrition Workshop Series Pediatric Program, Vol. 53, pp. 153–177,
Nestec Ltd.; Vevey/S. Karger AG, Basel, © 2004.

The Role of Bacteria in the Development of Intestinal Protective Function

N. Nanda Nanthakumar and W. Allan Walker

Harvard Medical School and Developmental Gastroenterology Laboratory of the Combined Program in Pediatric Gastrointestinal and Nutrition, Massachusetts General Hospital, Charlestown, Mass., USA

Introduction

The primary function of the gastrointestinal tract is to complete the digestion and absorption of nutrients so as to provide a source of energy and substrate for growth and maintenance of the complete organism. Therefore, diseases that affect intestinal function have a major impact on body systems [1, 2]. This challenge is further compounded by the fact that the gut is directly in contact with a microbial and nutritional rich external environment. Under normal circumstances, a large number of bacterial species reside in the intestinal lumen in a symbiotic relationship with the host [3]. In addition, the gut is continuously exposed to foreign antigens, derived from luminal microbes, diet and ingested toxic substances [4]. In contrast to other organ systems, with the exception of skin, the gut is continually exposed to this external environment with an epithelial surface juxtaposed between the lumen and the interstitium and circulation. Unlike the skin, the intestinal epithelium is made up of a single polarized monolayer [2]. The apical surface of the epithelium is exposed to luminal contents including commensal flora [2, 3] but these substances are restricted from the basolateral surface by tight and adherent junction proteins [5]. These two junctional complexes are specialized structures unique to polarized cells and provide not a rigid structure, but an active flexible surface that allows migration of activated polymorphonuclear cells [6] during infection and access by dendritic cells to sample foreign antigen in the lumen [7].

Structure and Function of the Intestine

The intestinal epithelium which separates luminal contents from the underlying mucosa consists of absorptive enterocytes (93–95% of cells), mucus-secreting goblet cells (3–5% of cells) and gastrointestinal hormone-producing enteroendocrine cells (1–2% of cells) [2]. Unlike the colon, the surface area of the small intestine is increased by invagination into 'tongue-like' structures called villi. Mucus produced by the goblet cells is secreted as a layer of highly glycosylated proteins onto the intestinal surface and functions as a lubricant and protective layer on the epithelial surface. Undifferentiated proliferative cells including stem cells exit in a pit-like structure called the crypts of Lieberkühn both in the small intestine and colon [8, 9]. However, only in the small intestine unique cells called paneth cells are located at the bottom of each crypt [10]. Paneth cells produce a number of unique antibacterial proteins which act to protect nearby stem cells from microbial damage. The crypt epithelium is also polarized but only acquires microvilli, also known as the brush border, on its apical surface as cells migrate from the crypt to villus [2, 8, 9]. As these cells emerge from the crypts and undergo epithelial differentiation they begin to express specialized apical proteins such as digestive enzymes and transporters [1, 2]. These glycoproteins, anchored on the apical surface of the epithelium, are responsible for the digestive and absorptive functions of this tissue. These highly glycosylated proteins and glycolipids that enrich the apical surface of the epithelium can also function as receptors for commensal microflora that begin to colonize the gut lumen shortly after birth [11, 12].

In addition to the multi-lineage epithelial cells described, the epithelial monolayer infrequently displays a dome-like surface called the follicle-associated epithelium (FAE) [2, 13]. Unlike the villus epithelium, the epithelial surface of those domes display, with varying frequency, a unique type of epithelial cell called the microfold cell (M cell). In humans and rodents 10% of FAE are made up of M cells [2, 13]. These cells have no lysosomes and are capable of invaginating upon attachment of microorganisms and large proteins. The M cells are a specialized lineage of epithelium dedicated to antigen sampling [13]. Unlike the adjacent enterocytes, M cells have fewer and shorter microvilli on their apical surface and the basolateral surface display numerous invaginations in which mucosal lymphocytes reside [14]. M cells are never seen on differentiated villus epithelium. The FAE and M cells appear above aggregates of lymphocytes in Peyer's patches [14]. Since a single stem cell resides in each crypt, how these two lineages are derived during epithelial differentiation is not known, because the lack of a suitable in vitro model system has precluded the elucidation of the mechanism of this form of epithelial differentiation. However, recently exciting in vitro studies have shown that a differentiated enterocyte cell line can trans-differentiate into M cells under the influence of luminal pathogens and basolateral exposure of B cells suggesting that luminal microbial attachments and paracrine action by B cell may be responsible for M-cell differentiation [15].

Development of the Small Intestine

Morphological development, cytodifferentiation and enterocyte-specific differentiation are established by the end of the first trimester in humans [16] and at birth in rodents (rats and mice) [2, 8]. Gestation is 21 days in rodents, whereas it is 40 weeks in humans. The functional maturation of the gut is divided into 2 periods. Details of the development of the gastrointestinal tract is beyond the scope of this review and provided in several recent reviews [1, 2, 9, 16].

By the end of the first trimester the epithelium begins to form a monolayer and a crypt–villus architecture appears. The epithelium starts to differentiate and tissue-specific markers appear [2]. Proliferating epithelium is confined to the crypts where multiple stem cells reside [9, 16]. This phase of development occurs during the second and third trimester in humans and during the first 2 weeks of postnatal development in rodents [2, 9]. The early phase of functional maturation of the small intestine can be defined using differentiation-specific enterocyte markers [1, 2]. For example, disaccharidases are first detected with initial cytodifferentiation of the enterocytes, but the levels of disaccharidases vary depending on species. In humans, lactase remains low in utero but sucrase is high during this period, e.g. equivalent to levels found in infants [16]. In contrast, in rodents sucrase is undetectable with high-lactase activity until weaning [2].

The second and final phase of development begins at birth for humans and at the time of weaning (3rd postnatal week) in rodents [2]. During this period, lactase activity rapidly declines to the levels seen in adult rodents but in humans this enzyme increases and reaches a maximal level in the newborn [16]. In rodents the expression of sucrase increases to adult levels by the end of weaning [2]. At the same time, most of the enzymes and transporters responsible for digesting solid food are rapidly established at mature levels. Terminal maturation of the small intestine temporally coincides with weaning in rats and mice. These changes, coinciding with 'hard-wired' development of enzymatic expression, reflect the adaptive process necessary for survival on solid food [1, 2].

Regulation of Intestinal Development

The functional development of the gut is regulated by a number of factors. To unravel the complex mechanism(s) of development, extensive studies have been done in the rodent model [1, 2, 16]. However, little objective data are available for human gut development because of the inaccessibility of human tissues and inadequate intestinal models. The regulators of intestinal development can be either extrinsic (luminal) factors such amniotic fluid, colostrum/milk and microbial flora or intrinsic factors such as circulating growth factors, e.g. glucocorticoids, intrinsic timing mechanisms (a biological clock), and/or epithelial–mesenchyme interactions. The role of these divergent regulators are briefly discussed below.

Colostrum and Mature Milk

Colostrum and mother's milk are complex biological fluids that contain many substances which provide nutrition but also protect and stimulate cell turnover including proteins such as casein, micelles, membranes, membrane-bound globules, and viable cells [4]. A complete description of the macro- and micronutrients in milk has been published recently [17]. However, in this review we will focus only on trophic factors present in colostrum/breast milk that play a critical role in intestinal development. These factors are present in physiologic quantities and their role(s) in intestinal development is not fully understood, again in part because of lack of availability of a model that recapitulates the newborn human gut.

Commensal Flora

At birth, commensal bacteria begins to colonize the gastrointestinal tract [18]. The composition of the flora changes at the time of weaning [19]. This is in part due to the changing luminal environment contributed to by diet and the epithelium itself. However, a symbiotic relationship likely exists between microbes and the developing gut and will be discussed in detail later. Studies with germ-free rats and mice show no difference in the final stage of development [20], but in the absence of microbes the proliferation rate and epithelial migration are significantly reduced [9]. When germ-free animals are conventionalized to a normal environment, proliferation and migration return to mature levels within 2 weeks. Therefore, maturation of the small intestine at weaning in rodents, an event similar to changes in the human at birth, is a complex process likely involving both secondary hormonal stimuli and alterations in the composition of the luminal microbial flora.

Circulating Growth Factors

Thus far, several factors have been implicated as potential growth factors regulating the development of the small intestine [1, 2]. Among them, only glucocorticoids appear to have a primary influence on the developing intestine. The other factors that have been studied are thyroxine, insulin, gastrin, epidermal growth factor, transforming growth factors (TGF-α and TGF-β). In rodents both endogenous as well as the exogenous glucocorticoids have a potent effect on the rate of intestinal maturation [2]. These effects can be recapitulated in both in vitro and in vivo model systems. They appear to regulate all facets of intestinal maturation, enabling precocious development of digestive absorptive function and activation, proliferation as well as epithelial migration from the crypt to the villus. These effects, however, are restricted to a narrow period of 2 weeks in the rodent and after the 3rd postnatal week the intestine loses its responsiveness to glucocorticoids [2]. Indirect evidence in the human suggests that a similar period of glucocorticoid sensitivity might exist during the third trimester (details will be discussed below). Non-circulating autocrine or paracrine factors may also play a role in the ontogeny of the intestine. As in vitro models and human intestinal cell lines have been established [21], the additive role of other growth factors, e.g. epidermal growth factor, TGF-β, etc., in concert with corticosteroids can be determined and the effect of these growth factors at other phases of development understood. This information may provide not only a better understanding of gut development but also can be used in gut repair after resection or vascular insufficiency and necrosis.

The Intrinsic Timing Mechanism (a Biological Clock)

A number of investigators have sought to determine the intrinsic factors controlling terminal maturation of the rodent small intestine, but these changes are not primarily dependent on hormones. Using intestinal isografts, studies have established an intrinsic timing mechanism that initiates the development of the gut at a precise time [22]. A similar hypothesis for other intrinsic timing mechanisms has been proposed in other organ systems. The existence of a 'hot-wired local trigger' mechanism in the small intestine has been proposed [23] but the cellular basis and the molecular nature of this biological clock is unknown and remains to be elucidated.

Epithelial–Mesenchyme Interactions

The importance of epithelial–mesenchymal interactions during intestinal development has been extensively analyzed [24]. The data suggest an instructive role for the epithelium and a permissive role for mesenchyme in epithelial cytodifferentiation, i.e. mesenchyme is necessary but not sufficient for development. For example, glucocorticoids most likely mediate their effect on the epithelium via epithelial–mesenchymal interactions [25]. However, the mechanism of mesenchyme action in hormonal regulation is not completely understood. It has been postulated that corticosteroids may affect direct cell interaction via specific extracellular matrix components [25]. However, new techniques such as immortalized, non-malignant human cell lines are needed to help answer this question. Unfortunately, the role of epithelial–mesenchymal interaction in the development of the mucosal immune system remains an unknown process.

Development of the Mucosal Immune System

The epithelial barrier of the gut separates luminal antigens and microbes from underlying lymphoid elements and acts as a first responder in the mucosal immune system [26]. Generally, food antigen and commensal microbes do not elicit an immune response but instead evoke oral tolerance [27]. However, when an immune reaction occurs in response to these stimuli in lamina propria lymphocytes, the activation can lead to food intolerance and intestinal inflammation. In contrast, enteric pathogens can stimulate a self-limited mucosal and systemic immune inflammatory response after breaching the epithelial barrier by using various adaptive techniques as an attempt to eliminate these pathogens [6, 28]. Depending on the pathogen, intestinal damage may vary from mild inflammation to full-fledged tissue damage. This ability to distinguish nutrients and luminal commensal bacteria from enteric pathogens and their toxins is an important feature of the normal mucosal immune response and generally results in intestinal immune homeostasis [6, 26]. The development of this balance is initiated during fetal maturation but requires initial bacterial colonization [18]. The luminal environment changes from a sterile surface bathed in amniotic fluid to bacterially contaminated food sources, initially milk and then solid foods, during the adaptation to the extrauterine environment [17]. Briefly the elements of the mucosal immune system are described below, but details can be obtained from recent reviews [4, 14, 26, 27].

As stated, a polarized epithelial monolayer exists as a tight barrier that prevents movement of various molecules from the lumen to the interstitium [5]. Direct sampling of luminal food and bacterial antigens is carried out by M cells which act as a conduit to underlying antigen-presenting cells, e.g. macrophages and dendritic cells that lie beneath the epithelium directly in contact with M cells [13, 26]. The lamina propria also contains mast cells, and various lymphocytes, particularly IgA-producing B cells. Moreover, the epithelium rather than being simply a physical barrier to antigens is also an active participant in the mucosal immune response by releasing cytokines and by transcytosing dimeric IgA produced by B cells via the polymeric immunoglobulin receptor. IgA acts on luminal bacteria to prevent their adherence to the enterocyte surface. In addition, specialized T cells, known as intraepithelial lymphocytes and juxtaposed between the epithelium at the basolateral surface, recognize bacterial antigens and/or immune-activated epithelial surface molecules so that they could respond rapidly upon stimulation [29].

The epithelium, together with these components of the immune system, modulates luminal antigen and bacterial activation of the peripheral immune system [26, 27]. This physical and functional barrier constitutes the mucosal immune system of the gut that continuously samples the luminal environment without disrupting the digestive and absorptive function of the gut as well as modulating a systemic immune response that can be muted or lead to excessive inflammation and tissue damage. These cells constitute the innate and adoptive immune system of the gut that is defined as a rapidly responding antigen nonspecific response and a delayed, antigen-specific memory cell response, respectively [26, 27, 30]. These two arms of the mucosal immune system initiate a self-limited inflammatory response by recruiting activated neutrophils and monocytes into the lamina propria from blood vessels but yet does not sustain a chronic inflammatory response.

The intestinal epithelium is closely associated with several cell types involved in innate immunity that include macrophages, dendritic, mast and paneth cells [4, 7, 10, 26, 27]. The developmental response of these cells has not been well studied. Macrophages are the major resident phagocytic lymphoid cell in the gut. They exist diffusely in the lamina propria, but mainly in Peyer's patches. In human fetal intestine, macrophages can be detected from about 12 weeks of gestation onwards, although specific subpopulations differ with gestational age and location in the gut. Of particular interest to this review is that lamina propria macrophages lack CD14, a cell surface co-receptor for lipopolysaccharide binding, and therefore these cells are hypo-responsive to endotoxin [31]. This regional difference in the macrophage may be important in preventing inappropriate activation of inflammatory signals in response to gram-negative bacteria continuously present in the gut lumen and potentially available to penetrate the epithelial barrier. Antigen-processing dendritic cells function at the interface between innate and adaptive immunity. Immature dendritic cells rapidly sample luminal food and microbial antigens and then become activated, migrate to regional lymph nodes where they present the processed antigen to T cells with co-stimulatory signals under the influence of regulatory cytokines [7, 26]. How they discriminate pathogenic and commensal bacteria is as yet not known. Recently dendritic cells from the intestinal lamina propria have been shown to protrude as cytoplasmic extensions across tight junction barriers into the lumen presumably to sample luminal antigens [32]. This is done without disrupting the polarized epithelium. The development of these mucosal dendritic cells is unknown. Mast cells which are present in significant numbers in the intestinal mucosa are considered to be effector cells in IgE-mediated allergic responses, but also play a role in defense against intestinal parasites and enteric bacterial pathogens via pathogen-induced tumor necrosis factor-α release [33]. However, the development as well as the mode of distribution of these mast cells in the intestinal mucosa is not completely understood.

The role of the epithelium in the development of the mucosal immune system is better characterized than other lymphoid cells in the mucosal immune system [26]. Tight and adherent junctions are formed during the second trimester [2, 5]. However, the functional property of transepithelial resistance and the passage of macromolecular markers during the second and third trimester of development is not known. Recently, the major proteins in the junctional complex, e.g. occludin and claudins, have been identified [34] but their developmental regulation functions have not been elucidated. Possibly because of incompletely developed tight junctions in newborn infants, immature enterocytes have the potential to translocate macromolecules such as maternal antibodies and trophic factors from colostrum and mother's milk [35] to function passively and act in initial mucosal defense. This process is partially facilitated by lower gastric acidity and pancreatic enzymes in the lumen preventing destruction of these bioactive molecules before reaching the small intestine for translocation into the mucosa [35, 36]. Gradually, within weeks, this capacity is lost and the gut becomes less permeable. This process has been termed 'closure', and the period of this uptake is well characterized in rodents, ending just before weaning [2, 36]. Exogenous glucocorticoids are capable of accelerating closure precociously along with terminal maturation in the developing rodent intestine. Though it is believed to be developmentally regulated, the mechanisms by which bioactive macromolecules are taken up, e.g. phagocytosis versus pericellular transport, by the small intestine is not known.

The ability to produce chemokines that can recruit activated polymorphonuclear cells to the site of inflammation may be developmentally regulated. Using intestinal explants of 20-week-old fetal intestine and biopsies of infants, we were able to demonstrate an excessive IL-8 response to endotoxins and endogenous pro-inflammatory stimuli [37]. The highest amount of IL-8 was produced in the epithelium in the developing gut and these results were confirmed using human fetal intestinal epithelial cell lines. This difference may in part be responsible for initiating the excessive inflammatory response in the premature infant gut seen in diseases such as necrotizing enterocolitis, which will be discussed below.

Sampling of luminal antigens are carried out by M cells so that the adaptive immune system can be tolerized to food and unknown bacterial antigens [26, 27]. M cells begin to appear by 17 weeks of gestation in the human, after lymphoid aggregates begin to appear [2]. This temporal sequence of events is of some significance since mice lacking B cells have either completely or partially impaired development of Peyer's patches, FAE and M cells [12, 38]. Though other lymphoid cells beside B cells have recently been shown to induce M-cell differentiation, antigenic macromolecules and a few pathogenic bacteria, viruses and protozoans preferentially penetrate the M-cell epithelial barrier by endocytosis or phagocytosis [4, 26]. M cells facilitate the sampling of these pathogens and luminal antigens by the mucosal and systemic immune system via the subepithelial lymphocytes [26, 27]. Unfortunately, the mechanism(s) by which either the macromolecules or pathogens penetrate the cells is not know and remains an active area of investigation.

Bacterial Colonization and the Role of Glycosylation during Gut Development

The lumen of the gut contains a complex ecosystem of microbial flora composed of an excess of 500 species with 100-fold more anaerobes than aerobes [3, 11, 18]. However, about 30–40 species comprise 99% of the total bacteria. These microbes facilitate colonic function, such as absorption, secretion of electrolytes and water, as well as storage and excretion of waste materials. The gut microflora plays an important role in tissue homeostasis because of fermentation which results in the production of compounds that have a positive and a negative influence on gut function. For example, the fermentation of residual undigested complex carbohydrate content (such as fiber) to short-chain fatty acids can provide an energy source for the colon while pathogenic species may produce toxic compounds.

The human gut is a complex microbial ecosystem in a multiplicity of different microhabitats and metabolic niches [11, 17, 18]. This observation has largely arisen by analyzing the bacteria content in feces. Gram-negative anaerobes of the genus bacteroides are the most prevalent microbe in the gut (30% of the total fecal flora). Other predominant groups are gram-positive rods (bifidobacteria, eubacteria, clostridia, lactobacilli) and gram-positive cocci (ruminococci, peptococci, peptostreptococci). Chief among these are the bifidobacteria, which may constitute as much as 25% of total fecal contents. A number of other groups exist in lower proportions, including enterococci, coliforms, methanogens and dissimilatory sulfate-reducing bacteria (fig. 1). More recently molecular techniques have been used to identify previously unknown bacteria. However, the unique microenvironment in which these microbes grow could not be recapitulated in vitro, thus preventing comprehensive identification of these bacteria and elucidating their role in microbial homeostasis in the lumen of the gut. Functionally, these bacteria are divided into species that exert either harmful or beneficial effects on humans (fig. 1). The pathogenic consequences of an imbalance in bacterial content include diarrhea, inflammation, necrosis, ulceration and intestinal perforation. Growth inhibition of harmful bacteria may promote better health by stimulating appropriate immune functions, decreasing gas production, improving digestion and absorption of essential nutrients as well as the synthesis of vitamins B and K.

At birth the gut is initially exposed to maternal bacteria that are present in the vagina and maternal colon. However, a delayed colonization occurs if the infant is delivered by cesarean section. The newborn intestine is first colonized with enterobacteria and their number attains 10^9/g of feces. On day 6, bifidobacteria become the predominant microbe in the breast-fed infants, exceeding enterobacteria by a ratio of 1,000:1, whereas enterobacteria remain predominant in formula-fed infants, exceeding bifidobacteria by 10:1 (fig. 2). By the end of a month, bifidobacteria are the predominant organism in both fed groups. However, these organisms in formula-fed infants are approximately one tenth that of breast-fed infants, presumably the breast milk creates an environment favoring the development of a simple flora such as bifidobacteria and few other anaerobic and small numbers of facultatively anaerobic bacteria. In contrast, formula-fed infants have complex microbiota,

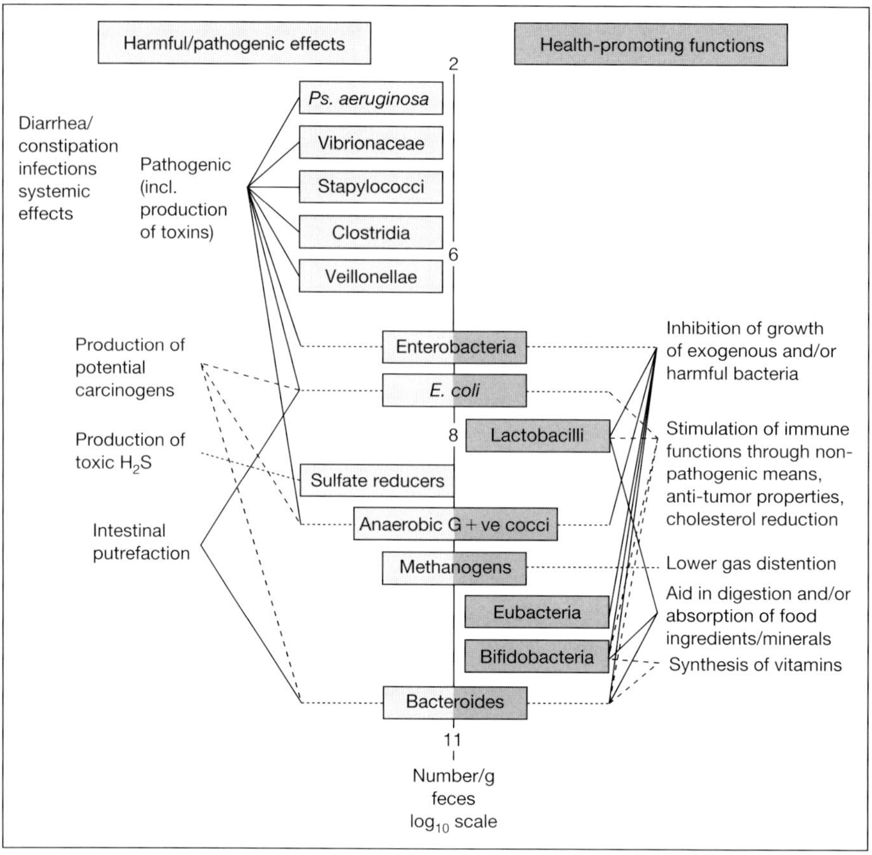

Fig. 1. Generalized scheme of the human gut microbial composition. The different bacterial groups are divided on the basis of whether they exert properties that are potentially damaging or health-promoting for the host. The central vertical line gives approximate number in feces. H_2S = Hydrogen sulfide. Adapted from Fuller and Gibson [40].

with bifidobacteria, bacteroides, clostridia and streptococci all prevalent (fig. 2). The introduction of solid foods to breast-fed infants caused a major re-disturbance of the microbial ecology of the colon as numbers of enterobacteria and enterococci colonized by *Bacteroides* spp., clostridia and anaerobic streptococci occurs. This was not observed when formula-fed infants began to take solids. Instead, counts of facultative anaerobes remain high while colonization by anaerobes other than bifidobacteria continue. By the end of a year the composition of the anaerobic bacteria of healthy infants in both groups resemble that of adults with a corresponding decrease in the number of facultative anaerobes [17, 39]. The incidence of pure cultures of aerobic bacteria is higher in the stool of the premature neonate and critically

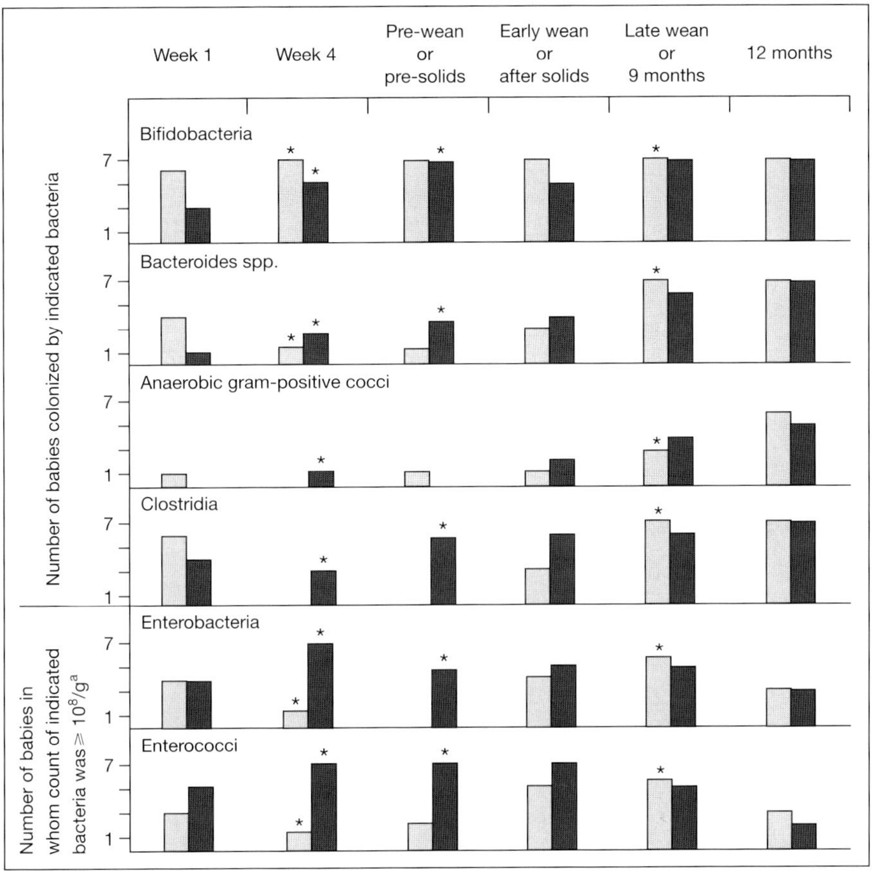

Fig. 2. The succession of bacterial colonization of specific bacteria in the large intestine of breast-fed (■) and formula-fed infants (□). *When fewer than 7 babies were examined the results were corrected to a fraction of 7. [a]Counts of facultative anaerobic bacteria $\geq 10^8$/g feces are raised in comparison to counts in normal adults. Adapted from Stark and Lee [39].

ill infants than in normal full-term infants [18, 39]. The composition changes in colonization of these bacteria differ in other locations in the world reflecting sanitary condition, differences in diet, other feeding patterns and antibiotic treatment during the newborn period. The method of feeding has a profound influence on the composition of the gut microbiota (fig. 2).

Differences in the fecal flora of breast-fed and formula-fed infants are not fully understood but believed to be related to the type of protein ingested (whey vs. casein), the availability of iron, e.g. bifidobacteria and lactobacilli do not need iron whereas bacteroides species and enterobacteria require iron

Table 1. Microbial glycoconjugate receptors on the brush border membrane of the gut epithelium

Organisms	Carbohydrate structure
Bacteria	
E. coli CFA/1	NeuAc(α2–8)–
E. coli K99	NeuGc(α2–3)Galβ4Glc
Staphylococcus epidermidis	Gal(β1–4)GlcNAc(β1–3)Gl(β1–4)Glc
Bacterial toxins	
V. cholerae (CT)	GM1 Galβ1–3GalNAcβ–4(NeuAcα2–3)GalB1–4GlcB1–1Cer
Shigella (Shiga toxin)	Gb3 Galα1–4Galβ1–4Glcβ1–1Cer
E. coli (heat-labile toxin)	GM1 Galβ1–3GalNAcβ1–4(NeuAcα2–3)Galβ1–4Glcβ1–1Cer
E. coli (heat-stable toxin)	Glycoprotein (determinant unknown)
E. coli (Shiga-like toxin)	Gb3 Galα1–4Galβ1–4Glcβ1–1Cer
C. difficile (toxin A)	nLc5Cer Galα1–3Galβ1–4GlcNAcβ1–3Galβ1–4Glcβ1–1Cer
X antigen	Galβ1–4(Fucα1–3)GlcNAcβ1–4Glc
Y antigen	Fucα1–2Galβ1–4(Fucα1–3)GlcNAcβ1
I antigen	Galβ1–4GlcNAcβ1–3(Galβ1–4GlcNAcβ1–6)Galβ1–4Glc

for growth, the composition of oligosaccharides in the milk and the pH in the gut lumen. The pH level of stool in breast-fed infants was 5.1 at age 7 days, whereas it is as high as 6.5 in formula-fed infants [18]. The low pH level favors the growth of bifidobacteria and lactobacilli but inhibits other bacteria proliferation.

Even though the composition of the gut microflora varies between individuals or between an individual at different times, it is composed of both resident and transient species [11, 40]. The resident microflora use specific glycoconjugates on the intestinal surface as receptors to colonize a region of the gut (table 1). These sugar moieties can facilitate adhesion by these resident bacteria. Glycoconjugate specificity depends on the region and on the developmental stage of the intestine. This is due to a developmental regulation of enzymes that are responsible for adding glycoconjugates to glycoprotein and glycolipids on the intestinal epithelium. As apical proteins are processed through the Golgi complex, they are glucosylated by specific glycosyltransferases at N- and O-linked sites. In the developing rodent intestine, glycoproteins on the apical surface contain high terminal sialic acid/fucose ratio whereas in the adult this ratio is reversed. This is due to developmental regulation of sialyl- and fucosyltransferase activities [11, 12, 20, 41]. The developmental decline in surface sialylation of glycoconjugates is due to a decline in α-2,6-sialyltransferase activity in the mouse small intestine but in the colon this decline is compensated by a reciprocal increase in α-2,3-sialyltransferase activity in the epithelium. Furthermore, a specific change in terminal sialylation in the mucosa was observed suggesting that coordinate changes in glycoconjugate expression occurs in both enterocytes and goblet cells. During the same developmental period, an increase in terminal fucosylation is predominantly found in the brush border membrane of the mature intestine. In a manner similar to fucosyltransfease activity galactosyltransferase activity is also developmentally regulated with highest activity found in the adult gut. Unlike sialyltransferase activity the changes in fucosyl- and galactosyltransferases were observed in both the small and large intestine, with an increasing gradient from the proximal to distal axis [20]. The developmental profiles of these three enzymes are precociously induced by glucocorticoids in suckling mice. It is worth noting that, in 75% of the mice, a disruption at the β-1,4-galactosyltransferase allele (knockout mice) is lethal at the time of weaning [42]. Studies are currently underway in this laboratory to elucidate the role of these enzymes and the regulation of glycoconjugate expression in response to commensal and enteric pathogens in the developing intestine and their role in modulating changing microflora in this and other mutant mouse models. We have recently reported that germ-free mice retain the immature high sialic acid/fucose ratio but rapidly revert to the mature pattern with colonization. Thus, the initial colonization of the intestine may determine the nature of colonizing bacteria (pathogens vs. commensal) via developmental regulation of glycoconjugates.

Major bacterial-binding sites on enterocytes are surface glycoconjugates because they are the most abundant structure exposed to the microbes [11, 12]. These glycoconjugates have a common structural backbone but often have tissue- and age-specific differences in their composition providing a diversity and selectivity to allow tropism which may lead to infection. Glycoproteins are found on cell surfaces as well as in the secretions, whereas glycolipids are strictly confined to the membrane except when the cells are shed at the top of the intestinal villus epithelium. Due to technical difficulties, our understanding of glycolipids has lagged behind glycosylation of proteins. But specific examples of changes in glycosylation of specific gangliosides in binding has been demonstrated [3]. For example, the GM1 ganglioside is a receptor for cholera toxin binding (table 1). Terminal sialic acid (NeuAc) galactose is equally effective in binding but adding NeuAcα8 to NeuAc reduces activity 50-fold. In like manner, removing terminal Galβ reduces activity 2,000-fold and a reduction in binding is also observed when Fucα or β GalNAcβ4 are added as the terminal moiety of Galβ3 in GM1 ganglioside. Therefore it is conceivable that modification by glycosylation may provide an opportunity for commensal flora as well as pathogens to dock on the surface of the intestinal lumen, enabling colonization and invasion of this epithelial barrier.

Pattern Recognition Receptors

In addition, there are specific proteins synthesized by the host that would recognize the diverse molecules of microbial flora. These receptors are called pattern recognition receptors [43]. Ten members of the Toll-like receptors (TLRs) belong to this family. For example TLR-4 is a receptor for the gram-negative bacterial cell wall component lipopolysaccharide, TLR-2 is the receptor for gram-positive bacterial cell wall components such as lipotheichoic acid and peptidoglycan and TLR-5 is the receptor for bacterial flagellin [28]. These transmembrane proteins are glycoproteins and upon dimerization are bound to these bacterial components. Pattern recognition receptors activate specific signal transduction pathways leading to the expression of specific inflammatory responses in various cells in the host intestine. The specificity of the glycosylation pattern on these receptors have not been defined. However, developmental expression of these proteins may play a role in the initial inflammatory response in the premature infant gut, whereas in adult non-responsiveness could be due to a lack of receptors or receptor desensitization in the intestinal epithelium. However, these receptors discriminate components of commensal flora from those of pathogens and prevent an inappropriate response to new microbial residents during the succession of bacterial colonization. The mechanisms of this variable response are not known. Apart from these cell surface receptors, eukaryotes have cytosolic receptors for gram-positive and negative bacterial cell wall components. These proteins have recently been identified and are called NOD-1 and NOD-2. Again, these proteins belong to a large family of caspase-activating and recruitment domain containing proteins, and elucidation of the function of other family members may yield more clues as to how mucosal immune cells cleave these bacterial cell wall components by producing activating caspases [44]. Furthermore, NOD-1 and 2 have been implicated in infection by shigella as well as an inheritable form of Crohn's disease. The ontogeny of these proteins are not known for humans or mice.

Exotoxin Responses

Apart from direct binding, enteric pathogens produce and secrete exotoxins that are bound to various cell surface receptors. Specificity of *Vibrio cholerae* and *Clostridium difficile* toxins binding to their receptors have been shown to be under developmental regulation leading to diarrheal disease (see below; table 1) [11, 45, 46]. Newborns are more susceptible to cholera toxin and *Escherichia coli* heat-stable toxin-induced diarrhea, but are less susceptible to *C. difficile* toxin and shiga toxin. As described above, the action of the exotoxin of *V. cholerae* is significantly altered by glycosylation of its receptor. Since the pattern of glycoconjugate expression is developmentally regulated, it might be worth investigating the possibility of whether predominance of infant diarrhea caused by these exotoxins are due to a changing pattern of glycosylation on the intestinal surface.

Clinical Diseases Unique to the Neonatal Period

Necrotizing Enterocolitis

Necrotizing enterocolitis (NEC) leads to severe morbidity and mortality in premature infants, especially in the developing world. As smaller premature infants survive due to sophisticated medical care, this disease has become a major health problem in pediatric hospitals totaling 5% of the total cost in managing premature infants [11, 47]. Though the pathophysiology of NEC is still not understood, the major risk factors are prematurity (90% of all NEC cases occur in premature infants of <1,500 g birth weight), bacterial colonization, and initiation of formula feeding. These risk factors suggest that an immature epithelial barrier and mucosal immune function prematurely exposed to bacterial colonization lead to an inappropriate immune response resulting in inflammation and bowel necrosis. Previous studies have demonstrated that the immature epithelium of the fetal gut inappropriately responds to bacterial endotoxins and proinflammatory stimuli. In addition, the mucosal immune system most likely has not reached the protective levels of term infants. A case of 3-year-old twins illustrates the role of bacteria in the process. One infant was predominantly colonized with clostridium and other with bifidobacteria [48]. The former twin developed NEC and the latter did not. In an animal model, clostridium-induced colitis is prevented by bifidobacteria treatment as well as the prevention of gut inflammation. In newborn rats under asphyxic conditions, formula feeding leads to gut inflammation similar to that of NEC. This inflammation was prevented by pretreatment with bifidobacteria. The pathology in the rat model is age-dependent, implicating both the development of the epithelial barrier and the mucosal immune system in the inflammatory response. In addition, specific stains of klebsiella, enterobacter or *E. coli* colonization have been shown to precede the development of NEC. Even though bifidobacteria appears to have potential probiotic effects, a clinical trial in a premature intensive care unit in Columbia did not protect against NEC. This study suggests that, rather than providing a specific single species of bacteria to the premature, a conducive environment in the premature infant gut lumen which allows the succession of bacterial growth from the germ-free state to complete colonization with a variety of bacteria may be more protective against NEC. In addition, appropriate colonization may lead to successive development of mucosal defenses and protection against pathologic colonization. Complete understanding of the pathophysiology of NEC requires a proper model in which immature epithelium and mucosal immune cells can be shown to induce an inappropriate inflammatory response.

Diarrhea

Bacterial-induced diarrhea exerts a heavy toll on the infant population worldwide [49–51]. Despite identification of these bacteria, their mode of

Table 2. Symptoms of enteropathogenic bacteria and its epidemiology

	Diarrhea		Inflammatory diarrhea/ dysentery		Industrialized countries %	Developing countries %
	watery	bloody	ileitis	colitis		
E. coli (ETEC)	+					
E. coli (EPEC)	+		±			
E. coli (EaggEC)	+				2–5	14–17
E. coli (EIEC)		+		+		
E. coli (EHEC)		+		+		
Shigella spp.		+		+	1–3	5–9
Non-typhoidal salmonella	+	±		±	3–7	4–6
Salmonella typhi			±			
Yersinia enterocolitica	+	+	+		1–2	?
Vibrio cholerae	+				<1	0–3
Vibrio parahaemolyticus	+	+	±	±		
Campylobacter jejuni	+	+	±	+	6–8	7–9
Clostridium difficile					?	?
Aemonas, plesiomonas and edwardsiella					0–2	4–5

Modified from references 49, 50 and 51.

action and understanding the pathophysiology of infection in the intestinal epithelium is incomplete (table 2). Death caused by these organism remains unchanged. A brief description of these pathogens is provided below, and a comprehensive description was recently published.

Among these bacteria *V. cholerae* causes a rapid fatal diarrhea especially in the underdeveloped world. Recent sequencing of the *V. cholerae* genome should help elucidate the origin and pathophysiology of this enteric pathogen and an understanding of the biology of resistance, which may lead to development of novel treatments. *Salmonella typhi* is a pathogen which colonizes the human gut and can be acquired via close contact from a carrier or an individual affected with typhoid fever. Since 1970 the incidence of non-typhoidal salmonella diarrhea has risen sharply and is ascribed to the repeated use of antibiotic treatment resulting in infection of resistant strains of salmonella. The mode of colonization in the intestinal epithelium of salmonella is similar to shigella. Unlike salmonella, the human is the only host for shigella which is orally transmitted by ingestion of a few bacteria.

Unlike other enteric pathogens, campylobacter has a significantly higher incidence in developed countries, though it was not identified until the late 1970s. The reservoir for campylobacter is the intestine of a variety of domestic and wild animals. According to a recent US government survey, 75% of raw poultry and 5% of pork are contaminated with this pathogen. Yersinia attaches to the β-integrin receptor on the basolateral surface of the human intestinal epithelium, disrupts the cytoskeleton and tight junction proteins leading to breakdown of the epithelial barrier. *C. difficile* acts via two related cytotoxins (TxA and TxB) again altering the epithelial cytoskeleton and is the most leading cause of diarrhea in hospitalized patients' (nosocomial) infections. The miscellaneous species of aemonas, plesiomonas and edwardsiella have been known for a long time and have recently been implicated in diarrhea, but their mode of action is not well understood (table 2).

Among the enteric pathogens, *E. coli* is the most prevalent organism and may cause mild to profound diarrheal disease by a variety of strains (table 2). These strains of bacteria have devised every possible strategy to invade the intestinal epithelium. Five distinct groups of *E. coli* are considered enteric pathogens (table 2) and EPEC was the first to be identified. It directly attaches to the apical surface of the epithelium. Unlike EPEC, ETEC uses toxins to compromise the epithelial barrier; EIEC invades the barrier in a manner similar to shigella and is the major cause of *E. coli*-induced diarrheal outbreaks in the developing world. EHEC produces bacterial phage encoded toxins (shiga-like toxins) type I and II which cause diarrhea or hemolytic uremic syndrome. Though initially identified in United States, it is a global problem due to contaminated food. Another toxin producing *E. coli* is EIEC, which is defined by its pattern of aggregative adherence to the epithelial surface. This is one of the most prevalent diarrheal diseases in the developing world.

Probiotics in the Neonatal Clinical Diseases

A probiotic is defined as a non-pathogenic microorganism usually found in the lumen of the human gut that is resistant to antibiotics and provides a beneficial effect by modulating the mucosal immune system [48, 52]. Among the plethora of such bacteria, the most extensively studied species are *Lactobacillus casei* GG (LGG), *Lactobacillus acidophilus, Bifidobacterium bifidum, Sacchromyces boulardii and Streptococcus thermophilus*. They have been used in clinical trials. Extensive discussion of probiotics can be found in other chapters of this book. A brief consideration of the role of probiotics in these neonatal diseases will be summarized below.

Probiotics have been tested against diarrheal diseases. *L. casei* GG, but not *L. acidophilus*, has been shown to be effective against viral-induced diarrhea, to shorten the duration of the diarrheal episode as well as to shorten the time required for recuperation either in hospital or at home. Though a positive therapeutic role has been observed for viral diarrhea, the mechanism of action is not known. Convincing data have also been observed against antibiotic-associated diarrhea by all these microorganism in various clinical trials. Since a fecal enema is the treatment of relapsing *C. difficile* toxin-induced diarrhea, it would be logical to treat with probiotics. *S. boulardii* inhibits clostridial toxin-induced destruction of the intestinal epithelium by secreting a protease that is able to cleave the toxin protein as well as its receptor. The treatment has a significant effect on inhibiting recurrence in patients with prior *C. difficile* toxin-induced diarrhea. However, the overall effects of probiotics in treating and preventing bacterial-induced diarrhea including traveler's diarrhea, with the exception of *C. difficile* toxin recurrent diarrhea, have been mixed.

Probiotics appear to be effective in an animal model of NEC. Very few clinical trials have been carried out using *L. acidophilus* and *Bifidobacterium infantis* in the neonatal intensive care unit. These results appear to be promising compared to other approaches. However, further studies using a placebo-controlled clinical trial are required to access the benefits of these bacteria in the premature infants as a preventative measure.

Acknowledgments

This work was supported by grants R37-HD12437, RO1-HD31852, PO1-DK33506, P30-DK043351 and P30-DK40561 from the National Institutes of Health, Bethesda, Md., USA. Due to space limitation, not all the primary articles have been cited.

References

1 Henning SJ: Functional development of the gastrointestinal tract; in Johnson LR (ed): Physiology of the Gastrointestinal Tract, ed 2. New York, Raven Press, 1987, pp 285–300.
2 Nanthakumar NN: Regulation of functional development of the small intestine; in Delvin E, Lentze MJ (eds): Gastrointestinal Functions. Nestlé Nutrition Workshop Series. Vevey, Nestlé/Philadelphia, Lippincott Williams & Wilkins, 2001, vol 46, pp 39–58.
3 Savage DC: Microbial ecology of the gastrointestinal tract. Annu Rev Microbiol 1997;31:107–133.
4 Sanderson IR, Walker WA: Uptake and transport of macromolecules by the intestine: Possible role in clinical disorders (An update). Gastroenterology 1993;104:622–629.
5 Mitic LL, Anderson JM: Molecular architecture of tight junctions. Annu Rev Physiol 1998;60: 121–142.
6 Galan JE, Bliska JB: Cross-talk between bacterial pathogens and their host cells. Annu Rev Cell Dev Biol 1996;12:221–255.
7 Rescigno M, Borrow P: The host-pathogen interaction: New themes from dendritic cell biology. Cell 2001;106:267–270.
8 Simon TC, Gordon JI: Intestinal epithelial cell differentiation: New insights from mice, flies and nematodes. Curr Opin Genet Dev 1995;5:577–586.
9 Wright NA: The development of the crypt-villus axis; in Delvin E, Lentze MJ (eds): Gastrointestinal Functions. Nestlé Nutrition Workshop Series. Vevey, Nestlé/Philadelphia, Lippincott Williams & Wilkins, 2001, vol 46, pp 1–22.

10 Ouellette AJ: Paneth cells and innate immunity in the crypt microenvironment. Gastroenterology 1997;113:1779–1784.
11 Dai D, Nanthakumar NN, Newburg DS, Walker WA: The role of oligosaccharides and glycoconjugates in intestinal host defense. J Pediatr Gastroenterol Nutr 2000;30:S23–S33.
12 Hooper LV, Gordon JI: Glycans as legislators of host-microbial interactions: Spanning the spectrum from symbiosis to pathogenicity. Glycobiology 2001;11:1R–10R.
13 Kraehenbuhl JP, Neutra MR: Epithelial M cells: Differentiation and function. Annu Rev Cell Dev Biol 2000;16:301–332.
14 McGee DW: Inflammation and Mucosal Cytokine Production; in Ogra PL, Mestecky J, Lamm ME, et al (eds): Mucosal Immunology. San Diego, Academic Press, 1999, pp 559–573.
15 Kerneis S, Bogdanova A, Kraehenbuhl JP, Pringault E: Conversion by Peyer's patch lymphocytes of human enterocytes into M cells that transport bacteria. Science 1997;277: 949–952.
16 Grand RJ, Watkins JB, Torti FM: Development of the human gastrointestinal tract. A review. Gastroenterology 1976;70:790–810.
17 Buescher ES: Host defense mechanisms of human milk and their relations to enteric infections and necrotizing enterocolitis. Clin Perinatol 1994;21:247.
18 Benno Y, Sawada K, Mitsuoka T: The intestinal microflora of infants: Composition of all flora in breast-fed and bottle-fed infants. Microbiol Immunol 1984;28:975–986.
19 Macfarlane GT, Macfarlane S: Human colonic microbiota: Ecology, physiology and metabolic potential of intestinal bacteria. Scand J Gastroenterol 1997;70:443–459.
20 Nanthakumar NN, Dai D, Newburg DS, Walker WA: The role of indigenous microflora in the development of murine intestinal fucosyl- and sialyltransferases. FASEB J 2003;17: 44–46.
21 Louvard D, Kedinger M, Hauri HP: The differentiating intestinal epithelial cell: Establishment and maintenance of functions between cellular structures. Annu Rev Cell Biol 1992;8: 157–195.
22 Yeh KY, Holt PR: Ontogenic timing mechanism initiates the expression of rat intestinal sucrase activity. Gastroenterology 1986;90:520–526.
23 Diamond JM: Developmental physiology. Hard-wired local triggering of intestinal enzyme expression. Nature 1986;324:408.
24 Kedinger M, Duluc I, Fritsch C, et al: Intestinal epithelial-mesenchymal cell interactions. Ann NY Acad Sci 1998;859:1–17.
25 Kedinger M, Simon-Assmann P, Alexandre E, Haffen K: Importance of a fibroblastic support for in vitro differentiation of intestinal endodermal cells and for their response to glucocorticoids. Cell Differ 1987;20:171–182.
26 Brandtzaeg P: Development, regulation and function of secretory immunity; in Delvin E, Lentze MJ (eds): Gastrointestinal Functions. Nestlé Nutrition Workshop Series. Vevey, Nestlé/Philadelphia, Lippincott Williams & Wilkins, 2001, vol 46, pp 91–114.
27 Nagler-Anderson C, Shi HN: Peripheral nonresponsiveness to orally administered soluble protein antigens. Crit Rev Immunol 2001;21:121–131.
28 Gewirtz AT, Madara JL: Periscope, up! Monitoring microbes in the intestine. Nat Immunol 2001;2:288–290.
29 Hayday A, Theodoridis E, Ramsburg E, Shires J: Intraepithelial lymphocytes: Exploring the third way in immunology. Nat Immunol 2001;2:997–1003.
30 Wills-Karp M, Santeliz J, Karp CL: The germless theory of allergic disease: Revisiting the hygiene hypothesis. Nat Rev Immunol 2001;1:69–75.
31 Smith PD, Smythies LE, Mosteller-Barnum M, et al: Intestinal macrophages lack CD14 and CD89 and consequently are down-regulated for LPS- and IgA-mediated activities. J Immunol 2001;167:2651–2656.
32 Rescigno M, Urbano M, Valzasina B, et al: Dendritic cells express tight junction proteins and penetrate gut epithelial monolayers to sample bacteria. Nat Immunol 2001;2:361–367.
33 Gurish MF, Boyce JA: Mast cell growth, differentiation, and death. Clin Rev Allergy Immunol 2002;22:107–118.
34 Anderson JM: Molecular structure of tight junctions and their role in epithelial transport. News Physiol Sci 2001;16:126–130.
35 Lebenthal E, Lee PC: Alternate pathways of digestion and absorption in early infancy. J Pediatr Gastroenterol Nutr 1982;3:1–3.

36 Teichberg S, Wapnir RA, Moyse J, Lifshitz F: Development of the neonatal rat small intestinal barrier to nonspecific macromolecular absorption. II. Role of dietary corticosterone. Pediatr Res 1992;32:50–57.
37 Nanthakumar NN, Fusunyan RD, Sanderson I, Walker WA: Inflammation in the developing human intestine: A possible pathophysiologic contribution to necrotizing enterocolitis. Proc Natl Acad Sci USA 2000;97:6043–6048.
38 Finke D, Kraehenbuhl JP: Formation of Peyer's patches. Curr Opin Genet Dev 2001;11: 561–567.
39 Stark PL, Lee A: The microbial ecology of the large bowel of breast-fed and formula-fed infants during the first year of life. J Med Microbiol 1982;15:189–203.
40 Fuller R, Gibson GR: Modification of the intestinal microflora using probiotics and prebiotics. Scand J Gastroenterol Suppl 1997;22:28–31.
41 Schachter H, Roseman S: Mammalian glycosyltransferases; in Lennarz WJ (ed): The Biochemistry of Glycoproteins and Proteoglycans. New York, Plenum Press, 1980, pp 3–160.
42 Asano M, Furukawa K, Kido M, et al: Growth retardation and early death of beta-1,4-galactosyltransferase knockout mice with augmented proliferation and abnormal differentiation of epithelial cells. EMBO J 1997;16:1850–1857.
43 Medzhitov R: Toll-like receptors and innate immunity. Nat Rev Immunol 2001;1:135–145.
44 O'Neill L: Crohn's disease gene is given the NOD. Trends Immunol 2001;22:418–419.
45 Pothoulakis C, Lamont JT: Microbes and microbial toxins: Paradigms for microbial-mucosal interactions. II. The integrated response of the intestine to *Clostridium difficile* toxins. Am J Physiol Gastrointest Liver Physiol 2001;280:G178–G183.
46 Lencer WI, Chu SW, Walker WA: Differential binding kinetics of cholera toxin to intestinal microvillus membrane during development. Infect Immun 1987;55:3126–3130.
47 Claud EC, Walker WA: Hypothesis: Inappropriate colonization of the premature intestine can cause neonatal necrotizing enterocolitis. FASEB J 2001;15:1398–1403.
48 Teitelbaum, JE, Walker WA: Nutritional impact of pre- and probiotics as protective gastrointestinal organism. Annu Rev Nutr 2002;22:107–138.
49 Keusch GT, Acheson DW: Invasive and tissue-damaging enteral pathogens: Bloody diarrhea and dysentery bacteria: 'Secretory' (watery) diarrhea; in Schaechter M (ed): Mechanism of Microbial Diseases, ed 3. New York, Lippincott, 1998, pp 185–198.
50 Keusch GT, Acheson DW: Enteric bacteria: 'Secretory' (watery) diarrhea; in Schaechter M (ed): Mechanism of Microbial Diseases, ed 3. New York, Lippincott, 1998, pp 176–184.
51 Fasano A: Toxins and the gut: Role in human disease. Gut 2002;50(suppl 3):III9–III14.
52 Fuller R, Gibson GR: Modification of the intestinal microflora using probiotics and prebiotics. Scand J Gastroenterol Suppl 1997;22:28–31.

Discussion

Dr. Bindslev-Jensen: I was very intrigued about your findings on sialic acid in the intestine because we showed more than 15 years ago that sialic acid in the mast cell and the basophile regulates the calcium influx, meaning that if you remove sialic acid from the basophile you make them responsive at a very low calcium level and vice versa if you increase. I can understand that in the newborn it is very wise for the child to have a lot of sialic acid because intrauterally you would then prevent binding of bacteria to the underlying carbohydrates. You should also have some repelling effects due to the negativity of the sialic acid as the last carbohydrate moiety. But to my knowledge only bacillus and *Vibrio cholerae* and the influence of viruses containing this enzyme neuroimmunidase can cut sialic acid off from the intestine. Are there other types of neuroimmunidases today that can account for that or is that the link between bacillus and the colonization in the intestine, the presence of neuroimmunidase?

Dr. Walker: For editorial purposes I covered a huge area of research, e.g., glycobiology and how carbohydrate moieties affect receptors is an enormous field.

For example, you can remove a sialic acid from GM1 and the cholera toxin response is decreased with regard to binding and the cAMP response. Thus there are many areas to investigate. We are not ourselves studying organisms producing sialyl transferase. We are interested in mechanisms which modulate surface glycoconjugates and how that affects colonization. The effect may be mediated through release of an enzyme from a bacteria. However, we are studying the epithelial surface. As I pointed out with work that Schiffrin et al. [1] did a decade ago, what might be happening is that the immaturity of the expression of these glycoconjugates may affect both adherence and translocation. But this is preliminary because there is considerable work to be done on receptors and carbohydrate moieties which affect either up- or downregulation.

Dr. Bindslev-Jensen: We also worked with sialyl transferases. The funny thing about it is that in order to ensure that you can look at the amount of bound sialic acid in the carbohydrate moieties, you have to measure the amount in both the carbohydrate moieties of the glycoprotein and also the glycolipids. The gangliosides present there might be very important for that. I look very much forward to following the progression of your work.

Dr. Walker: Your point is extremely well taken. What we are actively working on is determining the extent to which modification of glycoconjugates affects colonization. We are using cellular intestinal knockouts for fucosyl transferase to see if in fact this manipulation affects the attachment because this may be an epiphenomenon and there may not be an association. We are trying to answer this question.

Dr. Saavedra: One of the things I think would be important for the interpretation of these very nice and elegant studies that you are showing is the definition of colonization and commensal bacteria, because we tend to think immediately of colonization in the human versus the kind of animal or cell line studies that you are showing. The word colonization comes from colony not from colon. A lot of what we are talking about here is bacteria in the small bowel. You showed nice differences, for example, in terms of sialic and fucose expression in the small bowel versus colon, but we don't always interpret those things as such. So I wanted to first get your definition of what colonization is in this kind of experiment, and what colonization is when we are talking about an individual acquiring its own flora which then becomes its commensal bacteria. It is difficult to interpret something such as immature gut and commensal flora to which it is exposed, because if it is immature by definition it would not have established flora, and if it has established flora then it would be commensal but not immature.

Dr. Walker: First of all my review covered the entire colonization process and requires a number of steps including the nature of the bacteria in the lumen and how they utilize a substrate within the human gut, the genetic predisposition to the expression of certain types of surface molecules, etc. There are several reasons why we were interested in the small gut. There was an observation that the fermentation of bacteria in the small bowel producing short-chain fatty acids, particularly butyrate, can upregulate the IL-8 response, this may be a factor in what is happening in necrotizing enterocolitis (NEC). The other reason is that unlike the mature intestine of a full-term infant at 2 years of age, the premature and neonate have bacteria in the small intestine, so we wanted to determine if a different process occurs because butyrate in the colon functions as a source of energy, rather than an inflammatory stimulant. What I mean by adherence with colonization is the attachment of an organism to a surface molecule of the intestine. We determine adherence by isolating cells, removing mucus, or by isolating the microvillus membrane. To try to show a cause and effect relationship we are now starting to study fucosyl transferase knockouts of various enzymes to see if in fact that affects its activation. What is a commensal, what is a non-commensal? This is a very complex topic to discuss. We think of commensals as non-pathogens, and you think of commensals more as probiotics which means not only do they not cause disease but they have a positive protective effect. We know very little about commensal–epithelial interaction, that is why I said earlier that this is now becoming an extremely interesting area of investigation. Let me give you some examples. An article in the *Journal of Biological Chemistry* [2] showed that lactobacillus GG can affect apoptosis. Mack et al. [3] have shown that a commensal bacteria can stimulate the genes in the goblet cell to release mucus which is an important protective substance, and these are just a few of the observations on mechanisms. Thus this is a very hot area of investigation.

Dr. Saavedra: Just one cautionary comment about extrapolating what we believe, what we call colonization in the clinical arena in terms of a whole gut becoming adapted and adopting a particular flora as opposed to this kind of experiment. From the commensal point of view, as you say non-pathogen versus pathogens being used as a stimulant for this. I think when it comes to probiotics, as you mentioned, one of the things that we always had problems with is the difficulty or the potential difficulty that they are probiotics just because they are part of the flora we are not stimulating. But again this is the difference when we are talking about small bowel versus colon.

Dr. Walker: What happens in human studies is that you cannot remove the membrane as we can in cell lines and animal studies. That is why we are doing this so that it can be applied. What you mean by colonization is that a probiotic is given orally and over time it colonizes the gut. However, you are measuring feces, not at the actual binding site. You are assuming that it is colonized. This is what you mean about the clinical definition.

Dr. Guesry: In light of the knowledge about the importance of early colonization and the difference between babies born by vaginal delivery or cesarean section, do you think it would be time to make recommendations for allergic reasons against the usage of cesarean section for convenience? We know that in industrialized countries the vast majority of cesarean sections are made for the convenience of the surgeon or the mother rather than for good obstetrical indications.

Dr. Walker: We are close to suggesting that perhaps these babies should be given a probiotic supplement. There are some very interesting experimental and human studies [4] suggesting that bifidobacteria, for example, can prevent NEC. At this point I think our studies in human models are closer to the actual clinical state. We have to do some clinical studies or get our clinical investigators onto this.

Dr. Bedford-Russell: I am a neonatologist from London and I just want to make a comment first: I think that is slightly unfair on the obstetric colleagues. There is a maternal and infant mortality reason behind the increasing cesarean section as well as the desire on the part of the mother and the obstetrician, but I agree with your comment about prevention. The thing that I really wanted to ask about is if you have any data on the gut flora in US babies. If we look at the article by Schrag et al. [5] in the *New England Journal of Medicine* from last August, it seems that in some institutions around 50% of mothers get prophylaxis with ampicillin antenatally because of group-B streptococci. The consequence of which has been a dramatic reduction in group-B streptococci infection but no overall change in the early onset of neonatal sepsis as a result of a massive increase in coliform sepsis which additionally is resistant to ampicillin. I am just wondering whether you have any data on the consequences for the babies, whether you have been following the gut flora and the patterns in the gut flora, and whether that has an impact on immunological health in the United States?

Dr. Walker: First of all we are not doing clinical studies. All I can do is quote the literature. However, there are some studies suggesting that when antibiotics are given, there is a much less diverse flora and the infant is much more susceptible to environmental activity, i.e. the nature of flora that exist, so they are much more susceptible to the introduction of something that can cause a NEC. What I was trying to identify in a general way is that that type of colonization is perhaps not in the best interest of the baby and maybe that is something we should study further to try to modify the colonization process in babies born under those circumstances, cesarean section, premature and antibiotic use.

Dr. Bedford-Russell: What is your opinion on the obsession of some neonatologists with delaying enteral feeds, particularly in the most vulnerable population?

Dr. Walker: This is another Nestlé symposium. I am not a neonatologist but the neonatologist has strong feelings that (1) expressed mother's breast milk should be used to feed the baby, and (2) to provide some protection but not enough to sustain the baby nutritionally, so they need to be supplemented with peripheral or enteral nutrition by getting something into the gut to get it stimulated to start working. However, at least in the United States, from one center to another, there are different protocols and different patterns, than may be true in the UK.

Dr. Bedford-Russell: What I was specifically getting at was that you may hear comments on day notes or day 1 feeds within the first hours of birth.

Dr. Walker: Many centers are using much lower quantities of breast milk. Low feeds are used because it is more to protect than to provide nutrition. But I am not a neonatologist, so I just give you a point of view.

Dr. Marini: This is a very tricky point about the prevention of NEC and diet and all the problems. I would stress that many years ago we had a lot of experience in preterm infants with lysate pathogen germs, and we found that there was reduced bad colonization in the stools, and the babies grew better [6]. Then we did a series of experiments with different kinds of probiotics and ensured a very good concentration in the stools in the first few days. But subsequently even when we continued to give them probiotics the colonization went down and there was an increase in IgA and IgM specifically against these probiotics. These babies had a change in the intestinal flora with a decreasing aerobic:anaerobic ratio and an increasing gram-positive:gram-negative ratio. Recently we did a study with prebiotics and found that the administration of prebiotics in preterm infants is able to increase bifidobacteria significantly. Analyzing the stools of these preterm babies we also found that a number of pathogens that were present before the administration of prebiotics declined in the group who received prebiotics in comparison to the control group that stayed at the same level [7]. The question I would like to ask you, is it due to the fact that we have an increase in bifidobacteria or is it related to prebiotics and not only to the increase in bifidobacteria?

Dr. Walker: It is a hard question to answer not only because of the fermentation change in the intraluminal milieu which favors bifidobacteria growth. Prebiotics also compete with the surface glycoconjugate for the organisms so they can modulate colonization there. What is happening is that you are increasing the amount of good bacteria present, and all the mechanisms that have been eluded to for probiotics, e.g. prevention of colonization, release of antibiotic material, tightening of intracellular junctions, increasing IgA, are probably operational. It is very interesting to see that prebiotics actually are that effective because there was a study using prebiotics which was not all that effective and was reported in the *American Journal of Clinical Nutrition* [8]. The question I ask you is why not use mother's breast milk because it contains prebiotics, it can facilitate the same process and also has other protective factors. Therefore it is more protective.

Dr. Marini: We use a blend of GOS-FOS and, from the laboratory point of view, this blend was more effective in increasing the development of bifidobacteria [9]. Another question I would like to ask you is about the nucleotides that are present in human milk. Some people said that the nucleotides are good food for lactobacilli. What is your opinion about that?

Dr. Walker: I don't know that but I know that nucleotides have other effects, they augment the immune response and so forth. I reviewed a paper for *Pediatric Research* a couple of months ago where organisms isolated from babies with NEC were inoculated into germ-free quail. To me it was very impressive because there is no specific organism that causes NEC, but it underscores the principle that, in the absence of bacteria to balance the negative effect of pathogens, these animals develop NEC. Whereas if you take a conventional animal at the same age and provide that organism, it doesn't cause disease. We can learn a little bit from that observation. The studies showing that there was scarce colonization without the diversity you get with the full-term, vaginally delivered infant is another observation that we can learn from. Thus continue to use prebiotics, but I would favor mother's breast milk and also perhaps the use of probiotics.

Dr. Marini: If I remember well, 20 years ago a neonatologist from the United States said that good prevention of NEC is to give acid to a baby in order to increase gastric acidity, and it actually works.

Dr. Holt: There is increasing epidemiology showing isolation of a super antigen producing staphylococci which is something that is reasonably new. We know that these molecules have devastating effects on the immune system at the periphery, but what do we know about what they might do in the gastrointestinal tract, in particular how they bind?

Dr. Walker: I don't know, maybe Dr. Murch would know. I am aware that there are lots of questions that need to be answered and we need to go and look into this more carefully. Are you aware of any studies, Dr. Murch, on the super antigen in terms of the gut?

Dr. Murch: We used staphylococcal endotoxin in a human fetal organ culture model. Using an isolated loop of fetal intestine and administering endotoxin intraluminally, β-restricted polyclonal T-cell activation and enteropathy were induced, and thus it can potentially induce intolerance. There have been some studies in monkeys and dogs where endotoxin did not just cause diarrhea but also caused mucosal inflammation. At ESPGAN we presented a series of infants who had persistent small bowel enteropathy in response to toxin-producing staphylococci, toxins G and I. It begins to look as if these are potentially capable of inducing inflammatory reactions. The mucosal defenses in infants and all reported cases, under about 10 weeks old, are clearly less common. The family members just had a brief diarrheal illness. They are certainly capable of modulating host responses, and there is no literature on whether they play any kind of a role in initial priming.

Dr. Walker: In the last years we have published a number of articles [10, 11] suggesting that if a human fetus, anywhere between 12 and 18 weeks, is transplanted into the subcutaneous capsule of a SCID mouse, allowed to reepithelialize and revascularize, and then followed over an about 24-week period, and then the enzymes known to be expressed in the third trimester of pregnancy are measured, the gut of the premature infant can be reproduced in this model. We don't have the immune cells to study because this is a SCID mouse, but we can begin to study epithelial–microbial interaction. This technique answers questions that neonatologists need to know: e.g. do protective nutrients, prebiotics, or probiotics interfere?; can we affect bacterial interactions?, etc. Thus we have begun to get some answers that can be used for clinical trials.

References

1 Schiffrin EJ, Carter EA, Walker WA, et al: Influence of prenatal corticosteroids on bacterial colonization in the newborn rat. J Pediatr Gastroenterol Nutr 1993;17:271–275.

2 Yan F, Polk DB: Probiotic bacterium prevents cytokine-induced apoptosis in intestinal epithelial cells. J Biol Chem 2002;277:50959–50965.

3 Mack DR, Michail S, Wei S, et al: Probiotics inhibit enteropathogenic *E. coli* adherence in vitro by inducing intestinal mucin gene expression. Am J Physiol 1999;276:G941–G950.
4 Claud EC, Walker WA: Hypothesis: Inappropriate colonization of the premature intestine can cause neonatal necrotizing enterocolitis. FASEB J 2001;15:1398–1403.
5 Schrag SJ, Zell ER, Lynfield R, et al., Active Bacterial Core Surveillance Team: A population-based comparison of strategies to prevent early-onset group B streptococcal disease in neonates. N Engl J Med 2002;347:233–239.
6 Marini A, Negretti F, Boehm G, et al: Pro- and pre-biotics administration in preterm infants: Colonization and influence on fecal flora. Acta Paediatr 2003;(suppl 441):80–82.
7 Boehm G, Lidestri M Casetta P, et al: Supplementation of a bovine milk formula with an oligosaccharide mixture increases counts of fecal bifidobacteria in preterm infants. Arch Dis Child Fetal Neonatal Ed 2002;86:F178–F181.
8 Duggan C, Gannon J, Walker WA: Protective nutrients and functional foods for the gastrointestinal tract. Am J Clin Nutr 2002;75:789–808.
9 Boehm G, Lidestri M Jelinek J, et al: Effect of increasing number of intestinal bifidobacteria on the presence of clinically relevant pathogens (abstract 226A). Proc ESPGHAN Prague 2003.
10 Nanthakumar NN, Fusunyan RD, Sanderson I, Walker WA: Inflammation in the developing human intestine: A possible pathophysiologic contribution to necrotizing enterocolitis. Proc Natl Acad Sci USA 2000;97:6043–6048.
11 Nanthakumar NN, Klopcic CE, Fernandez I, WA Walker: Normal and glucocorticoid-induced development of the human small intestinal xenograft. Am J Physiol 2003;274:R1220–R1227.

Isolauri E, Walker WA (eds): Allergic Diseases and the Environment.
Nestlé Nutrition Workshop Series Pediatric Program, Vol. 53, pp. 179–198,
Nestec Ltd.; Vevey/S. Karger AG, Basel, © 2004.

Human Colonic Microbes: Ecology, Physiology and Metabolic Potential of Intestinal Bacteria

George T. Macfarlane and Sandra Macfarlane

University of Dundee, MRC Microbiology and Gut Biology Group, Department of Molecular and Cellular Pathology, Ninewells Hospital Medical School, Dundee, UK

Introduction

Humans live in close association with vast numbers of microorganisms that are present on the skin, in the mouth and in the genital and gastrointestinal tracts. In many cases, an intimate relationship exists between the host and its microflora that has developed as humans as a species have evolved. The best example of this is the complex assemblage of bacteria that constitutes the microbiota of the large intestine. Although fecal bacteria were first observed microscopically more than 300 years ago, the sheer scale of colonization of the lower intestinal tract by microorganisms was not appreciated until relatively recently. Savage [1] observed that while there are approximately 10^{14} cells associated with the human body, 90% of these are microorganisms, the majority of which reside in the colon. Viewed in another way, at any given time, 1 g of large intestinal contents contains about 150 times more bacteria than there are people on earth. Perhaps not surprisingly, therefore, the metabolic potential of the human colonic microflora is formidable, and because it plays an important role in digestion, and in many other aspects of host physiology and metabolism, it is tempting to view the microbiota as an organ in their own right.

The Upper Gut

In healthy individuals living in Western countries, viable bacterial counts progressively increase from the proximal to the distal small bowel. In the upper small gut, viable bacterial counts are usually less than 10^4/ml, and consist mainly of gram-positive facultative anaerobes and aerotolerant species such as streptococci, staphylococci and lactobacilli. Gastric acid is important in restricting entry of bacteria to the small intestine, while rapid peristaltic movements and transit of digesta through this part of the digestive tract (2–4 h) does not allow time for stable bacterial communities to establish [2]. Bacteria are also found in the biliary tract, particularly aerobes and facultative anaerobes. Although few bacteria can be recovered from the duodenum, jejunum and upper ileum, stasis of digestive material at the ileocecal valve results in a qualitative and quantitative increase in bacterial numbers [3, 4], and anaerobes increase, as pH and redox potential drop. Small bowel overgrowth can occur as a result of disorders in gut motility, achlorhydria, drugs, antibiotic treatment, radiation therapy, cirrhosis, strictures, diverticulae and small bowel resection.

The Large Gut: Physiologic and Anatomical Characteristics

In persons living in Western countries, the main area of permanent colonization of the gastrointestinal tract is the large bowel. The main reason for this is that the flow of material through the gastrointestinal tract slows markedly, providing time for stable bacterial populations to develop. Large intestinal transit times vary considerably between individuals, but usually range from about 20 to 120 h, with a mean of about 60 h [5].

The colon is an open system in the sense that food residues from the small bowel enter at one end, and feces are excreted at the other. The adult large gut is typically over 1 m in length, with an internal surface area in the region of 1,300 cm^2, and a total volume of about 500 ml. Fecal excretion in persons living in industrialized Western communities is approximately 120 g/day, but fecal output in Third World and other underdeveloped countries is considerably higher. Although feces are mainly water, bacteria are a major component, comprising 55% of fecal solids [6].

From anatomic, microbiological and environmental perspectives, the proximal bowel (cecum, ascending colon) and distal gut (descending colon, sigmoid/rectum) are quite different from each other. When digestive residues from the ileum enter the cecum, they encounter a pool of partially digested foodstuffs and bacteria, which rapidly begin to utilize simple carbon and nitrogen sources, and initiate the breakdown of complex carbohydrates and proteins. Due to production of fermentation acids, pH is reduced to about 5.5 or less in the proximal colon [7]. Due to high levels of substrate availability, the cecum and ascending colon are sites of the most intense microbial activity in the gut, but because of substrate utilization and water absorption, bacterial cell population densities increase distally through the colon [8].

Interactions with the Host

The microbiota play an important role in establishing and maintaining normal gut structure and function. Bacteria interact with the intestine in many ways, for example, bacterial cell mass stimulates peristaltic movement, thereby facilitating the passage of digestive residues through the bowel, while studies with germ-free animals indicate that small intestinal uptake of sugars, amino acids, minerals and vitamins is more efficient than in animals with a conventional microflora [9]. The role of bacterial metabolites in providing fuels for the colonic epithelium will be discussed later, but the influence of the microbiota on gut structure is seen in germ-free rodents, where the cecum is greatly distended, while lymphoid tissue and the lamina propria are atrophied. The cecal mucosa is also thinner than in normal animals, and gross alterations in cellular morphology are evident [10].

Host Defenses

While there is evidence that bacteria can translocate from the colon into portal blood and the liver, the invasion of body tissues by colonic organisms is prevented by a number of host and microbiological controls. The peristaltic action of the gut, pH of contents in the stomach and cecum, bacterial metabolites, bile salts, mucous layers and gastrointestinal epithelia, as well as host immune processes, all serve in one way or another to protect the host. In general, bacteria can only pass through the gut wall when its permeability is increased or its integrity compromised.

Mucins are high molecular mass glycoproteins secreted by cells lining the digestive tract, and they are amongst the most important host defenses. In the colon, mucus is secreted by goblet cells in the epithelium, forming a viscoelastic gel covering the gut surface. It acts as a physical barrier against luminal bacteria and many of their toxins and secretory products. Antigen–antibody complexes stimulate secretion of mucus, which anchors secreted antibody onto enterocytes, where antigens may be bound and subsequently degraded by adsorbed pancreatic and bacterial peptidases. This may be important in preventing internalization of antigens. Because many microorganisms in the large bowel degrade mucus, the colonic epithelium needs to produce glycoprotein at a faster rate than the bacteria can break it down, and a balance must therefore exist between mucin production and its destruction by the microbiota.

Host immune processes probably have little effect on ecologic events in the colonic lumen. However, interactions between intestinal bacteria and the immune system occur at the mucosal surface, and full structural and developmental expression of the intestinal immune system depends on continued exposure to bacterial antigens from the gut lumen.

Ecology

The vast majority of microorganisms in the healthy large intestine are bacteria. Yeasts are sometimes detected in low numbers, but protozoa are seldom found. While some gram-negative species occur in high numbers in the gut, the predominant organisms in the large bowel appear to be gram-positive anaerobic rods and cocci [11]. Several hundred different bacterial species and strains have been isolated from fecal material [12], but surprisingly little is known of the metabolic interactions that occur between different groups of microorganisms in the large gut, or of the ecology and multicellular organization of the microbiota as a whole. While culturing studies have shown that the ecosystem contains large numbers of phylogenetically and physiologically distinct microorganisms, molecular analysis of the microflora indicates that many intestinal bacteria are not being cultured [13]. Indeed, it is thought that only about 40% of the bacteria in the human large bowel are culturable [14].

Bacterial species diversity in the gut largely derives from the multiplicity of different carbon and energy sources available for growth, and the principal host factors regulating the microbiota in health are probably substrate availability and colonic transit time. Moreover, competition (e.g. for nutrients or space) and cooperative interactions (e.g. polymer breakdown) between individual groups of bacteria are also important in defining community structure in the microbiota.

The microbiota is a stable and immensely complex entity, which is to a large extent self-regulating. Although many microorganisms are able to infect the gastrointestinal tract, through competitive exclusion, indigenous species afford a degree of protection to the host by acting as a barrier to invading pathogens; however, the effectiveness of this process is frequently diminished during illness, or by antibiotic treatment [15].

The Gut Microbiota and Resistance to Disease

Many different types of microorganism including bacteria, viruses, fungi and protozoa are agents of disease in the gastrointestinal tract. Bacteria indigenous to the colon play an important role in preventing colonization of the gut by pathogenic organisms. Studies with germ-free or antibiotic-treated animals illustrate the protective effects of indigenous bacteria, since these animals are more susceptible to salmonella, campylobacter and shigella infections. Moreover, colonization of the gut by anaerobic pathogens such as *Clostridium difficile*, the primary etiologic agent of pseudomembranous colitis, and possibly, *Clostridium botulinum*, is prevented by normal gut microbiota. The barrier effects exerted by indigenous bacteria have also been demonstrated in human studies in which patients with pseudomembranous colitis and ulcerative colitis have been treated, to some effect, with rectal enemas containing slurries of feces from healthy donors [16].

The significance of colonization resistance to pathogens is sometimes seen in patients undergoing antibiotic therapy, which can have serious side effects on the gut microbiota, and the inadvertent removal of protective species may allow invaders to establish, as in pseudomembranous colitis [17, 18]. Clindamycin, tetracycline, chloramphenicol, and orally administered ampicillin have been associated with the onset of this disease [19]. Other pathogens may also establish during antibiotic treatment, including enterotoxigenic *Clostridium perfringens*, while overgrowth of facultative anaerobes such as yeasts, enterobacteria and pseudomonads may also be seen.

Biofilms in the Large Gut

Intestinal microorganisms occupy many different microhabitats and metabolic niches on the mucosa, in the mucous layer and on the surfaces of food residues in the colonic lumen [20]. These microcosms are continuously in a dynamic state of change, as resources are consumed or recycled. Intestinal bacteria are unlikely to exist as individuals in the gut, and probably occur in microcolonies, in complex associations with other species. Particle-associated and mucosal bacterial populations are likely to be components of highly evolved assemblages, analogous to those in oral biofilm communities [21]. Close spatial relationships between bacterial cells growing in gut biofilms may be important in relation to metabolic communication between microorganisms in the microbiota. Their ecological significance is that they reduce potential growth-limiting effects on bacterial cross-feeding populations, such as those involving mass transfer resistance [22]. Another characteristic of bacterial biofilms in the large bowel is that species colonizing surfaces in the gut lumen are directly involved in the digestion of complex insoluble polymeric substances, imparting a significant competitive advantage in the ecosystem [23].

Physiology

Growth Substrates and Nutrition of Intestinal Bacteria

Large intestinal microorganisms exist by digesting dietary residues (mainly carbohydrates and proteins) and a range of other substrates that are produced by the body itself. The anaerobic breakdown of organic matter in the colon is termed fermentation. Bacteria gain energy, carbon and nitrogen for cell growth from fermentation, and produce a variety of waste products, that are absorbed from the gut, and which are often of physiological importance to the host.

Carbohydrate Breakdown

Pancreatic amylase is the only polysaccharide-degrading enzyme secreted into the digestive tract in humans, despite this, starch is the most important dietary carbohydrate to reach the colon [24]. Evidence that this polymer is incompletely digested in the small gut comes from several sources, including intubation, breath hydrogen and ileostomy studies. For a variety of reasons, several types of starch are resistant to pancreatic amylase, but they are hydrolyzed by bacterial amylases in the large bowel. The other major group of complex carbohydrates fermented by colonic bacteria are the non-starch polysaccharides, or dietary fiber. They are structural components of plant cell walls, and include cellulose, hemicelluloses, pectins, inulin and various gums. They are not digested by mammalian enzymes, but intestinal bacteria produce an extensive range of polysaccharidases and glycosidases that degrade these polymers and make their constituent monomers available for fermentation [25]. Microbiologically, breakdown of complex polysaccharides in the colon is both a cooperative and competitive process, involving many different groups of organisms; however, bacteria belonging to the genera bacteroides and bifidobacterium seem to play a key role in depolymerization of these substrates [26–28]. Although dependent on diet and host intestinal transit time, fermentable carbohydrate is often limiting in the distal large bowel, due to its utilization by bacteria in the proximal gut. This has important consequences for the host, because the digestion of complex carbohydrates is a beneficial process in the large bowel that reduces the formation of putrefactive metabolites [29, 30].

Proteolysis

Unlike carbohydrate availability, there is no shortage of proteins and peptides in the distal large bowel [31]. It is estimated that between 3 and 25 g of these substances enter the colon every day [32–34], partly in the form of dietary residues (e.g. plant, sarcoplasmic and myofibrillar muscle proteins), although a significant proportion comes from the host's upper gastrointestinal tract. The large intestine is also a source of proteins, such as bacterial secretions and lysis products, colonic mucins and desquamated mucosal cells [35]. However, in quantitative terms, hydrolytic enzymes elaborated by exocrine cells of the pancreas, including proteases (trypsin, chymotrypsin, elastase), lipases, amylase and nucleic acid hydrolases are amongst the most important sources of protein in the large bowel [36].

The human large intestine is one of the most proteolytic natural environments known. Measurements of protease activity in small intestinal contents and in material taken from the proximal and distal colons show that proteolysis progressively declines as digestive materials move through the gut [37]. This occurs because pancreatic proteins are broken down by bacteria in the large bowel, while host antiproteases inhibit pancreatic endopeptidases in the gut [38, 39]. The role of bacteria in degrading these enzymes is shown in animal studies, where pancreatic protease activities are considerably higher in the feces of germ-free rats compared with conventional animals [40]. In humans, fecal trypsin increased 100-fold in patients treated with antibiotics, although chymotrypsin and elastase activities were only 2–3 times higher [38]. Pancreatic endopeptidases probably undergo autodigestion in the colon, and there may be synergistic effects with bacterial proteases [37, 41].

Fermentation

Anaerobic chemoheterotrophic populations in the colon include organisms that carry out anaerobic respiration, as well as fermentative bacteria, that produce adenosine triphosphate (ATP) through substrate level phosphorylation reactions. Fermentative bacteria predominate in the gut. In fermentation, the electron acceptors are metabolic products derived from the original substrate, consequently fermentation reactions are self-balancing, with the redox differential between substrates and products determining the amount of energy that can be produced. Compared to oxidative metabolism, fermentations are energetically inefficient processes that give low ATP yields. Large amounts of substrate are therefore required for growth in fermentative bacteria, which results in large quantities of metabolic end-products being formed. Fermentations are governed by the need to maintain redox balance, mainly by the reduction and oxidation of ferredoxins, flavins and pyridine nucleotides. This affects the flow of carbon through bacteria, the energy yield obtained from the substrate, and the metabolic end-products. Short-chain fatty acids (SCFAs) are the main fermentation products produced in the large intestine, while formation of reduced substances such as hydrogen gas, lactate, succinate, butyrate and ethanol is used to effect redox balance [42].

SCFAs

Acetate, propionate and butyrate are the principal products of carbohydrate and protein fermentation in the large bowel [42]. The vast majority of SCFAs (>95%) formed by gut microorganisms are absorbed and metabolized by the host [43]. This allows salvage of energy from food that is not digested in the upper gastrointestinal tract, and can account for up to 9% of the hosts energy requirements [44]. SCFAs have a wide range of physiological functions in the body, including colonocyte metabolism [45], cell growth and differentiation [46], epithelial cell transport [47], metabolism of lipids and carbohydrates in the liver [48], intestinal motility [49], as well as energy generation in muscle, kidney, heart and brain [50]. SCFAs also inhibit phagocytic cell function [51, 52]. Butyrate is believed to be protective against colon cancer, and has been shown to arrest cell growth early in G1 and induce cell differentiation, while stimulating cytoskeletal organization and alterations in gene expression [53–56]. The arrest of cell growth by butyrate is associated with differentiation which occurs in many human cell lines. Butyrate modulates the expression of many different genes and differentiation in tumor cells, and is linked to changes in their cytoskeletal architecture and adhesion properties [57].

Gas Production

Gas is a major product of carbohydrate and protein fermentation in the large bowel. Gas formation is diet-related, but the total amount formed each day can amount to as much as 4 liters. Foodstuffs such as beans, brussels sprouts, some fruit juices and some types of soluble dietary fiber can generate large amounts of fermentation gases, principally, hydrogen, carbon dioxide, and in some individuals, methane. Approximately 80% of fermentation gas produced in the large intestine is excreted as flatus, where the major gases are nitrogen (64%), hydrogen (19%) and carbon dioxide (14%) [58]. Nevertheless, considerable variation occurs, and between 10 and 20% of colonic gas is absorbed and excreted in the breath [24, 50]. A significant amount of hydrogen produced in the colon is sequestered by specialized groups of bacteria to produce either methane (methanogenesis), hydrogen sulfide (dissimilatory sulfate reduction) or acetate (acetogenesis). The organisms involved derive energy from these processes, and they can occur in high numbers in the large bowel [42]. By reducing the partial pressure of hydrogen in the gut, hydrogenotrophic species have important ecologic and physiologic roles in the microbiota [42, 59, 60].

Metabolic Potential

Products of Putrefaction

Not all of the metabolic activities of intestinal microorganisms are benign. The absorptive capacity of the large intestine is considerable, and many bacterial metabolites are toxic to host tissues, particularly those resulting from protein breakdown and amino acid fermentation, such as ammonia, amines, phenols and indoles [36]. Moreover, several sulfur-containing organic compounds are formed by anaerobic bacteria from the S-containing amino acids methionine and cysteine. Methanethiol and mercaptoacetate, in particular, are strong reducing agents that are toxic to isolated colonocytes in vitro [61]. Normally the products of protein digestion are detoxified in the mucosa and liver, by sulfate or glucuronide conjugation, but in some circumstances, their production in the large intestine exceeds the body's abilities to effect their disposal.

Ammonia

Fecal ammonia concentrations range from about 3 to 44 m*M* [62], and in the large bowel, concentrations of this metabolite increase distally through the gut, but this is not as marked as with other products of amino acid fermentation, particularly phenols and branched chain fatty acids. It is still unclear how much ammonia results from urea hydrolysis; however, studies in which human volunteers were infused with ^{15}N-labeled urea indicated that most ammonia in the gut results from deamination of amino acids [63]. The physiologic significance of ammonia formation is that low concentrations (<10 m*M*) can alter the morphology and intermediary metabolism of intestinal cells, while increasing DNA synthesis and reducing their lifespan [64].

Amines

Amines are major products of dissimilatory amino acid metabolism in the gut, and their excretion in urine is directly related to protein intake. Histamine, piperidine, pyrrolidine, cadaverine, putrescine, agmatine, tyramine, 5-hydroxytryptamine, methylamine, dimethylamine and propylamine are all produced by gut microorganisms, and are rapidly absorbed from the bowel, whence they are detoxified by mucosal and liver monoamine and diamine oxidases. However, hypertensive symptoms and migraine have been linked to amines produced in the large gut [36]. Many of these metabolites such as histamine, putrescine, tyramine and cadaverine are pharmacologically active, variously functioning as pressor or depressor substances, and as stimulators of gastric secretion or vasodilators [65]. Amine formation in the large bowel is therefore important because of the pervasive effects of these metabolites on different organ systems in the body.

Phenols and Indoles

The abilities of bacteria to produce phenolic and indolic metabolites is widespread in the colonic microbiota. These products of aromatic amino acid metabolism are formed in a series of deamination, transamination, decarboxylation and dehydrogenation reactions [29]. Levels of tyrosine breakdown products, such as phenol and *p*-cresol, increase markedly in the distal bowel, further showing that protein breakdown becomes more significant in this region of the gut. After absorption from the gut, phenols and indoles are detoxified and excreted from the body as sulfate or glucuronide conjugates. Little is known of the physiologic and environmental factors that control aromatic amino acid metabolism in the large intestine, but long colonic transit times result in reduced carbohydrate availability and more protein breakdown in the distal bowel. This was seen in feeding studies with human volunteers, where phenol excretion was related to both carbohydrate and protein intake, and where increasing the availability of fermentable carbohydrate reduced phenol formation due to saccharolytic bacteria sequestering tyrosine for biosynthetic purposes [66].

Phenols and indoles have been linked to cancer [67], but they also have other effects on host physiology. For example, the tryptophan metabolite skatole is associated with malabsorption, anemia and schizophrenia [68, 69]. In some animals, skatole causes tryptophan-induced acute bovine pulmonary emphysema, whereas in weanling pigs, *p*-cresol acts as a growth depressant [69, 70].

Hydrogen Sulfide

Dissimilatory sulfate reduction is an important route of hydrogen disposal in the large gut [71]. Sulfate-reducing bacteria (SRB) use sulfate as a terminal electron acceptor in metabolism, producing hydrogen sulfide, which is normally detoxified by the colonic mucosa. SRB can out-compete other

Table 1. Biochemical activities of gut microorganisms that affect host metabolism

Activity	Examples	Effect on host
Metabolism of neutral steroids	Chemical modification of steroid hormones, cholesterol and plant sterols	Reduction of cholesterol to coprostanol and coprostanone Reabsorption and recycling of reduced corticosteroids, progesterone, estrogens Possible role in breast cancer
Bile acid metabolism	Deconjugation and dehydroxylation of bile acids, desulfation of bile acid sulfates	Absorption of secondary bile acids Possible promoting activity in colon cancer
Detoxication of mutagens	N-Dehydroxylation of N-hydroxyacetyl-aminofluorene Reduction of nitropyrene to its less toxic derivative aminopyrene Breakdown of N-nitroso compounds such as diphenylnitrosamine, nitrosopyrrolidine, dimethylnitrosamine	Protective
Transformations of xenobiotics	Activation/inactivation of drugs Exemplified by conversion of the drug sulfasalazine to the active form, 5-aminosalicylic acid, which is used in treatment of inflammatory bowel disease. Release of cyanide from amygdalin. Desulfation and deconjugation of drugs excreted in bile	Prolonged enterohepatic circulation of foreign compounds Direct toxic effects on body tissues
Lignan and phytoestrogen metabolism	Substances occur naturally in some plants. Conversion to enterodiol, enterolactone and equol	These compounds have estrogenic and anti-estrogenic effects. May affect fertility and breast cancer

Table 2. Formation of genotoxic, mutagenic or carcinogenic agents, and precursor compounds by the colonic microbes

Toxic compound or precursor molecule	Metabolic significance
Fecapentaenes	Plasmalogens (polyunsaturated ether lipids) are converted to mutagenic fecapentaenes by some bacteroides
Diacylglycerol	Metabolism of phosphatidylcholine (dietary lipid) in conjunction with bile acids
Azo compounds	Azo dyes used as food colorings. Other azo compounds used in pharmaceuticals and cosmetics. Mutagenic and possibly carcinogenic after chemical reduction to primary aromatic amines by intestinal anaerobes
Secondary bile acids	Toxic, co-mutagenic and co-carcinogenic activities. Formed by breakdown of glycine and taurine conjugates by bacterial hydrolases, 7 α-dehydroxylation and other reactions
Nitrated polycyclic aromatic hydrocarbons (nitro-PAHs)	Toxic, mutagenic and carcinogenic in laboratory animals. Toxicity usually results from reduction of a nitro group on heterocyclic and aromatic nitrocompounds to an amine group by bacterial nitroreductase
Cholesterol metabolites	Bind to DNA in vitro. Bacterial catalytic mechanisms unclear. Cholesterol α-epoxide is tumorigenic in animals
Various plant glycosides	Toxic aglycones produced by bacterial glycosidase activity towards glycoside conjugates, e.g. hydrolysis of cycasin by β-glucosidase to release the carcinogen methylazoxymethanol
	Others include potentially mutagenic hydroxylated anthraquinones found in a number of plants, including rhubarb
Phenolic compounds	Possible co-carcinogens formed by metabolism of tyrosine
Indoles	Bladder co-carcinogen produced from tryptophan. Other metabolites of this amino acid reported to be genotoxic
Ammonia	Formed by amino acid fermentation. Affects DNA synthesis and reduces lifespan of colonic epithelial cells. More toxic to normal than transformed cells. May select for neoplastic growth
Amines	Mainly result from decarboxylation of amino acids and N-dealkylation of choline
N-Nitroso compounds	Produced by condensation of nitrite with a secondary amine (e.g. dimethylamine piperidine) or tertiary amine

hydrogenotrophic microorganisms in the colon for hydrogen, and people who have high numbers of SRB in their gut usually have low numbers of methanogenic archae [60]. Sulfate availability strongly affects the outcome of competition because most SRB have an obligate growth requirement for inorganic S-containing electron acceptors. SRB are not able to breakdown proteins and carbohydrates by themselves, and have an obligate dependence on other bacteria in the microbiota to produce substrates for their growth. However, hydrogen consumption by SRB can have profound effects on fermentation processes, by increasing acetate formation and lowering the production of electron sinks and other reduced metabolites [72].

Production of Genotoxic Substances

The gut microbiota displays considerable metabolic potential and diversity, in addition to its activities in relation to carbohydrate and protein metabolism (table 1). Bacteria in the colon deconjugate bile acids and modify steroids, which affects their enterohepatic circulation. In addition, intestinal microorganisms are able to chemically transform drugs and other xenobiotic compounds [73], as well as producing and detoxifying mutagenic and carcinogenic substances. There is also strong evidence for their involvement in the etiology of colon cancer (table 2). The colon is the second commonest site of cancer in humans, and this disease is a major source of morbidity and mortality in developed countries [74]. The Ames test indicates that feces from many individuals in Western populations are mutagenic [75], and there is a good correlation between the excretion of fecal mutagens and large bowel cancer. Although there is no general agreement concerning the etiology of colon cancer, a number of factors have been implicated, such as diet, the environment and genetics. The gut microbiota clearly has a role in the initiation of these diseases, possibly by converting nontoxic precursor compounds to substances with mutagenic or carcinogenic potential (table 2). A number of bacterial enzymes are thought to be involved in activating mutagens, including β-glucosidase, β-glucuronidase, azoreductase and nitroreductase [76]. They have been extensively studied in relation to diet, and the results have shown that high levels of meat and fat increase their synthesis by the bacteria. However, it is not clear whether this by itself leads to an increased cancer risk.

References

1 Savage DC: Microbial ecology of the gastrointestinal tract. Annu Rev Microbiol 1977;31: 107–133.
2 Gorbach SL: Population control in the small bowel. Gut 1967;8:530–532.
3 Borriello SP: Microflora of the gastrointestinal tract; in Hill MJ (ed): Microbial Metabolism in the Digestive Tract. Boca Raton, CRC Press, 1986, pp 1–19.
4 Cummings JH, Macfarlane GT, Drasar BS: The gut microflora and its significance; in Whitehead R (ed): Gastrointestinal and Oesophageal Pathology, ed 1. Edinburgh, Churchill Livingstone, 1992, pp 201–219.

5 Cummings JH, Bingham SA, Heaton KW, Eastwood MA: Fecal weight, colon cancer risk, and dietary intake of nonstarch polysaccharides (dietary fiber). Gastroenterology 1992;103: 1783–1789.
6 Stephen AM, Cummings JH: The microbial contribution to human faecal mass. J Med Microbiol 1980;13:45–56.
7 Cummings JH, Pomare EW, Branch WJ, et al: Short chain fatty acids in human large intestine, portal, hepatic and venous blood. Gut 1987;28:1221–1227.
8 Macfarlane GT, Gibson GR, Drasar BS, Cummings JH: Metabolic significance of the colonic microflora; in Whitehead R (ed): Gastrointestinal and Oesophageal Physiology. Edinburgh, Churchill Livingstone, 1995, pp 249–274.
9 Abrams GD: Impact of the intestinal microflora on intestinal structure and function; in Hentges DJ (ed): Human Intestinal Microflora in Health and Disease. New York, Academic Press, 1983, pp 291–310.
10 Norin E, Midtvedt T: Interactions of bacteria with the host. Microb Ecol Health Dis 2000; (suppl 2):186–193.
11 Holdeman LV, Cato EP, Moore WEC (eds): Anaerobic Laboratory Manual, ed 4. Blacksburg, Virginia Polytechnic Institute Anaerobe Laboratory, 1977.
12 Finegold SM, Sutter VL, Mathisen GE: Normal indigenous intestinal flora; in Hentges DJ (ed): Human Intestinal Microflora in Health and Disease. New York, Academic Press, 1983, pp 3–31.
13 Hold GL, Pryde SE, Russell VJ, et al: Assessment of microbial diversity in human colonic samples by 16S rDNA sequence analysis. FEMS Microbiol Ecol 2002;39:33–39.
14 Wilson KH: Molecular phylogeny of the human colon: An ecological approach to nosocomial diseases. Biosci Micro 1997;16:22.
15 Tannock GW: Modification of the normal by diet, stress, antimicrobial agents, and probiotics; in Mackie RL, White BA, Isaacson RE (eds): Gastrointestinal Microbiology. New York, Chapman & Hall, 1995, vol 2, pp 434–456.
16 Bennet JD, Brinkman M: Treatment of ulcerative colitis with implantation of normal colonic microflora. Lancet 1989;I:164.
17 Tedesco FJ: Clindamycin-associated colitis. Review of the clinical spectrum of 47 cases. Dig Dis 1976;21:26–32.
18 Cohen MB, Giannella RA: Bacterial infections: pathophysiology, clinical features and treatment; in Phillips SF, Pemberton JH, Shorter RG (eds): The Large Intestine: Physiology, Pathophysiology and Disease. New York, Raven Press, 1991, pp 395–428.
19 Bartlett JG: Pseudomembranous colitis; in Hentges DJ (ed): Human Intestinal Microflora in Health and Disease. New York, Academic Press, 1983, pp 447–479.
20 Macfarlane S, Cummings JH, Macfarlane GT: Bacterial colonisation of surfaces in the large intestine; in Gibson GR, Roberfroid M (eds): Colonic Microflora, Nutrition and Health. London, Chapman & Hall, 1999, pp 71–87.
21 Kolenbrander PE: Surface recognition among oral bacteria: Multigeneric coaggregations and their mediators. Crit Rev Microbiol 1989;17:37–59.
22 Conrad R, Phelps TJ, Zeikus JG: Gas metabolism evidence in support of the juxtaposition of hydrogen-producing and methanogenic bacteria in sewage sludge and lake sediments. Appl Environ Microbiol 1985;50:595–601.
23 Macfarlane S, McBain AJ, Macfarlane GT: Consequences of biofilm and sessile growth in the large intestine. Adv Dent Res 1997;11:59–68.
24 Macfarlane GT, Cummings JH: The colonic flora, fermentation and large bowel digestive function; in Philips SF, Pemberton JH, Shorter RG (eds): The Large Intestine: Physiology, Pathophysiology and Disease. New York, Raven Press, 1991, pp 51–92.
25 Englyst HN, Hay S, Macfarlane GT: Polysaccharide breakdown by mixed populations of human faecal bacteria. FEMS Microbiol Ecol 1987;95:163–171.
26 Salyers AA, Leedle JAZ: Carbohydrate metabolism in the human colon; in Hentges DJ (ed): Human Intestinal Microflora in Health and Disease. New York, Academic Press, 1983, pp 129–146.
27 Macfarlane GT, Macfarlane S, Gibson GR: Co-culture of *Bifidobacterium adolescentis* and *Bacteroides thetaiotaomicron* in arabinogalactan-limited chemostats: Effects of dilution rate and pH. Anaerobe 1995;1:275–281.
28 Degnan BA, Macfarlane GT: Arabinogalactan utilization in continuous cultures of *Bifidobacterium longum*: Effect of co-culture with *Bacteroides thetaiotaomicron*. Anaerobe 1995;1:103–112.

29 Smith EA, Macfarlane GT: Enumeration of human colonic bacteria producing phenolic and indolic compounds: Effects of pH, carbohydrate availability and retention time on dissimilatory aromatic amino acid metabolism. J Appl Bacteriol 1996;81:288–302.
30 Smith EA, Macfarlane GT: Studies on amine production in the human colon: Enumeration of amine forming bacteria and physiological effects of carbohydrate and pH. Anaerobe 1996;2:285–297.
31 Smith EA, Macfarlane GT: Enumeration of amino acid fermenting bacteria in the human large intestine: Effects of pH and starch on peptide metabolism and dissimilation of amino acids. FEMS Microbiol Ecol 1998;25:355–368.
32 Gibson JA, Sladen GE, Dawson AM: Protein absorption and ammonia production: The effects of dietary protein and removal of the colon. Br J Nutr 1976;35:61–65.
33 Chacko A, Cummings JH: Nitrogen losses from the human small bowel: Obligatory losses and the effect of physical form of food. Gut 1998;29:809–815.
34 Wrong OM: Bacterial metabolism of protein and endogenous nitrogen compounds; in Rowland IR (ed): Role of the Gut Flora in Toxicity and Cancer. New York, Academic Press, 1988, pp 227–262.
35 Christensen J: Gross and microscopic anatomy of the large intestine; in Phillips SF, Pemberton JH, Shorter RG (eds): The Large Intestine: Physiology, Pathophysiology and Disease. New York, Raven Press, 1991, pp 13–35.
36 Macfarlane S, Macfarlane GT: Proteolysis and amino acid fermentation; in Gibson GR, Macfarlane GT (eds): Human Colonic Bacteria: Role in Nutrition, Physiology and Pathology. Boca Raton, CRC Press, 1995, pp 75–100.
37 Macfarlane GT, Cummings JH, Macfarlane S, Gibson GR: Influence of retention time on degradation of pancreatic enzymes by human colonic bacteria grown in a 3-stage continuous culture system. J Appl Bacteriol 1989;67:521–527.
38 Bohe M, Genell S, Ohlsson K: Protease inhibitors in plasma and faecal extracts from patients with active inflammatory bowel disease. Scand J Gastroenterol 1986;21:598–604.
39 Catassi C, Cardinalli E, D'Angelo G, et al: Reliability of random fecal α_1-antitrypsin determination on non dried stools. J Pediatr 1986;109:500–502.
40 Genell S, Gustafsson BE, Ohlsson K: Immunochemical quantitation of pancreatic endopeptidases in the intestinal contents of germfree and conventional rats. Scand J Gastroenterol 1978;12:811–814.
41 Macfarlane GT, Macfarlane S: Utilization of pancreatic trypsin and chymotrypsin by proteolytic and non-proteolytic *Bacteroides fragilis*-type bacteria. Curr Microbiol 1991; 23:143–148.
42 Macfarlane GT, Gibson GR: Microbiological aspects of short chain fatty acid production in the large bowel; in Cummings JH, Rombeau JL, Sakata T (eds): Physiological and Clinical Aspects of Short Chain Fatty Acid Metabolism. Cambridge, Cambridge University Press, 1995, pp 87–105.
43 Cummings JH: Short chain fatty acids; in Gibson GR, Macfarlane GT (eds): Human Colonic Bacteria: Role in Nutrition, Physiology and Pathology. Boca Raton, CRC Press, 1995, pp 101–130.
44 Hume ID: Flow dynamics of digesta and colonic fermentation; in Cummings JH, Rombeau JL, Sakata T (eds): Physiological and Clinical Aspects of Short Chain Fatty Acid Metabolism. Cambridge, Cambridge University Press, 1995, pp 119–132.
45 Roediger WEW: Role of anaerobic bacteria in the metabolic welfare of the colonic mucosa of man. Gut 1980;21:793–798.
46 deFazio A, Chiew Y-E, Donoghue C, et al: Effect of sodium butyrate on estrogen receptor and epidermal growth factor receptor gene expression in human breast cancer cell lines. J Biol Chem 1992;267:18008–18012.
47 del Castillo JR, Muniz R, Sulbaran-Carrasco MC, Pekerar S: Cellular metabolism of colonocytes; in Binder HJ, Cummings JH, Soergel KH (eds): Short Chain Fatty Acids. London, Kluwer Academic, 1994, pp 180–191.
48 Demigne C, Remesey C: Short chain fatty acids and hepatic metabolism; in Binder HJ, Cummings JH, Soergel KH (eds): Short Chain Fatty Acids. London, Kluwer Academic, 1994, pp 272–282.
49 Cherbut C, Blottiere H, Kaeffer B, Galmiche JP: Short-chain fatty acids: A luminal modulatory signal for gastrointestinal motility; in Malkki Y, Cummings JH (eds): Dietary Fibre and Fermentation in the Colon. Brussels, European Commission, 1996, pp 203–208.

50 Cummings JH, Macfarlane GT: The control and consequences of bacterial fermentation in the human colon. J Appl Bacteriol 1991;70:443–459.
51 Eftimiadi C, Tonetti M, Cavallero A, et al: Short-chain fatty acids produced by anaerobic bacteria inhibit phagocytosis by human lung macrophages. J Infect Dis 1990;161:138–142.
52 Tonetti M, Cavallero A, Botta GA, et al: Intracellular pH regulates the production of different oxygen metabolites in neutrophils: Effects of organic acids produced by anaerobic bacteria. J Leuk Biol 1991;49:180–188.
53 Prasad KN, Sinha PK: Effect of sodium butyrate on mammalian cells in culture: A review. In Vitro 1976;12:125–132.
54 Kruh J: Effects of sodium butyrate, a new pharmacological agent, on cells in culture. Mol Cell Biochem 1980;42:65–82.
55 Fregeau CJ, Helgason CD, Bleackley RC: Two cytotoxic cell proteinase genes are differentially sensitive to sodium butyrate. Nucleic Acids Res 1992;20:3113–3119.
56 Hague A, Elder DJE, Hicks DJ, Paraskeva C: Apoptosis in colorectal tumour cells: Induction by the short chain fatty acids butyrate, propionate and acetate and by the bile salt deoxycholate. Int J Cancer 1995;60:400–406.
57 Wilson JR, Weiser MM: Colonic cancer cell (HT29) adhesion to laminin is altered by differentiation: Adhesion may involve galactosyltransferase. Exp Cell Res 1992;201:330–334.
58 Macfarlane GT, Cummings JH: Diet and the metabolism of intestinal bacteria; in Brostoff J, Challacombe SJ, Kniker WT (eds): Food Allergy and Intolerance, ed 2. London, Saunders, 2002, pp 321–343.
59 Macfarlane GT, Gibson GR, Cummings JH: Comparison of fermentation reactions in different regions of the human colon. J Appl Bacteriol 1992;72:57–64.
60 Gibson GR, Macfarlane S, Macfarlane GT: Metabolic interactions involving sulphate-reducing and methanogenic bacteria in the human large intestine. FEMS Microbiol Ecol 1993;12:117–125.
61 Roediger WEW, Duncan A, Kapaniris O, Millard S: Reducing sulfur compounds of the colon impair colonocyte nutrition: Implications for ulcerative colitis. Gastroenterology 1993; 104:802–809.
62 Macfarlane GT, Cummings JH, Allison C: Protein degradation by human intestinal bacteria. J Gen Microbiol 1986;132:1647–1656.
63 Wrong OM, Vince AJ, Waterlow JC: The contribution of endogenous urea to faecal ammonia in man, determined by ^{15}N-labelling of plasma urea. Clin Sci 1985;68:193–199.
64 Visek WJ, Clinton SK, Truex CR: Nutritional and experimental carcinogenesis. Cornell Vet 1978;68:3–39.
65 Drasar BS, Hill MJ: Human Intestinal Microflora. London, Academic Press, 1974.
66 Cummings JH, Hill MJ, Bone ES, et al: The effect of meat protein and dietary fiber on colonic function and metabolism. Part II. Bacterial metabolites in feces and urine. Am J Clin Nutr 1979;32:2094–3001.
67 Bryan GT: The role of bacterial tryptophan metabolites in the etiology of bladder cancer. Am J Clin Nutr 1971;24:841–847.
68 Dalgliesh CE, Kelley WEC, Horning EC: Excretion of a sulphatoxyl derivative of skatole in pathological studies in man. Biochem J 1958;70:13P.
69 Carlson JR, Yokoyama MT, Dickinson EO: Induction of pulmonary edema and emphysema in cattle and goats with 3-methylindole. Science 1972;176:298–299.
70 Yokohama MT, Tabori C, Miller ER, Hogberg MG: The effects of antibiotics in the weanling pig diet on growth and excretions of volatile phenolic and aromatic bacterial metabolites. Am J Clin Nutr 1982;35:1417–1424.
71 Gibson GR, Macfarlane GT, Cummings JH: Occurrence of sulphate-reducing bacteria in human faeces and the relationship of dissimilatory sulphate reduction to methanogenesis in the large gut. J Appl Bacteriol 1988;65:103–111.
72 Newton DF, Cummings JH, Macfarlane S, Macfarlane GT: Growth of a human intestinal *Desulfovibrio desulfuricans* in continuous cultures containing defined populations of saccharolytic and amino acid fermenting bacteria. J Appl Microbiol 1998;85:372–380.
73 Rowland IR: Interactions of the gut microflora and the host in toxicology. Toxicol Pathol 1988;6:147–153.
74 Cummings JH, Macfarlane GT: Bacteria in the pathogenesis of colorectal cancer; in Scheppach W, Scheurlen M (eds): Exogenous Factors in Colonic Carcinogenesis. Dordrecht, Kluwer Academic, 2002, pp 180–191.

75 Gibson GR, Macfarlane GT: Intestinal bacteria and disease; in Gibson SAW (ed): Human Health: The Contribution of Microorganisms. London, Springer, 1994, pp 53–62.
76 Wilkins TD, Van Tassell RL: Production of intestinal mutagens; in Hentges DJ (ed): Human Intestinal Microflora in Health and Disease. New York, Academic Press, 1983, pp 265–288.

Discussion

As the authors of this paper were unable to join the workshop, the presentation and the discussion were conducted by Florence Rochat, Switzerland.

Dr. Guesry: First of all Dr. Rochat I would like to congratulate you on this magnificent presentation, knowing that you had less than 24 h to prepare, but I have also two questions. You pointed out the difference between breast-fed and bottle-fed infants, the first showing bifidus bacteria, the second bacteroide, as the predominant flora. But do you have any data on a baby who would be bottle-fed with the mother's own expressed milk, to try to see the difference between the mere composition of the milk and the important contact between the baby and the skin of the breast?

Dr. Rochat: I have no data on such an experiment and I am not aware of such data in the literature comparing the groups in the same study. It would be very interesting to have this approach, but all 3 models of feeding are needed to compare the results.

Dr. Guesry: Dr. Marini, maybe you have data like that?

Dr. Marini: We are not experts on this. But I would like to ask about the problem of pasteurized human milk which is used a lot in preterm units simply because there is a risk with human milk of cytomegalovirus (CMV) infection, there is reactivation during pregnancy and in very small preterm babies there could be a risk. We have seen cases of sepsis due to CMV infection acquired since birth through human milk. What is happening with pasteurized milk, because we know that fresh human milk is the best for protection?

Dr. Rochat: But certainly we lose an important part in this pasteurized milk because of the structure of carbohydrate, many important compounds will be changed during pasteurization, and this is the fourth group in the proposed experiments.

Dr. Guesry: It is not only pasteurization; the cells disappear when you put breast milk into a bottle. The cells stick to the glass.

Dr. Rochat: To the glass yes, and so the container is really important to consider.

Dr. Marini: I would like to make a comment about hydrolysate and colonization. We have done a study in guinea pigs from birth up to 20 days of age with different kinds of feeding, not extensively hydrolyzed protein, intact protein and mother's milk [1]. We have found that with hydrolyzed protein there is a pattern of biliary acid secretion similar to human milk, and this can also be a factor in good colonization because we know that the bile is not only for digestion but it also has some antibacterial effect, at least in the ileum and jejunum. It has also been demonstrated that oligosaccharides can influence biliary secretion.

Dr. Rochat: The guinea pig is a very interesting model for gut alteration. There is only one limitation, we know there is no perfect model but for us one of the limitations to be perfect or closer to the human is the intestinal microflora because it is quite different from the human, there is no bifidobacteria, and that is why there is some limitation to this approach.

Dr. Salminen: Thank you for your nice presentation, I think it very nicely covered all the different areas that are currently of interest. I would like to put one specific question to you. In your slides you pointed out the work that is done on bifidobacteria and prebiotics, and we saw how bifidobacteria are promoted by prebiotics. Do you have any information on the species composition? We have worked on that area and shown with Dr. Isolauri that there is very different species composition in allergic and nonallergic infants.

Dr. Rochat: We are finalizing the analyses from one of our studies. In a study done with different prebiotics, we have observed the increasing bifidobacteria, but we do not have the results right now.

Dr. Salminen: I think it is of crucial importance if you think about infants and prebiotics, because by defining what kind of microbiota he or she receives, more adult type or elderly type, compared to healthy infants, you really do have the question there.

Dr. Rochat: It is true, it is really important for infants and for the moment I think there are few data with prebiotics in infants. For the time being there are few data demonstrating the impact of the prebiotics on the gut intestinal microbiota in the infant.

Dr. Walker: Dr. Rochat, you did a wonderful job of covering this topic. Several studies have suggested that as formula has changed, the differences in colonization between breast-fed and formula-fed infants are becoming similar. One observation that you made is the increase in bifidobacteria with both. There have been some studies that suggest that peptides have a bifidogenic effect as well as oligosaccharides [2]. I wonder if anyone has looked at the breakdown of the protein content of formula in the context of the peptides to discover if they have a bifidogenic stimulatory effect? Do you know of any studies?

Dr. Rochat: I know that this is one possible explanation for the change that we observed in many studies, and we have more bifidobacteria. It is true that the appearance of bifidobacteria in bottle-fed babies is more important, but there are still some other changes that remain: the diversity, the difference in the pH. So this is not very close for the moment. But the peptide and also some changes in the production of formula may influence the promotion of bifidobacteria.

Dr. Papageorgiou: Was there any difference in the degree of hydrolysis in your rat experiments in terms of effect, which has some relevance on the size of peptides?

Dr. Rochat: This was quite extensively hydrolyzed protein.

Dr. Marini: I think it was about 700 if I read correctly.

Dr. Bedford-Russell: Just the question you asked about the raw breast milk. Virtually all the long-term epidemiological studies on this have been done on either a mixture of formula and breast milk or breast milk, and some of that breast milk was pasteurized and some of it was frozen. So it is very interesting whether raw milk has all the immunological factors. What I can say about CMV though is that there was an article published in the *Lancet* some years ago in which babies were given raw breast milk in a neonatal unit and the CMV incidence was found to be about 25%. We looked at our own babies and published a study a couple of years ago [3]. Our practice often is to freeze the breast milk and our own rate was significantly reduced by that because of course freezing gets rid of about 98% of CMV, but we don't know what effect it had on getting rid of the other goodies in the breast milk.

Dr. Rochat: It is interesting for me also to see that, depending on the country, there are different procedures. A few months ago it was quite new to me that there is not a single procedure for the treatment of breast milk: in some countries it is pasteurized, and in others it is frozen.

Dr. Bindslev-Jensen: I am not a neonatologist or a pediatrician so I was rather astonished to learn that the fetal pH is 1.6 units. The neuroimmunidases and the sialyl transferases in contrast to the fucosyl transferases don't work at a pH above 6.5. So there might be a connection to what is going on if there is such a big difference in the fetal pH. Is it present already at birth? What is the pH in the fetus at birth and what constitutes this pH acidity?

Dr. Rochat: The pH is not so low at birth but it changes when the bacteria appear. There are a lot of changes when the bacteria colonize the gut, and this is also part of the important changes which will determine which bacteria will stay after that in the digestive tract.

Dr. Hill: What is known about bacterial flora in totally breast-fed infants who present with atopic dermatitis in the first month of life compared to nonatopic dermatitis breast-fed infants? Is there a difference in the bacterial flora?

Dr. Rochat: A difference was described.

Dr. Vandenplas: I have two questions, the first one regards the floral development in formula-fed infants. The liquid formula is sterile, powdered infant formula is not sterile, mineral water is also not sterile. Do you know if there is a different floral development whether liquid formula or powdered formula is used?

Dr. Rochat: I don't know. I have no data.

Dr. Vandenplas: The second question is the role of gastric pH because gastric acid is probably important. A lot of infants who have gastroesophageal reflux are treated with antacids or acid-blocking drugs. Does anyone know about the role of having no gastric acid on floral development or the flora that you have?

Dr. Rochat: We know that the pH is really important because we can easily correlate the pH and certain bacterial compositions. But there is a difference between the pH in the upper part of the digestive tract and the fecal pH. We know that when there is a less acidic condition we have a chance to have more bacterial growth in the upper part of the digestive tract.

Dr. Neijens: By studying the microbes from the gut so intensely, did you take the opportunity to analyze the interaction between specific bacteria and the way they might more specifically influence the spectrum of mediators, and secondly is there interaction between the various strains?

Dr. Rochat: The exchange of genes was studied mainly by people working on antibiotic treatment to see if there is a possible transfer from antibiotic resistance from one bacteria to another. As to the first part of your question on the interaction between the bacteria, some studies have been done, and gnototibiotic animals are really a useful model for this because we can place in competition two different types of bacteria, two different species, and see the interaction. This is the case in the work done by Corthier et al. in which they demonstrate the interaction between the bifidobacteria and the *Clostridium difficile*. But here again a lot of work needs to be done on this because there are so many species, and firstly we were working with quite well-known bacteria, quite easy to cultivate. I am sure that we have to be more deeply interested in bacteria such as peptostreptococci or eubacteria which are really the main components in the digestive tract. So these will be really important bacteria to study. That is why I also mentioned that in the future some people will start to work with mono-associated mice with specific bacteria to see what the effects are on the genome. We have to do the same with pluri-associated mice, but this is a big job. In my opinion there is a lack of knowledge at present.

Dr. Neijens: Gene interaction will be very important because it might have several effects: it might have a beneficial effect but also a risk because there is a risk that they change antibiotic-resistant strains between them, so that should be carefully studied.

Dr. Rochat: That is true, and there is interaction between the bacteria and the host also.

Dr. Sorensen: If I understood you correctly you said that only 40% of the flora can be cultivated. So is that 40% of all the species or of the total bacterial load? If 60% is not detected then are you looking at the right bacteria?

Dr. Rochat: This is a good question. This is 40% of the total bacteria that we can easily enumerate. But the other part is also really interesting and we have a poor knowledge today of these bacteria, we know that they play a role in colonization resistance. Here we are talking about strict anaerobe bacteria because they are very complicated to cultivate, as the peptostreptococci or eubacterium for example, and it will be very interesting to investigate the role of these bacteria further. That is why when I showed one of the first graphs prepared by Gibson demonstrating the dichotomy between healthy bacteria and harmful bacteria, I said that probably in the future we will also have some changes because we will understand the interrelation between these types of bacterial species better.

Dr. Marini: It is about the problem of gastric pH. Ten years ago we did a study comparing gastric pH and total acid output in the stomach of near-term babies who were divided into 3 groups: one was fed mother's milk; one was fed not extensively hydrolyzed protein, and the third one was fed intact protein. We also had another group with a low chloride content in the formula. We found that the babies fed the hydrolyzed protein behave the same as those fed mother's milk, and the babies who received the formula with low chlorine content have less gastric acid output [4]. One of the problems is why the babies fed mother's milk do not have a very low gastric pH during the whole feeding time. This is important to me because you can save IgA, IgM and IgG from the mother's milk for the protection of the gut.

Dr. Rochat: And this also gives the infant the chance to be in sufficient contact with exogenous bacteria to make its 'own choice' for the final colonization of its digestive tract.

Dr. Marini: Of course in mother's milk there are two things: there is a high gastric pH and also a defense system like IgA, IgM, IgG. When artificial feeding is given, the pH level is perhaps the same as that of the hydrolysate, but protection is less because there is no IgA, IgM and so on.

Dr. Guesry: In your study with baby rats bottle-fed with extensive hydrolysate or intact protein, in which part of the intestine did you measure the bacterial overgrowth, and did you also measure the nitrogen residue at this same level? I ask this because the very small peptides of the extensive hydrolysate should have been totally absorbed in the jejunum, whereas for the intact protein you probably have a nitrogen residue coming down to the colon. So I think it is very important to correlate the two.

Dr. Rochat: Unfortunately I don't have the results on the nitrogen residue but the effect was observed mainly in the upper part of the digestive tract, in the jejunum and ileum. On the cecum level there was no difference between the 3 groups.

Dr. Vandenplas: I just wanted to react to the hypothesis of the gastric acid and breast-feeding and formula-feeding. When you do gastric pH monitoring it is clear that mother's milk has a very rapid gastric emptying and 30–45 min after having fed mother's milk or hydrolysate you again have a pH of about 1–1.5 in the stomach, and when you give a casein-predominant formula it neutralizes the gastric acid for 2 h or even more. So I am not convinced that with breast-feeding you have less gastric acid in your stomach than with formula-feeding.

Dr. Marini: I am talking about the neonates. In the neonate you have very frequent feeding. Probably in your case you don't have frequent feedings, but we have intervals between feeding of about 2 h.

Dr. Vandenplas: We did that in premature newborns who were fed 8 times a day. Much more gastric acid was clearly present in those breast-fed than those formula-fed, certainly if it is a casein-predominant formula.

Dr. Marini: Did you also measure total gastric acid output?

Dr. Vandenplas: No, I said gastric pH monitoring.

Dr. Guesry: On this point, one of the very important differences between breast milk and formula for the pH of the intestinal content is the level of phosphate. Phosphate is a very important buffer which we studied a long time ago. When we give a low-phosphate formula we decrease the pH of the stool, whereas when we give a casein-predominant high-phosphate level, the pH remains neutral.

Dr. Schiffrin: We heard today that some of you have given prebiotics to preterm babies that generate a fermentation in short-chain fatty acids, and at the same time we had some concerns about butyrate and necrotizing enterocolitis or butyrate and the stimulation of inflammatory cytokines in enterocytes. Is there any concern about the administration of prebiotics in preterm babies?

Dr. Marini: We have experience with preterm babies and prebiotics, and they tolerate them very well. There was no problem. Actually indirectly we were able to show that they have a better calcium absorption from the gut.

Dr. Walker: What I was referring to is the observation that butyrate can activate or stimulate the inflammatory response in the small intestine. Therefore theoretically there is a concern because these may be increased levels of the fermented oligosaccharides in the small intestine based on bacteria, but I can only talk about this as a theoretical possibility.

Dr. Salminen: I am a little bit concerned about prebiotics in the infant right now because to my knowledge we don't really have very specific prebiotics yet, and so we don't know the long-term consequences in the gut microbiota development, especially thinking about species composition and bifidobacteria. So I may be wrong, but I am still a bit concerned.

References

1 Colombo C, Setchell KR, Crosignani A, et al: Influence of breast feeding, and adapted and hydrolyzed formulas on biliary acids in newborn guinea pigs. Biol Neonate 2003;83:36–41.
2 Duggan C, Gannon J, Walker WA: Protective nutrients and functional foods for the gastrointestinal tract. Am J Clin Nutr 2002;75:789–808.
3 Sharland M, Khare M, Bedford-Russell A: Prevention of postnatal cytomegalovirus infection in preterm infants. Arch Dis Child Fetal Neonatal Ed 2002;86:F140.
4 Marini A, Agosti M, Mosca F, Farina C: Dietary prevention programs for allergy: Some metabolic and nutritional remarks; in Allergy and Nutrition. New York, Parthenon, 1994, pp 7–12.

Isolauri E, Walker WA (eds): Allergic Diseases and the Environment.
Nestlé Nutrition Workshop Series Pediatric Program, Vol. 53, pp. 199–216,
Nestec Ltd.; Vevey/S. Karger AG, Basel, © 2004.

Does Breast-Feeding Protect from Allergies?

Renate L. Bergmann, K.E. Bergmann and J.W. Dudenhausen

Department of Obstetrics, Humboldt University,
Charité Virchow Hospitals, Berlin, Germany

The resurgence of breast-feeding in the Western world since the early 1970s is paralleled by a dramatic increase in the prevalence of allergic diseases (fig. 1) [1–3]. Breast-feeding and allergies are more prevalent in more advantaged people than in the poor, in higher social classes, and in persons of higher education [4]. Does a causal relationship exist between both phenomena? Does breast-feeding protect from allergies or rather promote them? Is the breast best for all infants?

Breast milk is a unique food which so far cannot exactly be imitated. The composition of breast milk is as complex and as particular as that of any organ or fluid in the human body. Breast milk is not only suited to provide the infant with energy and nutrients, but it also has innumerable constituents and agents which are important for the growth and normal development of the infant [5]. Whether all of them play a biological role under our living conditions has to be evaluated critically. Several prerequisites for a biological role were formulated by Bernd and Walker [6] in 1999: (1) the agent must be present in sufficient quantity; (2) it must be proven to reach its site of action, and (3) it must show an effect on the infant. Which factors in breast milk could influence immune function?

Human milk has the lowest protein content of all species, most of which is whey protein [7]. It should be assumed that protein produced by the mother is highly compatible to the infant's immune system. The casein in breast milk prevents microbial adhesion to the gastrointestinal mucosa, the proteolytic product K-casein is a growth factor for bifidobacteria [8]. Of the immunoglobulins present in human milk, polymeric IgA is predominant, consumption by the infant is 4 g on day 1, and after a few days it is about 1 g/day [8].

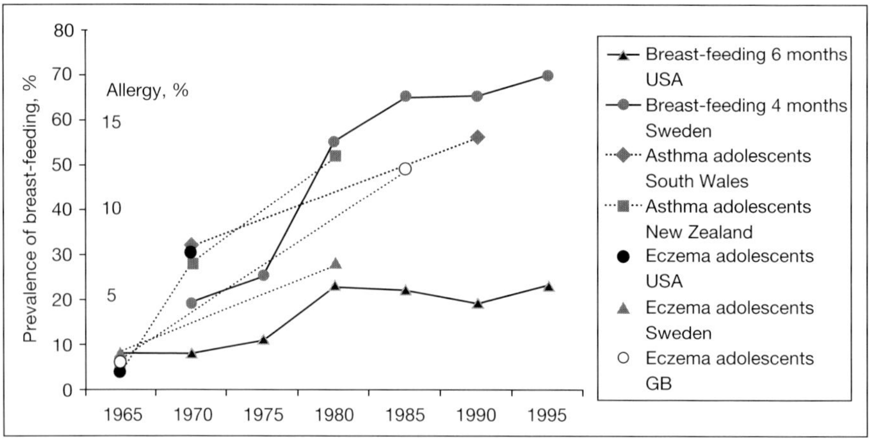

Fig. 1. The parallel rise in the prevalence of breast-feeding for at least 4 months in Sweden and at least 4 months in USA and the prevalence of some atopic disorders in adolescents. Adapted from the data of Ryan [2], Zetterström [3], and Burr et al. [64].

Specific IgA is resistant to low pH and proteolytic enzymes, 30% of it appears in the feces of the infant. In human milk, specific IgA antibodies have been found against pathogens and bacterial toxins, e.g. against *Clostridium difficile* [9]. Lactoferrin, an iron-binding protein, is present in high concentrations in human milk, is relatively resistant to digestion, and exerts immunomodulatory functions [6]. Nucleotides are nitrogen-containing nonproteins which promote the maturation of T lymphocytes, activate macrophages and enhance natural killer cells [10]. Lysozyme, an amino acid-containing glycoprotein, lyses mostly gram-positive and few gram-negative bacteria [8]. Oligosaccharides, glycoconjugates and lipids, most abundant components of human milk, protect infants from infections by many different mechanisms [8].

Milk lymphocytes (memory T cells) and macrophages are part of the host-defense strategies [6]. T lymphocytes and plasma cells producing IgA migrate from the lymphoid tissue of the intestine and the bronchial tree of the mother to the mammary gland, and are the excreted and consumed by the infant, They probably are able to traverse the baby's intestine [6, 8].

Anti-inflammatory components in human milk consist of vitamins, enzymes, prostaglandins, growth factors, cytokines and cytokine receptors [8]. Human milk contains many immunomodulating agents, but their physiologic function is still not totally clear [8] (table 1). Transforming growth factor-β (TGF-β), which is present in a high concentration in human milk, may play a role in the induction of tolerance [6].

Exclusively breast-fed newborns develop a specific flora. Because of prebiotic factors in breast milk, a flora predominant in lactobacilli and bifidobacteria is

Table 1. Immunomodulating agents in human milk [8]

Component	Function
IL-1	Production of defense agents
IL-3	–
IL-4	–
IL-5	–
IL-6	Regulates function of mammary gland
IL-8	Chemotactic for intestinal intraepithelial leukocytes
IL-10	Modulates epithelial barrier integrity
IL-12	Enhances production of inflammatory cytokines
IFN-γ	Modulates epithelial barrier integrity
TNF-α	Regulates function of mammary gland
TGF-β	Anti-inflammatory

established by 1 month [11]. Bifidobacteria play a role in the development of oral tolerance [12, 13].

The low allergen load as well as the anti-inflammatory and immunomodulating properties of human milk should prevent allergies in breast-fed infants. On the other hand, the anti-infective components and qualities of human milk prevent infections. Protection against diarrhea and (to a lesser extent) against acute respiratory infection in breast-fed children of less developed countries, especially in disadvantaged populations, was most pronounced during the first 6 months of life, but continued into the 2nd year [14]. Protection against gastrointestinal and upper respiratory infection is observed in developed countries even after control for confounding variables [15]. The protection is achieved in a dose-response manner [16]. It is possible that suppression of atopy depends on infection during a critical period, perhaps in early life with powerful and long-lasting effects on immunological development, consistent with an early 'programming' influence on allergic sensitization [17]. This would explain the phenomenon of the rising prevalence in Western countries, the higher prevalence in Western compared to Eastern Europe, in affluent families compared to poor, in small compared to large families and in first-born children [17]. The escape from certain microbial exposures in early life allows the immune system to mount unnecessary type-2 T-helper immune responses to allergens derived from innocuous environmental agents [18].

But human milk itself may have constituents that promote allergies. Macromolecules from the mother's food were demonstrated in her milk [19–22]. The concentration of biologically active agents shows individual differences. Total IgA levels in colostrum and human milk were significantly lower in mothers whose babies later developed cow's milk allergy [23]. Polyamine levels were higher in the milk of atopic mothers [24]. The fatty acid composition is different in the milk from atopic and nonatopic mothers, suggesting a disturbed metabolism of long-chain fatty acids [25]. This appears to influence the development of atopy in the infant [26]. The concentrations of IL-4, IL-8 and RANTES were higher in colostrum and milk from allergic than nonallergic mothers [27, 28]. The concentrations of TGF-β levels and the TNF-α production by breast milk leukocytes were lower in maternal colostrum and milk of breast-fed atopic infants [29, 30].

Human α-lactalbumin appeared 30–60 min after breast-feeding in the sera of the infants [20]. Specific IgE to human lactalbumin was found in the sera of breast-fed but cow's milk-allergic infants, which cross-reacted to cow's milk protein [31]. Food antibodies were detected in the sera of breast-fed infants with food allergy especially after challenge [32–34].

It is therefore not surprising that symptoms of food allergy were observed in exclusively breast-fed infants. Colic, erythema, urticaria, atopic eczema, and bloody stools as symptoms of cow's milk and multiple food allergies have been described in even exclusively breast-fed infants [32–39]. Symptoms improved or disappeared after an elimination diet of the mother or after breast-feeding of the infant was stopped, i.e. with causal treatment of the food-allergic infant. In view of these facts, is it justifiable to recommend breast-feeding to all infants for the prevention of allergy?

Naturally, so far breast-feeding cannot be randomly assigned, therefore evidence for the advantages of breast-feeding cannot be proven by a randomized double-blind placebo-controlled study. The short- and long-term effects of breast-feeding compared to bottle feeding a cow's milk-based infant formula on the development of atopic sensitization or manifestation have been derived from observational studies, which implies that other factors may confound the association (fig. 2).

The atopic march usually begins with food-associated allergies, e.g. atopic eczema. The publication by Grulee and Sanford [40] in 1936 begins: 'There is probably no subject in pediatrics, that has received so much attention in the last few years as that of infantile eczema. Both, external and internal factors have been studied, and some advances have been made in its treatment. We believe, however, that the effect of diet on these infants, once so stressed, has been largely lost sight of recently. In Chicago these two pediatricians followed up 22,000 babies during a 5-year period and observed that of those fed cow's milk seven times as many developed eczema than breast-fed infants and twice as many if partially breast-fed [40].

A review article by Kramer [41] appeared in 1988. He specifically developed 12 biologic and methodological standards for studies concerned with infant feeding and atopic disease, and then individually rated original research reports published through 1986 according to these standards [41] (table 2). Among the studies on atopic eczema the 9 claiming a protective effect of breast-feeding performed less well than the 12 not making such a claim. For the other atopic conditions, there were no important differences between positive and negative studies. 'What, if anything, can be concluded

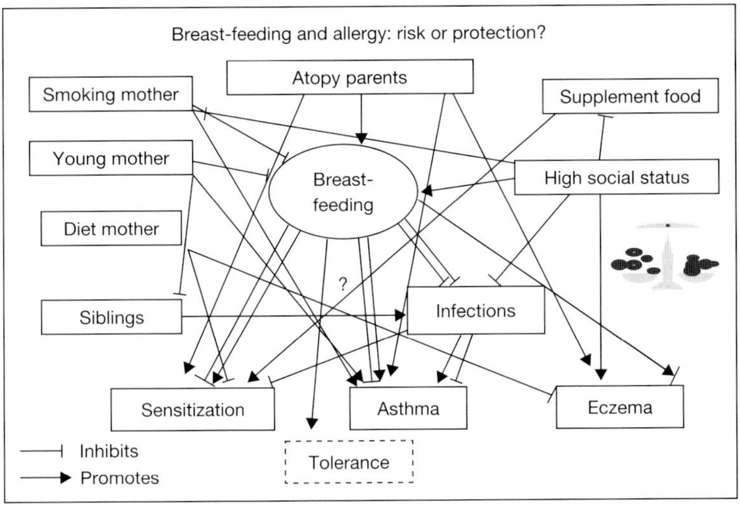

Fig. 2. Interaction of protective and risk factors, inhibitory and promoting influences in the development of allergies by breast-feeding.

Table 2. Twelve standards for studies on infant feeding and atopic disease [41]

Exposure	
1	Nonreliance on prolonged maternal recall
2	Blind ascertainment of infant feeding history
3	Sufficient duration of breast-feeding
4	Sufficient exclusivity of breast-feeding
Outcome	
5	Strict diagnostic criteria
6	Blind ascertainment of outcome
7	Severity of outcome
8	Age at onset of outcome
Statistical analysis	
9	Control for confounding
10	Assessment of dose-response effect
11	Assessment of effect in children at high risk
12	Adequate statistical power

about the prophylactic benefit of breastfeeding? Unfortunately, not much', he states. 'To avoid another 50 years of unresolved controversy, future studies should improve both, the biologic and methodologic aspects of the design analyses' [41].

To somehow increase statistical power (point 12 of Kramer's standards [41]), Gdalevich et al. [42] performed a meta-analysis of 18 prospective

Table 3. Number of preterm infants who developed eczema by 18 months after term according to a family history of atopy and initial diet [43]

Family history of atopy			No family history of atopy		
preterm formula (n = 37)	human milk (n = 38)	OR (95% CI)	preterm formula (n = 182)	human milk (n = 189)	OR (95% CI)
6 (16%)	15 (41%)	3.6 (1.2–11)	40 (21%)	29 (16%)	0.7 (0.4–1.2)

studies published between 1966 and 2000 on the influence of at least 3 rather than 2 months of exclusive breast-feeding, which had to fulfill 9 of the 12 Kramer criteria. This meta-analysis produced an overall effect on eczema prevalence with an odds ratio (OR) of 0.58 (95% confidence interval (CI) 0.41–0.92) for infants with a positive atopic family history, and an OR of 0.84 (95% CI 0.59–1.19) for infants with a negative family history [42]. An OR of 0.77 (95% CI 0.60–0.98) was estimated for all infants. Originally, of the 14 studies on infants with a positive family history only 4 had ORs and 95% CIs significantly below 1 (3 of these studies by the same Canadian team), and of the 7 studies in infants with a negative family history only 1 study showed a significant risk reduction.

Fortunately, 2 studies on the influence of breast-feeding on the development of eczema have a randomized assignment. A prospective, controlled study of preterm neonates randomly allocated to either human or cow's milk-based premature formula demonstrated that, beside other outcomes, exposure to cow's milk formula for at least 8 weeks increased the risk of developing atopic eczema by 18 months nearly fourfold in the subgroup with an allergic family history [43] (table 3). A cluster-randomized trial with a total of 17,046 mother–infant pairs conducted between 1996 and 1997 in Belarus by Kramer et al. [44] demonstrated that infants from the intervention sites were more likely than control infants to be exclusively breast-fed at 3 months, to have a significant reduction in gastrointestinal tract infections and atopic eczema with an adjusted OR of 0.54 (95% CI 0.31–0.91; table 4).

One of the confounding factors in observational studies on exclusive breast-feeding may be unnoticed neonatal exposure to cow's milk formula, the 'hidden bottle' in the newborn nursery. But it could be shown by prospective and proven by randomized studies that the development of atopic diseases was not influenced by these early supplements [45–49]. Another factor could be the presence of macromolecules in the breast milk from the mother's diet. Prescribing an antigen-avoidance diet to high-risk women as a measure for preventing eczema may reduce their child's risk of developing eczema [50, 51], but it is not recommended at this time because of the nutritional risks for mother and infant [52].

Table 4. Frequencies and odds ratios for atopic eczema and other rashes [44], adjusted for family atopic history

Outcome	Intervention group, %	Control group, %	Adjusted OR (95% CI)
Any rash	12.3	18.3	0.56 (0.38–0.81)
Atopic eczema	3.3	6.3	0.54 (0.31–0.95)
Non-eczematous rash	9.9	13.5	0.59 (0.38–0.92)
Non-eczematous, noninfectious rash	8.8	1.9	0.61 (0.40–0.93)

Table 5. Percentage with recurrent wheeze according to infant feeding category and maternal asthma status in the first 3 years of life and at 6–13 years of age [65]

	Total	Never BF	Exclusive BF	
			<4 months	≥4 months
Age ≤3 years				
Maternal asthma	18.4	27.3	19.2	14.3
No Maternal asthma	11.2	14.4	12.5	7.9
Age 6–13 years				
Maternal asthma	31.0	25.0	29.8	42.2
No Maternal asthma	15.5	20.1	13.7	15.7

BF = Breast-feeding.

In the real world atopic eczema is observed in breast-fed infants, and in observational studies, like the Multicenter Allergy Study in Germany [53], even after controlling for all possible confounders, including parental eczema, sensitization, social status and other atopic manifestations, it could be demonstrated that for each month of additional breast-feeding the risk of eczema increased by a predictable percentage. This exemplifies that even with the best statistical evaluation of an observational study, reverse causation cannot be excluded. Since the publication by Grulee and Sanford [40] in 1936, more infants of atopic, educated parents will be breast-fed, and continue to be breast-fed once they develop eczema. Therefore referral for allergy counselling is delayed in breast-fed infants [54].

The risk pattern for respiratory allergies is different from that of food-associated allergies. Genetic and environmental factors of the phenotypes only partly overlap, the atopic march begins with food-associated disorders, respiratory disorders follow later [55, 56]. Wheezing and asthma in preschool children are associated with infections, whereas in school-age children they are primarily associated with atopy [57]. In the Tucson Prospective

Observational Study, 60% of the transient early wheezers had stopped wheezing by the age of 6 years [58]. Sibling number and day care attendance were risk factors for wheezing at preschool age and protective factors from age 6 years on [59]. In the prospective German Multicenter Allergy Study [60] repeated episodes of runny nose significantly lowered the risk for asthma from 3 to 7 years.

Having 3 or more siblings (OR 0.16, 95% CI 0.04–0.71) and breast-feeding (OR 0.41, 95% CI 0.22–0.74) decreased the risk of asthma in Australian children aged 3–5 years [61]. In a prospective birth cohort study of 3,000 children in Western Australia, the introduction of milk other than breast milk before 4 months of age was a significant risk factor for asthma at 6 years of age [62]. In a population-based cross-sectional study in Italy on 16,000 children, 6–7 years old, breast-feeding for at least 6 months was found to be slightly protective against transient early wheezing (OR 0.82, 95% CI 0.68–0.97), whereas it was a moderate risk factor for late onset wheezing (OR 1.22, 95% CI 0.99–1.50 [63]). In South Wales, children who had ever been breast-fed, had a lower incidence of wheeze than those who had not, but the effect persisted to age 7 years only in nonatopic children [64]. In the Tucson study, while associated with protection against early wheeze, exclusive breast-feeding for at least 4 months was associated with an increased risk of asthma beginning at the age of 6 years, but only in children with asthmatic mothers, and significantly so ($p < 0.0001$) in atopic children with asthmatic mothers (table 4) [65]. In the New Zealand study, more children who were breast-fed were atopic at all ages from 13 to 21 years to cats, house dust mites and grass pollen, and more children reported current asthma at each assessment between age 9 and 26 years than those who were not [66].

In the Tucson study, Wright et al. [67] observed that among children whose mothers were in the two lower tertiles of IgE, breast-feeding was associated with lower total serum IgE at 6 years. But for children whose mothers were in the highest tertile of IgE, breast-feeding for 4 months or longer was associated with higher IgE levels in the child compared with those never breast-fed or breast-fed for less than 4 months.

We conclude that the relation between breast-feeding and the development of atopic disease is not yet settled. From the prospective studies published to date, those including a randomized design show an effect on eczema. The results of observational studies are contrasting, but a protective effect on wheezing is observed up to 6 years of age. The adverse effects on asthma beyond 6–7 years and probably on sensitization and total IgE could be the consequence of the lower rate of early infections in breast-fed infants. More asthma developed only in those children who became sensitized. These long-term respiratory allergies may have been preceded by atopic eczema, a predictor of respiratory allergies [68].

In view of the many health benefits of breast-feeding for the infant, for the mother, and for the mother–infant dyad, exclusive breast-feeding for

6 months should be recommended for all infants, and so far, even for infants with a risk of atopy.

References

1 Burr ML: Epidemiology of Clinical Allergy. Karger, Basel, 1993.
2 Ryan AS: The resurgence of breastfeeding in the United States. Pediatrics 1997;99:E12.
3 Zetterström R: Trends in research in infant nutrition, past, present and future. Acta Paediatr Suppl 1994;402:1–3.
4 Bergmann Rl, Edenharter G, Bergmann KE, et al: Socioeconomic status is a risk factor for allergy in parents but not in their children. Clin Exp Allergy 2000;30:1740–1745.
5 Neville MC: Anatomy and physiology of lactation. Pediatr Clin North Am 2001;48:13–34.
6 Bernd KM, Walker WA: Human milk as a carrier of biochemical messages. Acta Paediatr Suppl 1999;430:27–41.
7 Fomon SJ: Protein; in Fomon SJ (ed): Nutrition of Normal Infants. St Louis, Mosby, 1993, pp 126–127.
8 Hamosh M: Bioactive factors in human milk. Pediatr Clin North Am 2001;48:69–86.
9 Xanthou M: Immune protection of human milk. Biol Neonate 1998;74:121–133.
10 Barness LA, Carver JD: Dietary nucleotides with relation to immune response. Int Pediatr 1992;7:57–60.
11 Walker WA: Role of nutrients and bacterial colonization in the development of intestinal host defense. J Pediatr Gastroenterol Nutr 2000;30(suppl 1):S2–S7.
12 Strobel S, Mowat A: Immune responses to dietary antigens: Oral tolerance. Immunol Today 1998;19:173–180.
13 Sudo N, Sawamura S, Tanaka K, et al: The requirement of intestinal bacterial flora for the development of an IgE production system fully susceptible to oral tolerance induction. J Immunol 1997;159:1739–1745.
14 WHO Collaborative Study Team on the Role of Breastfeeding and the Prevention of Infant Mortality: Effect of breastfeeding in infant and child mortality due to infectious diseases in less developed countries: A pooled analysis. Lancet 2000;355:451–455.
15 Howie PW, Forsyth JS, Ogston SA, et al: Protective effect of breastfeeding against infection. BMJ 1990;300:11–16.
16 Scariati PD, Grummer-Strawn LM, Beck Fein S: A longitudinal analysis of infant morbidity and the extent of breastfeeding in the United States. Pediatrics 1997;99:1–5.
17 Strachan D: Socioeconomic factors and the development of allergy. Toxicol Lett 1996;86: 199–203.
18 Hopkin JM: The rise of allergy and links to infection. Allergy 2002;57:5–9.
19 Donnally HH: The question of the elimination of foreign protein (egg-white) in woman's milk. J Immunol 1930;19:15–19.
20 Jacobsson I: Food antigens in human milk. Eur J Clin Nutr 1991;45(suppl 1):29–33.
21 Kilshaw PJ, Cant AJ: The passage of maternal dietary proteins into human breast milk. Int Arch Allergy Appl Immunol 1984;75:8–15.
22 Shannon WR: Demonstration of food proteins in human breast milk by anaphylactic experiments on guinea pigs. Am J Dis Child 1921;22:223–226.
23 Järvinen K-M, Laine ST, Järvenpää A-L, Suomalainen H: Does low IgA in human milk predispose the infant to development of cow's milk allergy? Pediatr Res 2000;48:457–462.
24 Duchén K, Thorell L: Nucleotide and polyamine levels in colostrum and mature milk in relation to maternal atopy and atopic development in children. Acta Paediatr 1999;88:1338–1343.
25 Yu G, Duchén K, Björkstén B: Fatty acid composition in colostrum and mature milk from nonatopic and atopic mothers. Acta Paediatr 1998;87:729–736.
26 Duchén K, Yu G, Björkstén B: Atopic sensitization during the first year of life in relation to long chain polyunsaturated fatty acid levels in human milk. Pediatr Res 1998;44:478–484.
27 Böttcher MF, Jenmalm MC, Garofalo RP, Björkstén B: Cytokines in breast milk from allergic and nonallergic mothers. Pediatr Res 2000;47:157–162.
28 Böttcher MF, Jenmals MC, Björkstén B, Garifalo RP: Chemoattractant factors in breast milk from allergic and non allergic mothers. Pediatr Res 2000;47:592–597.

29 Järvinen KM, Laine S, Suomalainen H: Defective tumor necrosis factor-alpha production in mother's milk is related to cow's milk allergy in suckling infants. Clin Exp Allergy 2000;30: 637–643.
30 Kalliomäki M, Ouwehand A, Arvilommi H, et al: Transforming growth factor-β in breast milk: A potential regulator of atopic disease at an early age. J Allergy Clin Immunol 1999;104: 1251–1257.
31 Cantisani A, Giuffrida G, Fabis C, et al: Detection of specific IgE to human milk proteins in sera of atopic infants. FEBS Lett 1997;412:515–117.
32 Cavagni G, Paganelli R, Caffarelli C, et al: Passage of food antigens into the circulation of breast-fed infants with atopic dermatitis. Ann Allergy 1988;61:361–365.
33 Isolauri E, Tahvanainen A, Peltola T, Arvola T: Breast-feeding of allergic infants. J Pediatr 1999;134:27–32.
34 Järvinen K-M, Mäkinen-Kiljunene S, Suamalainen H: Cow's milk challenge through human milk evokes immune responses in infants with cow's milk allergy. J Pediatr 1999;135:506–512.
35 Barau E, Dupont C: Allergy to cow's milk proteins in mother's milk or in hydrolysed cow's milk infant formulas as assessed by intestinal permeability measurements. Allergy 1994;49:295–298.
36 De Boissieu D, Matrazzo P, Rocchiochioli F, Dupont C: Multiple food allergy: A possible diagnosis in breastfed infants. Acta Paediatr 1997;86:1042–1046.
37 Gerrard JW: Allergy in breast-fed babies to ingredients in breast milk. Ann Allergy 1979;42: 69–72.
38 Jacobsson I, Lindberg T: Cow's milk as a cause of infantile colic in breast-fed infants. Lancet 1978;ii:437–439.
39 Jacobsson I, Lindberg T: Cow's milk proteins cause infantile colic in breast-fed infants: A double-blind crossover study. Pediatrics 1983;71:268–271.
40 Grulee CG, Sanford HN: The influence of breast and artificial feeding on infantile eczema. J Pediatr 1936;9:223–225.
41 Kramer MS: Does breastfeeding help protect against atopic disease? Biology, methodology, and a golden jubilee of controversy. J Pediatr 1988;112:181–190.
42 Gdalevich M, Mimouni D, David M, Mimouni M: Breast-feeding and the onset of atopic dermatitis in childhood: A systematic review and meta-analysis of prospective studies. J Am Acad Dermatol 2001;45:520–527.
43 Lukas A, Brooke OG, Morley R, et al: Early diet of preterm infants and development of allergic or atopic disease: Randomized prospective study. BMJ 1990;300:837–840.
44 Kramer MS, Chalmers B, Hodnett ED, et al, for the PROBIT Study Group: Promotion of Breastfeeding Intervention Trial (PROBIT). A randomized trial in the Republic of Belarus. JAMA 2001;285:413–420.
45 Lindfors ATB, Danielsson L, Enocksson E, et al: Allergic symptoms up to 4–6 years of age in children given cow's milk neonatally. Allergy 1992;47:207–211.
46 De Jong M, Scharp-van der Linden VTM, Aaalberse R, et al: Randomized controlled trial of brief neonatal exposure to cow's milk on the development of atopy. Arch Dis Child 1998;79: 126–130.
47 Gustafsson D, Löwhagen T, Andersson K: Risk of developing atopic disease after early feeding with cow's milk based formula. Arch Dis Child 1992;67:1008–1010.
48 Juvonen P, Månsson M, Andersson C, Jakobsson I: Allergy development and macromolecular absorption in infants with differing feeding regimens during the first three days of life. A three year prospective follow-up. Acta Paediatr 1996;85:1047–1052.
49 Schmitz J, Digeon B, Chastang C, et al: Effects of early exposure to partially hydrolyzed and whole cow's milk proteins; in de Weck AL, Sampson HA (eds): Intestinal Immunology and Food Allergy. Nestlé Nutrition Workshop Series. Vevey, Nestec/New York, Raven Press, 1995, vol 34, pp 259–266.
50 Hattevig G, Sigurs N, Kjellman B: Effect of maternal dietary avoidance during lactation in children at 10 years of age. Acta Paediatr 1999;88:7–12.
51 Kramer MS: Maternal antigen avoidance during lactation for preventing atopic disease in infants of women at high risk. Cochrane Database Syst Rev 2003;1:ISSN 1464–780X.
52 Zeiger RS: Dietary aspects of food allergy prevention in infants and children. J Pediatr Gastroenterol Nutr 2000;30(suppl 1):S77–S86.
53 Bergmann RL, Diepgen TL, Kuss O, et al, for the MAS Group: Breastfeeding duration is a risk factor for atopic eczema. Clin Exp Allergy 2002;32:205–209.

54 Arvola T, Hvitfelt-Koskelainen J, Eriksson U-M, et al: Breastfeeding and allergy counselling: Theory and practice. Acta Paediatr 2000;89:365–374.
55 Bergmann RL, Wahn U, Bergmann KE: The allergic march from food to pollen. Environ Toxicol Pharm 1997;4:79–83.
56 Marsh D, Blumenthal M (eds): Genetic and Environment Factors in the Development of Allergy. Minneapolis, University Minnesota Press, 1990.
57 Silverman M: Out of the mouths of babes and sucklings: Lessons from early childhood asthma. Thorax 1993;48:1200–1204.
58 Martinez FD, Wright AL, Taussig LM, et al: Asthma and wheezing in the first six years of life. The Group Medical Associates. N Engl J Med 1995;332:133–138.
59 Ball TM, Castro-Rodriguez JA, Griffith KA, et al: Siblings, day-care attendance, and the risk of asthma and wheezing during childhood. N Engl J Med 2003;343:538–543.
60 Illi S, von Mutius E, Lau S, et al, the MAS Group: Early childhood infectious diseases and the development of asthma up to school age: A birth cohort study. BMJ 2001;322:390–395.
61 Haby MM, Peat GB, Woolcock AJ, Leeder SR: Asthma in preschool children: Prevalence and risk factors. Thorax 2001;56:589–595.
62 Oddy WH, Holt PG, Sly PD, et al: Association between breast feeding and asthma in 6 year old children: Findings of a prospective birth cohort study. BMJ 1999;319:815–819.
63 Rusconi F, Galassi C, Corbo GM, et al: Risk factors for early, persistent, and late-onset wheezing in young children. SIDRIA Collaborative Group. Am J Respir Care Med 1999;160: 1617–1622.
64 Burr ML, Limb ES, Maguire MJ, et al: Infants feeding, wheezing, and allergy: A prospective study. Arch Dis Child 1993;68:724–728.
65 Wright AL, Holberg CJ, Taussig LM, Martinez FD: Factors influencing the relation of infant wheezing and recurrent wheeze in childhood. Thorax 2001;56:192–197.
66 Sears MR, Green JM, Willan AR, et al: Long-term relation between breastfeeding and the development of atopy and asthma in children and young adults: a longitudinal study. Lancet 2002;360:901–907.
67 Wright AL, Sherill D, Holber CJ, et al: Breast-feeding, maternal IgE, and total serum IgE in childhood. J Allergy Clin Immunol 1999;104:589–594.
68 Bergmann RL, Edenharter G, Bergmann KE, et al: Atopic dermatitis in early infancy predicts allergic airway disease at 5 years. Clin Exp Allergy 1998;28:965–970.

Discussion

Dr. Szajewska: I have one comment and one question. You said that in your opinion early feeding in the early neonatal period doesn't make any difference later on. My conclusion from these studies when I analyze them, especially the Finnish study [1] and that of de Jong et al. [2] with a 5-year follow-up, was slightly different. As a matter of fact, I think it matters very much what the history of atopy was in the families. The conclusions from these studies, at least for me, are quite clear that if there is a family history of atopy, early feeding with hydrolyzed formula is extremely important. My question is: could you please speculate on what the plausible mechanism could be for breast-feeding that increases the risk of atopy as some studies suggest?

Dr. R. Bergmann: I think part of it is that in observational studies we have not been able to find out which is the cause and which is the consequence. So as I told you, children are more often breast-fed if they come from a higher socioeconomic class, which means they are at a higher risk of having atopic diseases.

Dr. Guesry: Thank you for bringing our level of confusion to a much higher level than before.

Dr. R. Bergmann: I thought it was clear.

Dr. Guesry: I think it is very useful that we start to ask questions about dogmas, it is always good in research. But you seem to favor the idea that the risk of breast-feeding would be higher from atopic mothers. Your study had a large population, did you look at this factor because it is very important? And particularly did you look at the IgA level in breast milk because, according to a rather old study from Machtinger and Moss [3], specific IgA was one of the protective factors in the breast milk of nonatopic mothers, that the specific IgA could block the allergen.

Dr. R. Bergmann: None of the epidemiological studies cited looked for this but other studies found a difference. We look at a landscape and then try to explain. It could be that specific IgA is a risk factor but I don't know how important it is and if it could explain all, it is just one factor. There are many other factors that could play a role.

Dr. Isolauri: To continue the comment that Dr. Szajewska just made. If we make recommendations particularly for atopic mothers to breast feed or not to breast feed, we need always to remember that these studies have only looked at the frequencies and the months of breast feeding and not the composition of the breast milk. In our country in particular, 60% of the atopic mothers are advised to eliminate specific foods from their diet, including fish and certain vegetables. Our data, as I will show later, are negative. It is harmful for these components which are protective in breast milk. So we cannot make a statement, because in one study breast-feeding was protective and in another study it was not. We are not comparing the same substances, we are comparing mothers who behave differently and their breast milk is not comparable at all.

Dr. R. Bergmann: It is true, I did not show the preventive effect of an elimination diet because I thought this might confuse things even more. In practice we made the experience that mothers eliminate everything until their children become malnourished, so we don't recommend this any longer. But when we recommend breast-feeding we recommend it usually for all infants, the total population. I am a member of the National Breast-Feeding Committee in Germany, so I am of course for breast-feeding. If the infant is becoming allergic and atopic to any of the compounds in the mother's food and to the mother's milk which has to be diagnosed, then a tailored diet should be recommended.

Dr. Zakiudin Munasir: I have two questions. In your slide showing the exclusively breast-fed babies with eczema and mothers on elimination diets, is it caused by food allergy? And the second question is, do you think that, if the mothers do not have any food allergy, the micromolecular allergen can enter the blood stream and be excreted in the breast milk?

Dr. R. Bergmann: I think it could, of course. It can cross the mammary barrier and enter the milk. This is the answer to the second question, and I did not understand the first.

Dr. Zakiudin Munasir: If the mothers do not have a food allergy, can the macromolecule of the allergen molecular protein enter the blood stream and be excreted in the breast milk?

Dr. R. Bergmann: Of course it can. What do you think Dr. Walker?

Dr. Walker: There are several studies that suggest that in the early infancy period proteins can in fact cross the mucosal barrier and enter the blood stream. Whether it has a positive or negative effects isn't clear.

Dr. Isolauri: This has also been studied clinically so there are data to support the comment you made [4]. The macromolecules cross the barrier in antigenic form, they can be detected in the blood stream as well as in breast milk. The concentrations in breast milk for β-lactoglobulin have been measured and there is no correlation to the dietary level of intake of that substance in the mother. It is not associated with an increase in permeability as measured by, for instance, the lactulose mannitol test and so on. So they do cross and they are detected.

Dr. Walker: I wanted to just comment briefly on what we heard from Dr. Guesry. This is a confusing topic but your presentation of it was very clear. You did a very good job of covering a difficult field. In every decade in medicine the same problems arise, and either the same or different conclusions are made. I have practiced for a long time and have been to multiple conferences like this. There was a study done in England many years ago in which breast-feeding seemed not to prevent allergy but to delay the expression of allergy which was found to be beneficial to both the baby and the mother [5]. That is one observation. Secondly, about atopic mothers who have higher levels of IgE in their breast milk: it has been my understanding that if they are actively atopic, e.g. if they are wheezing or if they have eczema or hay fever, that this might be a contraindication to breast-feeding because that is more likely to effect the baby. Is that a true statement?

Dr. R. Bergmann: I do not think that we should recommend this.

Dr. Walker: Can I make one final comment. The problem lies in part in our lack of understanding of how breast milk influences the infant's immune system because it is a very complex process. I go back to investigations that were done many years ago [6]. The theory was that early introduction of proteins actually protected rather than caused allergy. Thus the problem is that we don't quite understand how breast milk influences protection and the development of the infant's mucosal system. Those antibodies that were reported against breast milk proteins might be anti-idiotypic antibodies, which are antibodies against antibodies. I am not sure we can make that statement.

Dr. R. Bergmann: What we do not take into account are the different environments in which infants are breast fed. It probably makes a difference if it occurs in a developing country compared with our country.

Dr. K. Bergmann: I don't know whether you have got your point of reverse causation really across. The point is, and this is something you can conclude from the MAS data, that if a mother observed that her child had the first symptoms of eczema then she tended to breast-feed this child for longer and so finally you had more combinations of eczema and long-term breast-feeding in one group than in the other, and if the child was not symptomatic the mother tended to wean earlier, and so this is reverse causation. So the eczema caused the mother to breast-feed and not the breast-feeding caused the eczema, but in statistics you cannot discriminate between both, and this is the disadvantage of observational studies.

Dr. Lack: I have two comments and the first relates to the important point you made about reverse causation. I think the main problem is study design. It will never be ethical to do the real study which is to randomize children to breast-feeding or placebo.

Dr. R. Bergmann: We can randomize infants to human milk, but not to breast-feeding.

Dr. Lack: Yes, but there is always a process of self-selection in mothers who choose prolonged breast-feeding, and therefore you have factors like reverse causation. Together with Dr. Golding at the University of Bristol we looked at a cohort of 14,000 children and examined the relationship between breast-feeding and IgE-mediated peanut allergy later in life. It was found that prolonged breast-feeding is a risk factor for the development of IgE-mediated food allergies. However, in a regression analysis if you then take into account the early development of eczema the relationship disappears; this is simply because the mothers and their GPs decided to prolong breast-feeding in the children who develop eczema, so you find this reverse causation when you look at food allergy. The second point was simply that because of the possible protective effect in some studies on the development of eczema there is the assumption therefore that breast-feeding protects against food allergies. I think that is partly a problem relating to phenotypic definitions of atopic dermatitis and food allergy. We assume that if something is going to work in atopic dermatitis it will work in food allergy. Eczema and food allergies are distinct though eczema can be a manifestation of food allergy. To my knowledge, there is no really good evidence anywhere showing that breast-feeding protects against IgE-mediated food allergy.

Dr. Neijens: Is it possible to interpret all that information by accepting that breast-feeding does protect against the infections. This might obscure the information and the development and the effect of breast-feeding. If it is shown that breast-feeding protects against infections then it might be an advantage in the beginning, it may diminish atopic dermatitis and also nonatopic disease, but in the long run it might be a drawback. The study from Wright seems to suggest that. What is your opinion about that?

Dr. R. Bergmann: I agree, but I don't know if these children will develop allergy, so I would not advise the mother not to breast-feed.

Dr. Neijens: But you can breast-feed. By inviting all the children in the cohort together with those being breast fed. It is a social system which has been used for many centuries, and then you have the protective effect of breast-feeding and also the infections.

Dr. R. Bergmann: As for me I would like to protect them from infections although the risk for asthma is higher.

Dr. Neijens: But those children need activation of a microorganism just to diminish the development of sensitization and expression of atopic disease. In the long run then breast-feeding might be a drawback in the protective mechanism against infections.

Dr. R. Bergmann: But this is not the only protective factor, there are others.

Dr. Isolauri: It has been shown that, for instance, for rotavirus infection breast-fed infants do not have symptoms. We can detect rotavirus excretion, so they are not protected against the infection but they are protected against the clinical infection which is then important for preventive effects, and that is another story. So, again, by looking at the reported rates of infection we cannot make a statement that there is less infection, it protects against the disease. Duffy [7] I think from the US has shown that.

Dr. R. Bergmann: And the same is true for vaccination. It does not weaken the effect of vaccination, not even the survival of living microbes.

Dr. Hill: Can I ask you how much you think the long-term studies on the influence of breast-feeding on the development of eczema might be confounded by the failure of people to appreciate the different phenotypes associated with atopic dermatitis? For instance, in our experience a diet-related eczema is a phenomenon in the first 12 months of life. It seems unwise to then look for the effect of that at the age of 5 years because the development of eczema in the second year of life and later seems to be a completely different ideology. In addition we seem to be seeing the phenotypes in breast-fed infants, those infants who seem to develop the symptoms while being totally breast-fed, and those who seem to develop symptoms with the onset of coincidence, with the onset of solid feeding in the second 6 months of life. I am not familiar enough with the literature, but my impression is that people haven't understood these different phenotypic expressions and I don't see evidence that people have considered confounders like the introduction of solids and the effect in the range of solids in addition to bottle-feeding or breast-feeding. These were data which were examined by the New Zealand group some 10 years ago, demonstrating the emergence of eczema related to the introduction of solids.

Dr. R. Bergmann: In the study by Kramer 43% of the mothers were exclusively breast-feeding at 3 months in the intervention group compared to 6% in the control group, so this is a high-risk against a low-risk group in relation to breast-feeding. In most epidemiological studies there is no clear limit between one and the other group. It is usually a dark gray against a light gray zone.

Dr. Bindslev-Jensen: I want to take Dr. Hill's and also Dr. Lack's questions a little further. I think it is very important that we try to define further which kinds of patients we are talking about because in most of the data we are seeing there is a history of atopic predisposition in the mother, and in some cases it means that the patients have asthma but there is nothing about sensitization. In the other case it means that the patient had or has had atopic eczema and now has atopic dermatitis after having had atopic dermatitis. The third thing is that in many of the studies the diagnosis in the infant is made either by interview or by clinical examinations, but in very few cases have the gold standards really been followed to demonstrate that the child is in fact suffering from that disease from the clinical point of view. I still think that it would be possible using computer models, or something like that, and a meta-analysis on what has been published to try to figure out what are the truly important things and what are the very many confounders in this issue, but so far I don't think it has been done.

Dr. R. Bergmann: In our study we had a very strict definition of atopic eczema and we also looked at the sensitization of the mother. We asked many questions and then used an algorithm for this diagnosis, and still we did not find a protective effect.

Dr. Bindslev-Jensen: I just wanted to add one comment to that because I do think that the kind of recommendation that you are making should be pursued, and I think it has been pursued in some studies more rigorously than others, there is no question there. But one warning regarding just using meta-analysis for all those perfect studies, or as perfect as possible, we might find in the last 20 years. One other factor to add to the confusion is time, the secular trend. From the point of view of the changes made in daycare centers since the start of the HIV epidemic, it is difficult to compare a study made before this time to one now. Five years ago all the pediatricians in the audience here would have told the mother of an atopic child to continue breast-feeding, but today they might not be compelled to do so. Therefore the studies done 20 or 25 years ago, although excellent, may not be appropriate for analysis today.

Dr. R. Bergmann: It is true. Breast-feeding is a cultural development and we are part of this culture, our mind this part of this culture, and we act according to our knowledge.

Dr. Saavedra: We are a confounding variable.

Dr. Suyoko: Because breast-feeding is still the most important nutrition for the babies in our country, I have a question. For how long should we recommend that mothers breast-feed their babies to prevent allergic diseases, because you said that prolonged breast-feeding could increase the risk of eczema in babies.

Dr. R. Bergmann: We don't know.

Dr. Nieman: A question for Dr. Isolauri. There are some who would say that if you use an elimination diet for nursing mothers you can cause more harm than good. When you do that in your clinic, do you always involve dieticians or do you allow physicians to work by themselves?

Dr. Isolauri: I am presenting the backup for that in my talk later, but it is not what we recommend, it is not what we do, march in there and recommend it. It is something we try to advise not to happen. But that has been the practice, allergologists in our country started something like 20–30 years ago to try to eliminate atopic diseases from our country, and the method was to eliminate the exposure. Just as other people eliminated cats and dogs and house dust mite, we eliminated foods. In our country people usually follow the advice and they continue to do so even when you try to stop them, and we do try to stop them. Later I will present data showing that it is not only unnecessary but harmful.

Dr. Ham Pong: I would like to comment further on the role of breast-feeding and the development of IgE-mediated food allergies. About a decade ago in my practice I began to notice that children with peanut allergy had been breast-fed, and I have continued to follow this over the last 10 years. I had perhaps about 1,000 patients with peanut allergy and over 95% of those had been breast-fed. Breast-feeding in our area is probably less than 80% so I can't comment on what the relationship is, whether it is a causal relationship or just an association, but certainly a very high percentage of peanut-allergic patients in my practice have been breast-fed.

Dr. R. Bergmann: This fits to the whole landscape.

Dr. K. Bergmann: I think there is one basic consideration with respect to breast-feeding and eczema that I would like to share with you. I think the majority of people considering prevention of atopic manifestations more often end in the field of secondary prevention. So if you have early signs you start to do something and it appears to be quite effective for most of the manifestations, whereas with respect to primary prevention this appears to be somewhat disappointing. Everywhere some people thought that house dust mite elimination could do something but it apparently doesn't do anything, and some people thought that not having animals in the house was protective and now we see that perhaps it is protective to have cats in the house and so on. So one of the aspects would be breast-feeding and all together it appears that primary prevention is not very promising. On the other hand in this century we if we are talking about disease we are talking about something completely different from what it was in the last century. Prevention of early death was an important aspect of prevention in the past and today it is prevention of lack of quality of life that is not so much a concern in our preventive activities, and so in terms of quality of life I think breast-feeding contributes highly to quality of life. Then if we have symptoms of atopic manifestations we should take care of them in terms of secondary prevention.

Dr. R. Bergmann: I am not even sure that there isn't some reverse causation in many of the studies observing that elimination is not as good as exposure. In our MAS study parents who had asthma themselves removed cats and dogs and there was a low mite allergen load in the house.

Dr. Manjra: We have much bigger problems in that we have a very high HIV prevalence and we think that about 10% of the population is HIV-positive. As you know breast-feeding is not advised in mothers who are HIV-positive for the risk of transmitting it to the baby. However, the reality of the situation is that if these mothers don't breast-feed they cannot afford formula feeds. So we have to take a pragmatic view and advise them rather to breast-feed and take the risk of the child being infected or dying from a diarrheal disease or respiratory infections. So there is a completely different picture in poor countries, and we have other diseases that take priority. So allergy should not be the priority for the minority, otherwise the majority pays for the minority.

Dr. Isolauri: There are data on record of a positive association, so some might think that reducing the risk of allergic disease is not the most important question, even in industrialized countries.

Dr. Guesry: Yesterday I was asking that we revisit the work of Strobel and Ferguson [8] about the timing of the introduction of allergens. I wonder today, after listening to this very interesting presentation and discussion, if the Jarret hypothesis [9] should not be revisited in the light of modern immunology because what we are saying today reminds me of what was said 20 years ago about the importance of the quantity of allergens presented to the child.

Dr. van den Biggelaar: What is known about the cytokines that are present in breast milk and how are these determined? Since cytokines in the breast milk seem to create the microenvironment in which the early immune response of the children may be shaped, they seem very important. What is known about the regulation of these cytokines in the breast milk and do we know if there is a difference in these concentrations in Western compared to developing countries?

Dr. R. Bergmann: I have shown you what is published, I don't know more than that. Berthia said that she doesn't believe that this is a real cause for the different reactions of children, she meant making atopic diseases or not. It is probably a small contribution. What do you think?

Dr. Isolauri: In a recent issue of *Pediatric Research* [10] we looked at that question and found, for instance, that eicosanoids have an important regulatory effect and so there are many factors from the mother's diet that have one effect.

Dr. Murch: In terms of the pathogenesis of eczema there was an important study in the *New England Journal of Medicine* last autumn showing that defensing expression within the skin or reduced defensing was quite important in allowing the toxin staphylococcide to drive eczema. Now could you not invoke some kind of cutaneous harm of the clean child hypothesis to suggest that if a mother continues to give her own defenses in innate immune stimulation to the child then this is going to prevent the drive on the skin from the child's own gut flora? A bottle-fed baby will have no inhibition to defensing augmentation, whereas the mother who continues to breast-feed is actually going to be dumping down the response within the skin and thus maintaining defenses low and allowing then local skin infection to drive inflammation.

Dr. R. Bergmann: Kramer showed that infectious rashes were also less prevalent in the intervention group.

Dr. Murch: I think it all comes down to what type of infection and at what time they actually get it, and what modulatory factors are present. We know very little or less than we should about the cutaneous flora.

Dr. Bedford-Russell: Just a comment about dogs and cats. I think from my understanding of the studies that it depends on the timing of exposure. Certainly Strachan has produced data suggesting that if the animal is in the household before the baby is born it is protective but if the baby gets exposed afterwards by someone deciding they are going to have a puppy for their toddler, that is when it is more dangerous in terms of atopy. In the studies I have not seen much evidence in the data collected from the breast-fed babies, for example, about the effect of nipple creams being used and the practice of applying oils to the baby's skin. I do worry about some major confounding variable, because I still see babies in my follow-up clinic whose mothers are advised to apply almond oil to the skin and I have seen little of that in the studies that have been published. Of course, those of us who have breast-fed know that the nipples get a bit hard and painful, and the nurses often advise applying copious amounts of oils without knowing what is in them.

Dr. R. Bergmann: There are a lot of confounding factors that were not considered, e.g. we did not look at pesticides.

References

1 Saarinen KM, Juntunen-Backman K, Jarvenpaa AL, et al: Supplementary feeding in maternity hospitals and the risk of cow's milk allergy: A prospective study of 6,209 infants. J Allergy Clin Immunol 1999;104:457–461.

2 de Jong MH, Scharp-van den Linden VT, Aalberse R, et al: The effect of brief neonatal exposure to cows' milk on atopic symptoms up to age 5. Arch Dis Child 2002;86:365–369.

3 Machtinger S, Moss R: Cow's milk allergy in breast-fed infants: The role of allergen and maternal secretory IgA antibody. J Allergy Clin Immunol 1986;77:341–347.

4 Hoppu U, Kalliomäki M, Laiho K, Isolauri E: Breast milk – Immunomodulatory signals against allergic diseases. Allergy 2001;56:23–26.

5 Shah U, Walker WA: Pathophysiology of intestinal food allergy. Adv Pediatr 2002;49:299–316.

6 Spieckermann GM, Walker WA: Oral tolerance and its role in clinical disease. J Pediatr Gastroenterol Nutr 2001;32:237–255.
7 Duffy LC, Riepenhoff-Talty M, Byers TE, et al: Modulation of rotavirus enteritis during breast-feeding. Am J Dis Child 1986;140:1164–1168.
8 Strobel S, Ferguson A: Immune response to fed antigen in mie. Systemic tolerance of priming is related to age at which antigen is first encountered. Pediatr Res 1984;18:588–594.
9 Jarrett EE: Perinatal influences on IgE responses. Lancet 1984;ii:797–799.
10 Laiho K, Lampi AM, Hämäläinen M, et al: Breast milk fatty acids, eicosanoids and cytokines in mother with and without allergic disease. Pediatr Res 2003;53:642–647.

Isolauri E, Walker WA (eds): Allergic Diseases and the Environment.
Nestlé Nutrition Workshop Series Pediatric Program, Vol. 53, pp. 217–249,
Nestec Ltd.; Vevey/S. Karger AG, Basel, © 2004.

Protective Nutrients and Gastrointestinal Allergies

Christopher Duggan

Clinical Nutrition Service, Division of GI/Nutrition, Children's Hospital, Boston, Mass., USA

Introduction

The nutritional management of gastrointestinal (GI) allergic diseases has historically relied on the avoidance of dietary allergens. Among formula-fed infants, in whom food allergies are often transient and alternative sources of nutrients are plentiful, this approach is appropriate, safe, and often effective. Dietary avoidance of foods, however, entails nutritional risks and can be difficult to maintain if allergies are numerous or persistent. An alternative approach in treating GI diseases due to allergy, infection or others is the provision of some of a variety of nutrients that may actively exert healthful affects on the GI tract. Here a review is made of the evidence that standard approaches of dietary avoidance may be poorly designed for optimal health, as well as the possibility that so-called gut-protective nutrients may play a role in mediating intestinal inflammation.

Pitfalls of Dietary Avoidance of Suspected Food Allergens

Perhaps the most common drawback with the dietary therapy of food allergy is the fact that food allergies are often overdiagnosed by parents, patients, and physicians. As a result, food restrictions and dietary avoidance of perceived allergens can be performed without justification and with significant nutritional risk. For instance, in a case series of 9 children with multiple purported food allergies who were found to have few or no food allergies, significant undernutrition was documented [1]. Numerous case series have documented severe nutritional problems, including kwashiorkor and severe protein energy malnutrition, in children treated with severely restricted or misguided diets [2].

Once the diagnosis of food allergy is accurately made, the primary therapy is dietary avoidance. The most common form of food allergy in infancy and childhood, cow's milk allergy, is commonly treated with dietary avoidance of cow's milk protein. In the breast-fed infant, allergic colitis can often be managed with maternal dietary manipulation. This often means maternal avoidance of cow's milk protein, although sometimes more limited diets are recommended to avoid multiple possible allergens. Few studies have systematically evaluated the effects of these restrictive diets on maternal health, though these may be significant in the setting of increased nutrient needs during lactation [3].

In the formula-fed infant with cow's milk protein allergy, it is recommended that extensively hydrolyzed protein formulas be used. The widespread availability in developed countries of infant formulas free of cow's milk protein makes the nutritional management of cow's milk allergy in the formula-fed infant straightforward. However, data concerning the utilization of soy and protein hydrolysate formulas in the US suggest that these formulas are startlingly overused. Surveys show that 25–30% of infants less than 6 months of age in the US receive either a soy-based infant formula or a protein hydrolysate formula [4]. In contrast, the incidence of cow's milk protein allergy has been estimated at 2–5% in industrialized countries [5]. These patterns of special infant formula use are significantly higher than in previous years, and are out of proportion to the documented increase in atopic diseases noted recently.

Although the nutritional adequacy of these infant formulas has been generally well established, concerns have been raised about the long- and short-term significance of dietary restrictions for the treatment of food allergies in general as well as the specific use of these infant formulas. These have included studies of growth, nutrient absorption, and micronutrient adequacy.

Many studies have documented the importance of early nutrition on bone health. In one study, 27 young children (mean age 4 years) were studied who had had cow's milk allergy diagnosed by typical history, resolution of symptoms with dietary avoidance, and then confirmed by open challenge. Most of these received a soy or extensively hydrolyzed protein formula and avoided cow's milk protein for an average of 11 months. Compared to age-matched healthy control children, those treated with a cow's milk dietary avoidance had significantly higher serum concentrations of alkaline phosphatase and parathyroid hormone. Using single photon absorptiometry of the forearm, mean bone mineral density Z score of the allergic infants was −0.6; 10 of 27 had bone mineral density Z scores below −1.0 [6].

Another recent study [7] has underscored the association of cow's milk intake early in life with subsequent lower risk of osteopenia and fracture in adulthood. Using data from the third National Health and Nutrition Examination Survey, investigators evaluated the effect of diet from age 5 to adulthood on bone mineral content in adulthood (measured by dual-energy absorptiometry) among more than 3,000 non-Hispanic white women. Factors known to affect bone health, such as age, weight, height, menopausal status, smoking, alcohol use, physical activity, and medications including estrogen therapy, were also assessed. Among women aged 20–49 years, the bone mineral content of the hip was significantly lower (5.6%) among women who consumed <1 serving of milk/week during childhood compared to those who consumed more than 1 serving/day ($p < 0.01$), even when controlling for current calcium intake. The risk of bone fractures after age 50 was also increased with lower intakes of milk; the odds ratio for fractures was 2.25 (1.26–4.00) among those with a milk intake of <1 serving/week in childhood, compared to those who consumed more than 1 serving/day.

All of the currently available soy and protein hydrolysate formulas are lactose-free owing to the potential of cross-contamination of the carbohydrate source with cow's milk protein. The routine exclusion of lactose from the diet of infants, however, has potential health effects. For instance, routine exclusion of lactose from birth may result in false-negative neonatal screening for galactosemia. Lactose-free diets may alter the composition of the colonic flora, the implications of which are not yet clear but are of growing interest. Protein hydrolysate formulas have also been reported to have substandard nitrogen accrual rates compared to standard formulas [8, 9], and their use in premature infants has been discouraged for this reason [10]. Concern has also been raised that mineral absorption may be compromised in infants receiving soy-based, lactose-free formulas owing to the enhanced calcium absorption with lactose and the possibility that phytates present in soy formulas would reduce calcium and zinc bioavailability. Recent data using stable isotopes, however, seem to reduce this concern [11].

Investigators have also noted that the use of soy-based formulas may have long-lasting effects on health [12]. In a retrospective cohort study, women who as infants had been fed soy formula reported a slightly longer duration of menstrual bleeding and greater discomfort with menstruation compared to women fed cow's milk formulas as infants. Pubertal maturation and reproductive history were similar in the 2 groups. The authors hypothesized that infant exposure to phytoestrogens via soy isoflavones may in part be responsible for these outcomes, although more data in this field are needed.

More recently, amino acid-based formulas have gained increasing usage in treating food allergies, and these formulas have been extremely helpful in children with severe food allergies or those whose symptoms have not responded to protein hydrolysates [13]. However, we have reported on a child treated with an amino acid formula who developed multiple micronutrient deficiencies, including symptomatic scurvy [14]. This child had spastic cerebral palsy and was therefore fed an amount of formula adequate to meet his lower energy needs, but this lower volume lead to his receiving only 62% of his recommended dietary allowance of vitamin C and zinc, and 70% of the recommended dietary allowance for vitamin A. Despite this intake, he developed bone, skin and oral mucosal changes of vitamin C deficiency, and biochemical vitamin A and zinc deficiencies. Similar reports have been forthcoming [15, 16] and underscore the need for physicians recommending specialized enteral formulas to be vigilant that the nutrient needs of their patients are being met, especially since many elemental formulas provide lower amounts of micronutrients than do formulas with intact proteins.

A review of the available literature therefore suggests that while the nutritional management of cow's milk or other food allergies in infants and young children is commonly managed with dietary avoidance, there are several real and potential risks of poor nutritional and health outcomes if this is done cavalierly. Especially in growing toddlers and young children, dietary restriction can place patients at risk of undernutrition, and both long- and short-term nutritional problems can arise. The long-term effects of soy, protein hydrolysate, and elemental diets are still to be determined.

Definition of Protective Nutrients

Since dietary avoidance has disadvantages, it might therefore be reasonable to investigate whether the occurrence of allergy can be modified by active dietary therapy. Indeed, some foods or nutrients have an important physiologic effect on the body, separate and distinct from their nutritional role. These have been termed 'functional foods' [17, 18]. Certain classes of functional foods have been termed 'protective nutrients', whereby nutrients or other food components (e.g., prebiotics, probiotics) could exert a specific protective affect on the GI tract [19]. The postulated mechanisms through which these nutrients might be protective are many, and include acting directly as a nutrient for the rapidly turning over GI epithelia, as a stimulant to the growth of bifidobacter and other bacteria, acting in a way to stimulate mucosal and systemic immune function, and others. Multiple components of human milk may be classified as these types of nutrients (table 1).

The case of breast milk is of more than passing interest to the discussion of food allergies, since many studies have confirmed that breast-fed infants have lower incidence and/or delayed onset of many atopic diseases, including atopic dermatitis, food allergies, and asthma. Could these results be due to active components of breast milk and not just to the dietary avoidance of cow's milk proteins and other allergens? Observational studies cannot of course answer this question, and randomized clinical trials have been difficult to carry out. Furthermore, few studies have addressed the issue of whether 'immunostimulatory' protective nutrients may be helpful in intestinal

Table 1. Protective components of human milk

Proteins/amino acids
Lactoferrin
Lysozyme
Secretory IgA
Lactadherin
Creatine*
Glutamine*
Arginine*
Oligosaccharides and glycoconjugates*
Monoglycerides and fatty acids*
Growth factors
Epidermal growth factor
Polyamines
G-CSF
Cortisol
Cytokines
IL-10
TGF-β
TNF-α
Others
Nucleotides*
Antioxidants*
Vitamin C*
Vitamin A and β-carotene*
Zinc*

* Nutrients which may play a role in gastrointestinal protection.

inflammation due to allergies. A review of selected protective nutrients and their role in other types of intestinal disease may therefore be helpful.

Is Glutamine a Protective Nutrient?

The amino acid glutamine (Gln) has been widely touted as a protective nutrient since it is an important fuel source for rapidly turning over cells including GI epithelia, lymphocytes, fibroblasts, and reticulocytes [20]. A large amount of in vitro and animal data support the importance of Gln in GI function. Animals nourished with parenteral nutrition showed less mucosal atrophy when supplemented with Gln [21, 22]. Decreased intestinal permeability, as measured by the lactulose:mannitol ratio in urine, has also been shown with Gln treatment [23]. After ischemia and reperfusion, treatment with Gln helped preserve mucosal glutathione concentrations and reduced markers of lipid peroxidation [24]. Gln's specific role as a possible mediator of intestinal adaptation in short bowel syndrome has been indicated in some [25, 26] but not all [27] animal models.

A large number of human experiments have also been performed (table 2). These studies have documented a role for Gln in ameliorating the mucosal atrophy seen in prolonged states of parenteral nutrition [28, 29]; in the healing of GI mucosa after damage from either radio- or chemotherapy [30, 31]; in improving gut and systemic immune function [32–34]; in attaining nitrogen balance and transition from parenteral nutrition [35], and in reducing episodes of bacterial translocation [36, 37] and clinical sepsis [38, 39].

Some important negative trials have also been published. Oral rehydration solutions with added Gln have not proven more effective than standard solutions in correcting dehydration due to acute diarrhea [40]. In 6 patients with short bowel syndrome, the use of a Gln-containing isotonic rehydration solution resulted in lower sodium absorption compared to a glucose-containing solution [41]. In a large multicenter trial of intravenous Gln among 1,430 premature infants, there were no differences in sepsis, incidence of necrotizing enterocolitis (NEC), or mortality, despite an increase in the plasma Gln concentration in the supplemented group [42].

Table 2 summarizes a large number of randomized, blinded clinical trials of Gln supplementation that have been published. Some of these trials have been plagued by methodologic shortcomings, including inadequate sample size, incomplete description of blinding and randomization procedures, lack of control group, or lack of isonitrogenous control. Inclusion criteria are unclear in some papers, some studies have not followed intent-to-treat data analysis, and others have reported only subgroup analyses. A recent meta-analysis of 14 randomized trials in surgical and critically ill patients showed a lower rate of infection (RR 0.81, 95% CI 0.64–1.00) and a shorter hospital stay (mean −2.6 days, 95% CI −4.5, −0.7) with Gln supplementation, as well as a trend to reduced mortality. These findings were more apparent in trials that used high dose (>0.2 g/kg/day) Gln, compared to lower doses [43].

Although much data suggest that Gln is an important protective nutrient for the GI tract mucosa, larger, well-designed randomized trials are needed to fully confirm its role. At least one large trial among premature infants failed to support its role in reducing mortality; data among adult surgical patients are more promising. Important research issues include the selection of valid and reliable outcome variables that have biologic plausibility and can be routinely measured in study subjects.

Is Arginine a Protective Nutrient?

The amino acid arginine (Arg) plays important roles in nitrogen transport, storage, and excretion, polyamine synthesis, and the disposition of ammonia via the urea cycle [44]. Arg is a dietary precursor nitric oxide (NO), a molecule

Table 2. Randomized, blinded trials of glutamine (Gln) in patients at risk of gastrointestinal disease

References	Subjects	Gln dose and route	Comparison group	Outcomes of Gln group
38, 142–144	45 adult allogeneic BMT patients	0.57 g/kg/day i.v.	Isonitrogenous and isocaloric PN	Better N balance Fewer clinical infections Shorter LOS Lower hospital charges Less ECF expansion Increased total lymphocyte count Increased CD4 and CD8 counts
145	29 adult allogeneic and autologous BMT patient	0.57 g/kg/day i.v.	Isonitrogenous and isocaloric PN	Shorter LOS Less ECF expansion No decrease in clinical infections
28	20 adults requiring inpatient PN for 2 weeks	0.23 g/k/day i.v. via dipeptides	Isonitrogenous and isocaloric PN	Preserved villus height Lactulose:mannitol ratio preserved
29	12 adults requiring PN in intensive care	0.30 g/kg/day i.v. *L*-alanine-*L*-glutamine	Isonitrogenous and isocaloric PN	Higher area under the *D*-xylose time curve
146	28 adults in ICU with APACHE score >10 who received enteral nutrition by 48 h of admission	EN with 25% Gln	Isonitrogenous and isocaloric EN	Reduced phe:tyr ratio Transient rise in CD4:CD8 ratio
147	67 adult women with advanced breast cancer	30 g QD p.o.	Maltodextrin	No differences in diarrhea incidence
148	84 adults in ICU with APACHE II score >10	PN with 2.5% Gln	Isonitrogenous PN	Reduced mortality at 6 months
39	68 premature infants	Up to 0.31 g/kg/day in enteral formula	Unsupplemented formula	Fewer infections Better tolerance of enteral feeds

(continued overleaf)

Table 2. (continued)

References	Subjects	Gln dose and route	Comparison group	Outcomes of Gln group
149	193 BMT patients	1 g/m^2 BSA swish and swallow QID	Same dose of glycine	In auto BMT, Gln patients had less mouth pain and used opiates for fewer days (5 vs. 10) No differences in GVHD, antibiotic use, or LOS noted
150	34 adult BMT patients	50 g glycyl-Gln i.v.	Isonitrogenous PN	Protein C and serum albumin levels better maintained Markers of thrombin and plasmin generation not different
151	14 adults with severe acute pancreatitis	0.22 g/kg/d i.v.	Isonitrogenous PN	Lowered IL-8 release by mononuclear cells No changes in TNF or IL-6
152	72 adults with trauma and ISS >20		Isonitrogenous EN	Fewer episodes of bacteremia, pneumonia, and sepsis
153	28 adults with colon carcinoma or other reason	0.3 g/kg/day Ala-Gln i.v.	Isonitrogenous PN	Higher N balance Shorter LOS
154	24 adults with AIDS and abnormal lactulose:mannitol tests	4 (n = 8) or 8 (n = 8) g Gln p.o./day × 28 days	6 g sucrose	No changes in intestinal histology or lactulose:mannitol ratios
155	13 patients with advanced esophageal cancer	30 g/day p.o.	None	Less reduction in lymphocyte count with chemotherapy
156	9 infants in ICU with sepsis or respiratory failure	0.3 g/kg/day EN	Casein	No differences
157	24 adults with metastatic colon cancer receiving chemotherapy	0.4 g/kg glycyl-*L*-glutamine i.v.	Non-supplemented group	Less small bowel and gastric inflammation by EGD Higher villus to crypt ratio

158	14 patients with Crohn's disease and increased intestinal permeability	7 g p.o. t.i.d. × 4 weeks	Glycine	No change in intestinal permeability or Crohn's disease activity
159	50 adults in ICU with APACHE score >10 who tolerated EN by 48 h of admission	11–21 g/day in Gln-supplemented elemental formula	Isonitrogenous EN (glycine)	No differences in mortality, morbidity, ICU stay or LOS; Hospital costs lower
160	134 adults receiving 5-fluorouracil chemotherapy	4 g b.i.d. swish and swallow × 4 days	Identical-appearing placebo	No differences in oral mucositis scores
161	168 adults requiring PN	Gln-supplemented PN	Isonitrogenous PN	Shorter LOS in surgical patients only
162	66 adults undergoing allogeneic or autologous BMT	10 g p.o. t.i.d. or 0.57 g/kg i.v.	10 g glycine p.o. t.i.d. or isonitrogenous PN	No significant differences in mortality, LOS, engraftment, incidence of infections, or GVHD
163	26 HIV-infected adults with >5% weight loss	40 g/day × 12 weeks plus additional antioxidants	40 g/day glycine	Increased body weight, body cell mass, and intracellular water
164	18 children with active Crohn's disease	Polymeric EN with 7.9–8.3 g GLN/100 g formula	Isonitrogenous and isocaloric EN	Less improvement in Crohn's disease activity score
165	58 adults BMT patients	30 g Gln p.o. QD	30 g sucrose p.o. QD	No significant differences in mortality, LOS, engraftment, mucositis, or diarrhea

PN = Parenteral nutrition; EN = enteral nutrition; N = nitrogen; ECF = extracellular fluid; LOS = length of stay; ISS = injury severity score; BMT = bone marrow transplantation; GVHD = graft versus host disease; EGD = esophagogastroduodenoscopy; TNF = tumor necrosis factor; IL-8 = interleukin-8; IL-6 = interleukin-6.

Reproduced with permission from the *American Journal of Clinical Nutrition*. ©AM J Clin Nutr. American Society for Clinical Nutrition. Adapted from Duggan et al. [19].

with a wide range of functions [45]. Arg is converted to citrulline by the action of NO synthase (NOS), which combines the terminal guanidino N-atom of Arg with oxygen to form NO. The constitutive form of NOS (cNOS) produces the small amounts of NO that are necessary for certain cell functions in the nonpathologic state, such as neurotransmission and vascular relaxation. An inducible form of NOS (iNOS) is found in a wide variety of mammalian cells and its induction by the presence of inflammatory cytokines and bacterial endotoxin results in the production of larger amounts of NO. NO may have both anti- and proinflammatory effects; homeostatic, anti-inflammatory effects are observed with small amounts of NO produced by cNOS, while the pro-inflammatory effects are seen with iNOS's production of excessive amounts of NO. Excessive NO production in the setting of endotoxemia, septic shock and increased intestinal vascular permeability has been studied in a variety of animal and human experiments.

Many animal studies have examined the role of Arg and NO in immunity and inflammation. Arg supplementation leads to higher thymic weight, higher thymic lymphocyte content, and an increased response of T lymphocytes to mitogen stimulation [46]. Rats receiving Arg-supplemented parenteral nutrition had a more vigorous acute phase protein response when septic [47]. Tumor-bearing rats, when treated with parenteral nutrition high in Arg and branch-chain amino acids, show lower rates of tumor protein synthesis and higher rates of whole body protein synthesis, when compared to standard nutrition [48]. Higher muscle concentrations of Gln, Arg, and other amino acids were also reported with Arg-supplemented parenteral nutrition [49]. Animal data suggest that inhibition of cNOS by N^G-nitro-*L*-arginine methyl ester (*L*-NAME) increases small intestine permeability to smaller molecules [50]. Another study confirmed that *L*-NAME increased intestinal permeability as well as increased evidence of mast cell degranulation [51].

Arg and NO are both intestinal secretagogues, and inhibition of NOS can result in intestinal ischemia as well as increased fluid secretion [52]. Animal models of intestinal transplantation have also shown that Arg supplementation results in less disruption of GI structure when reperfusion occurs [53, 54]. Rats subjected to massive small bowel resection showed better preserved intestinal barrier function when treated with Arg [55]. Recovery from radiation enteritis has also been shown to be improved with Arg supplementation, as measured by increased mucosal thickness, villous height, number of villi per centimeter of small bowel, and gut barrier function [56].

Studies of Arg supplementation in humans have also been performed (table 3). In healthy subjects, NO formation can be increased by *L*-Arg administration in the range of 0.1–0.2 g/kg/day [57]. Premature infants who developed NEC were found to have lower serum concentrations of Arg and Gln both before and during an episode of NEC [58, 59]. In a trial of 152 premature infants, those receiving Arg-supplemented nutrition had a lower

Table 3. Summary of clinical studies of arginine (Arg) in patients at risk of GI mucosal disease

References	Study type	Subjects	Arg dose and route	Comparison group	Outcomes of Arg group
166	Randomized, double-blind, clinical trial	22 adult surgical ICU patients	12.5 g/l supplemented with nucleotides and n-3 FA	Isocaloric formula	Greater in vitro stimulation of peripheral blood lymphocytes
167	Randomized, double-blind, clinical trial	50 adult and pediatric patients with >10% BSA burn	5 g/l supplemented with n-3 FA	2 control groups; both isocaloric, isonitrogenous formulas	Decreased LOS, controlled for percent burn Lower incidence of wound infections
168	Randomized, clinical trial	85 adult surgical patients with upper gastrointestinal cancer	12.5 g/l supplemented with nucleotides and n-3 FA	Isocaloric formula	Fewer infectious and wound complications Decreased LOS
169	Randomized, double-blind, clinical trial	30 adult surgical patients with lower gastrointestinal cancer	20 g/day parenteral	Isocaloric, isonitrogenous parenteral mixed amino acid solution	No difference in postop complications Lower lymphocyte response to PHA stimulation on postop day 4 Higher percentage of CD3+ lymphocytes by postop day 7
170	Randomized, multicenter trial	114 adult ICU trauma patients with ISS ≥16 or ATI ≥18	15.4 g/l supplemented with nucleotides	Isocaloric formula	Lower incidence of intra-abdominal abscesses Lower multiorgan failure scores Higher total lymphocyte, CD3+ and CD4+ concentrations
171	Randomized, double-blind,	326 adult ICU patients with	12.5 g/l supplemented with nucleotides and	Isocaloric formula containing lower	Decreased mortality rate in analysis of successfully fed

(continued overleaf)

Table 3. (continued)

References	Study type	Subjects	Arg dose and route	Comparison group	Outcomes of Arg group
	multicenter trial	APACHE II ≥10 or TISS ≥20	n-3 FA	amount of nitrogen	subgroup
172	Randomized, clinical trial	60 adult surgical patients with upper gastrointestinal tract cancer	12.5 g/l supplemented with nucleotides and n-3 FA	Formula with higher protein, fat and calories	Shorter LOS Fewer infectious and wound complications Higher plasma concentration of n-3 FA at postop day 7
173	Randomized, double-blind, clinical trial	44 adult surgical patients with upper gastrointestinal cancer	12.5 g/l supplemented with nucleotides and n-3 FA	Isocaloric, isonitrogenous formula	Higher overall T-lymphocyte and CD4+, CD3+ and activated CD3+ subset concentrations by postop day 10 Higher B-lymphocyte concentration by postop day 7
174	Randomized, double-blind, clinical trial	42 adult surgical patients with upper gastrointestinal tract cancer	12.5 g/l supplemented with nucleotides and n-3 FA	Isocaloric, isonitrogenous formula	Faster decline of APACHE II scores Lower IL-6 concentrations on postop days 3 and 7
175	Randomized, double-blind, clinical trial	44 adult patients with upper or lower gastrointestinal tract cancer	12.5 g/l supplemented with nucleotides and n-3 FA Given from preop day 7 to postop day 7	Isocaloric formula from preop day 7 to surgery, then isonitrogenous to postop day 7	Lower CRP postop Higher serum NO concentration postop Higher mean Doppler intestinal blood flow Lower serum concentrations of intestinal alkaline phosphatase postop

					Higher phagocytic and respiratory burst activity postop
176	Randomized, clinical trial	60 adult surgical patients with upper gastrointestinal tract cancer	12.5 g/ supplemented with nucleotides and n-3 FA	(1) Isocaloric isonitrogenous enteral formula or (2) PN	Shorter postop LOS vs. PN group Lower postop sepsis score in patients with infectious complications Higher visceral protein concentrations at postop day 8 Lower plasma IL-6 concentration by postop day 8
177	Randomized, clinical trial	35 adult trauma patients with ATI ≥25 or ISS ≥20	14 g/l supplemented with nucleotides, n-3 FA and glutamine	(1) Isonitrogenous, isocaloric formula or (2) unfed trauma patients	Fewer infectious complications Shorter LOS
178	Randomized, clinical trial	41 adult surgical patients with upper or lower gastrointestinal cancer	12.5 g/l supplemented with nucleotides and n-3 FA	(1) Isocaloric enteral formula or (2) PN without protein	No overall differences demonstrated in mortality, LOS and infectious complications
179	Randomized, clinical trial	260 adult surgical patients with upper gastrointestinal	12.5 g/l supplemented with nucleotides and n-3 FA	Isocaloric, isonitrogenous (1) enteral formula or (2) PN	Shorter hospital LOS Faster decline of plasma IL-6 concentration, higher plasma prealbumin concentration and faster recovery of DHS by and neutrophil phagocytic function by postop day 8

(continued overleaf)

Table 3. (continued)

References	Study type	Subjects	Arg dose and route	Comparison group	Outcomes of Arg group
180	Randomized, clinical trial	195 adult surgical patients with upper gastrointestinal	12.5 g/l supplemented with nucleotides and n-3 FA	Intravenous crystalloid	No overall differences demonstrated in mortality, LOS or infectious complications
181	Randomized, clinical trial	18 adult surgical patients with lower gastrointestinal	30 g/day for 3 days preop in addition to standard hospital diet	Standard hospital diet	Higher percentage of CD16/CD56 cells found in tumor-infiltrating lymphocyte population
182	Randomized, double-blind, clinical trial	59 adult ICU trauma patients with ISS >13	6.6 g/l supplemented with n-3 FA, selenium, chromium, molybdenum, *L*-carnitine and taurine	Isocaloric, isonitrogenous formula	Faster recovery of LPS-stimulated monocyte TNF and PGE2 production by postop days 6 and 10, respectively Greater neutrophil oxidative burst activity by postop day 6
183	Randomized, double-blind,	50 adult and pediatric burn patients	14 g/l supplemented with nucleotides and n-3 FA	Isocaloric formula	No overall differences demonstrated in mortality, LOS and infectious complications
184	Randomized, double-blind, multicenter trial	164 adult surgical patients with upper gastrointestinal tract cancer	12.5 g/l supplemented with nucleotides and n-3 FA	Isocaloric, isonitrogenous formula	Fewer patients with complications occurring after postop day 5
185	Randomized, double-blind, clinical trial	398 adult ICU patients with APACHE II >10 and TISS >20	12.5 g/l supplemented with nucleotides and n-3 FA	Isocaloric, isonitrogenous formula	Decreased need for mechanical ventilation and decreased LOS in a priori subgroup (intake >2.5 liters by 24 h)

186	Randomized, clinical trial	166 adult surgical patients with upper gastrointestinal tract cancer	12.5 g/l supplemented with nucleotides and n-3 FA	Isocaloric, isonitrogenous (1) enteral formula or (2) PN	No difference demonstrated vs. EN control group Lower postop sepsis score vs. PN group Decreased LOS vs. PN group in patients <90% usual body weight
187	Randomized, clinical trial	30 adult surgical patients with gastric adenocarcinoma	12.5 g/l supplemented with nucleotides and n-3 FA, given only from preop day 7 to postop day 7	Same formula, given only for 7 days in postop period	Preop formula group had higher serum prealbumin concentration and lower plasma IL-6 concentration postop
188	Randomized, blinded, clinical	32 adult ICU trauma patients with ISS >20	12.5 g/l supplemented with nucleotides and n-3FA	Isocaloric, isonitrogenous formula	No overall difference demonstrated in mortality, LOS and infectious complications Fewer systemic inflammatory response syndrome days/patient Lower multiple organ failure scores
189	Randomized, double-blind, clinical trial	206 adult surgical patients with upper or lower gastrointestinal tract cancer	12.5 g/l supplemented with nucleotides and and n-3 FA, given from preop day 7 to postop day 7	Isocaloric, isonitrogenous formula	Decreased LOS and infectious complications
190	Randomized, double-blind, clinical trial	23 adult marathon runners	10 g t.i.d. for 14 days prior to marathon	Glycine 10 g t.i.d. for 14 days prior to marathon	No overall difference demonstrated

(continued overleaf)

Table 3. (continued)

References	Study type	Subjects	Arg dose and route	Comparison group	Outcomes of Arg group
191	Randomized, double-blind, clinical trial	58 adult surgical patients with upper or lower gastrointestinal	12.5 g/l supplemented with nucleotides and n-3 FA from preop day 7 to postop day 7	Isocaloric formula with (1) less protein for 7 days preop, and (2) equivalent amount of protein from surgery to postop day 7	Faster decline of plasma IL-6 concentration and higher serum visceral protein concentrations by postop day 1
192	Randomized, double-blind, multicenter	178 adult patients with upper gastrointestinal tract cancer	14.8 g/l for 5 days preop and 12.5 g/l postop supplemented with nucleotides and n-3 FA	Isocaloric formula for 5 days preop and isocaloric, isonitrogenous formula postop	Fewer infectious complications
193	Randomized, multicenter trial	181 adult ICU patients with sepsis and APACHE II score $\geq$10	12.5 g/l supplemented with nucleotides and n-3 FA	Nearly isonitrogenous, higher calorie formula	Lower overall mortality rate, especially in patients with lower APACHE II score Fewer episodes of bacteremia Fewer recurrent nosocomial infections
194	Randomized, single-blind, 2-center trial	15 adult surgical ICU patients	22.5 g/l parenteral	Isocaloric, isonitrogenous parenteral mixed amino acid solution	Higher plasma arginine, ornithine, and glutamine concentrations during infusion Decreased muscle protein catabolism
195	Randomized, clinical trial	212 adult patients undergoing pancreaticoduo-denectomy	12.5 g/l supplemented with nucleotides and n-3 FA	Isocaloric, isonitrogenous (1) enteral formula, or (2) PN	Lower sepsis score Fewer complications versus parenteral group Lower CRP, higher visceral protein stores and better

					neutrophil phagocytic ability by postop day 8
196	Randomized, clinical trial	44 adult head and neck cancer surgical patients	6.25 g/l	Isocaloric, isonitrogenous formula	Lower incidence of complications and LOS in malnourished subgroup
60	Randomized, double-blind, clinical trial	152 premature infants (gestational age <32 weeks and weight <1,250 g) in NICU	0.261 g/kg/day in PN or formula	Isocaloric, isonitrogenous PN or formula	Lower incidence of NEC Later onset of NEC
197	Randomized,	56 malnourished (>10% of body weight loss over preceding 6 months) head and neck cancer surgical patients	12.5 g/l	Two groups: (1) Isocaloric, isonitrogenous for 9 days preop and postop (2) No nutrition therapy preop and isocaloric, isonitrogenous postop	No difference

APACHE = Acute physiology and chronic health evaluation; ATI = abdominal trauma index; BSA = body surface area; CRP = C-reactive protein; DHS = delayed hypersensitivity score; EN = enteral nutrition; FA = fatty acids; ISS = injury severity score; LOS = length of stay; LPS = lipopolysaccharide; NEC = necrotizing enterocolitis; PGE2 = prostaglandin E2; PHA = phytohemagglutinin; PN = parenteral nutrition; TISS = therapeutic intervention severity score; TNF = tumor necrosis factor.

Reproduced with permission from the *American Journal of Clinical Nutrition*©: Duggan et al. [19].

incidence and a later median age at onset of NEC [60]. The precise value of Arg-supplemented nutrition among premature infants awaits larger trials.

Recent years have seen the marketing of a number of Arg-containing enteral formulas, and some have been combined with n-3 fatty acids, branch-chain amino acids, and nucleotides to have an 'immunostimulatory' effect (e.g., Impact, Novartis Nutrition; Immune-Aid, McGaw, Inc.). The justification for the precise formulation of these products is not well established, and the study designs employed to evaluate them have generally been lacking. These include not comparing formulas in an isonitrogenous, isocaloric manner and not following intention-to-treat analysis.

In a large systematic review [61] of 22 trials among 2,419 subjects, use of immunologically active formulas was associated with fewer infectious complications and reduced length of hospital stay. Those patients who were undergoing elective surgery had the most benefit from these formulas as compared to critically ill patients. Trials with a higher quality score actually showed a higher mortality rate among patients treated with the experimental formulas (RR = 1.19, 95% CI 0.99–1.43), although these studies also showed a reduction in infectious complications (RR = 0.53, 95% CI 0.42–0.68). Overall, it appears that Arg-containing formulas may reduce infectious complications in certain patient groups, particularly surgical patients. Further studies are needed to justify the use of Arg supplementation in other patient groups.

Zinc's Role in Gut Protection

The trace element zinc is a critical nutrient in literally hundreds of metalloenzymes, is an important component in cell membrane structure and function, functions as an antioxidant, and protects against lipid peroxidation [62]. Zinc's importance in protein synthesis and on transcription proteins, where zinc fingers are important in regulating gene expression, points to its importance among cells with a high rate of turnover such as GI epithelia and cells of the immune system. Zinc deficiency has also been associated with multiple important changes in immune function [63].

Although not all studies are in agreement [64, 65], some investigators have noted significant histologic evidence of intestinal damage in rat models of zinc deficiency, including ulcerations, inflammatory infiltration, and edema of the jejunum [66, 67]. Functional changes in the GI mucosa have also been demonstrated. Zinc-deficient rats were noted to have significantly negative sodium and water balance compared to pair-fed control and ad libitum-fed rats [68]. Zinc deficiency may predispose the intestinal tract to damage by free radicals [66] and increased NO activity [69].

Human studies of zinc deficiency have also suggested that this nutrient has an important protective effect on the GI tract. In acrodermatitis enteropathica, or congenital zinc deficiency, severe diarrhea and perianal skin breakdown are seen [70]. Several studies have linked diarrhea and abnormal zinc status [71], including increased stool zinc loss [72], negative zinc balance [73], and reduced tissue levels of zinc.

Numerous clinical trials of zinc supplementation have shown improved outcomes in children with GI diseases. The most significant improvements have been observed among patients whose diets are low in zinc and/or high in phytate. Zinc supplements also improved markers of intestinal permeability children with diarrheal diseases in Bangladesh [74]. A pooled analysis showed that zinc-supplemented children with acute diarrhea had a significant reduction in continuing diarrhea, and children with persistent diarrhea had a lower probability of continuing diarrhea, treatment failure or death [75]. A recent analysis of community-based trials of zinc interventions in infants and young children who received 5–10 mg zinc for 5 or 7 days/week for 12–54 weeks found that the pooled odds ratio for diarrhea incidence was 0.82 (95% CI 0.72–0.93) [76]. Since the publication of these 2 large reviews, several further trials have confirmed the beneficial effect of zinc [77–81].

Vitamin A and GI Function

Vitamin A plays a central role in epithelial cell integrity, immune function, and retinal function, and a number of studies have confirmed its important gut-protective properties. Vitamin A deficiency leads to reduced intestinal cell division and differentiation, and a reduced number of goblet cells in the crypt [82] and villus [83]. Histologic changes in the GI tract in vitamin A-deficient rats are mild, although with prolonged deficiency (<60 days) villus height was decreased [83]. When vitamin A deficiency is paired with an inflammatory or infectious insult, however, significant histologic abnormalities occur [84, 85].

The finding that periodic, high-dose vitamin A supplementation can reduce child mortality in susceptible populations by approximately 30% has been one of the most important public health advances in the past several decades [86]. Several studies determined that the prevalence and severity of diarrheal diseases are especially reduced with vitamin A supplementation. Studies showing improved GI outcomes with vitamin A therapy have been performed in Ghana [87], Bangladesh [88], Brazil [89], India [90, 91], and Tanzania [92, 93], among others.

Further studies which specifically assess the mechanism of action in humans are needed, especially since both immune and mucosal barrier effects are seen with vitamin A repletion in animal models. It is unclear, for instance, whether vitamin A is an important protective nutrient in populations who are not deficient in the nutrient. Although infectious diseases of even well-nourished (and presumably vitamin A-replete) children are associated with declines in serum vitamin A, intervention studies have not been widely performed in these settings.

Probiotics

Probiotics, defined as live microorganisms in fermented foods that promote good health through establishing an improved balance in intestinal microflora [94], have been termed the quintessential functional food. Microorganisms that are principally used as probiotics include various species of lactobacilli or bifidobacteria used individually or in combination. A non-pathogenic yeast, *Saccharomyces boulardii*, has also been used in both animal studies and clinical trials. Of all the protective nutrients summarized in this article, more data exist on the application of probiotics to the field of allergic disease than any other.

The principal purported health-promoting effect of probiotics are their enhancement of mucosal immune defenses [95]. Probiotics can compete for receptor sites on the intestinal surface, produce antibiotic substances, enhance host immune defenses and compete with pathogens for intraluminal nutrients [96, 97]. They can also affect other nonimmune intestinal host defenses including strengthening intestinal tight junctions, increasing mucous secretion, enhancing motility, and producing metabolic products (amino acids such as Arg and Gln, as well as short-chain fatty acids) which secondarily function as protective nutrients [98–100]. Probiotics have been studied in a number of animal models of gut inflammation, including those due to inflammatory bowel disease [101, 102], NEC [103], and colon cancer [104].

Probiotic supplemented formula induced a bifidogenic stool pattern [105] and has been shown to improve outcomes of rotavirus diarrhea [106–109]. Among undernourished Peruvian infants with a high burden of diarrheal diseases, lactobacillus GG was associated with fewer episodes of diarrhea, especially among non-breast-fed children [110]. Lactobacillus GG therapy was shown to dramatically reduce (RR 0.2, 95% CI 0.06–0.6) the incidence of nosocomial diarrhea among hospitalized children [111]. Several studies in both pediatric and adult populations with either lactobacillus GG or *S. boulardii* have shown a prevention in the recurrence of *Clostridium difficile* infection after initial antibiotic treatment [112–114]. In addition, probiotics have been used in conjunction with antibiotic therapy to prevent or lessen the severity of antibiotic-associated diarrhea in children [115, 116].

A number of studies over the past several years on probiotic therapy have come from the Isolauri group, with early studies focusing on the role of probiotics in the treatment or prevention of GI infections [107, 117, 118] and more recent studies focusing on the management of allergic diseases. For instance, compared to 14 infants with atopic dermatitis and cow's milk allergy treated with a hydrolyzed whey protein, 13 children receiving lactobacillus GG in addition to the formula had less symptoms of eczema and lower measures of intestinal inflammation (as measured by stool α_1-antitrypsin and tumor necrosis factor-α) [119]. In a randomized controlled study, breast-feeding infants with atopic dermatitis were weaned to protein hydrolysate formulas with or without probiotics. The extent and severity of the dermatitis was significantly lower in the probiotic-supplemented group, as were markers of allergic inflammation (serum-soluble CD4, urinary eosinophilic protein X) [120]. Kalliomaki et al. [121] have shown that lactobacillus GG given to pregnant mothers at risk of delivering infants with allergies and then to their newborns for the first 6 months of life was associated with a significantly decreased incidence of atopic dermatitis compared to mothers and infants given placebo. Finally, this group has recently reported that serum IgE concentrations correlated with fecal *Escherichia coli* and bacteroide counts among infants with atopic dermatitis, and that probiotic supplementation reduced these *E. coli* counts [122].

Taken together, these series of studies suggest a potential role for probiotics in the management or prevention of a wide variety of diseases, including allergies. However, the quality of some of the clinical studies has been questioned [123], and some of the studies have suffered from poorly specified inclusion criteria and inadequate control of possible confounding factors. Sample sizes have also been relatively low. As with other protective nutrients reviewed, larger, more rigorous clinical trials are needed.

Prebiotics

Prebiotics are defined as nondigestible food ingredients that beneficially affect the host by selectively stimulating the growth and/or activity of one or a limited number of bacteria in the colon [94]. Oligosaccharides in human breast milk are considered the 'proteotypic prebiotic' in that they facilitate the preferential growth of bifidobacteria and lactobacilli in the colon of exclusively breast-fed neonates [124–126]. Inulin and fructose oligosaccharides are the most widely studied prebiotics in the literature.

Data evaluating the protective nutrient aspects of prebiotics are more limited, compared to the wealth of data with probiotics, but are growing. Certainly it is clear that prebiotics induce a bifidogenic bowel pattern, with a preferential growth of bacteria such as bifidobacteria and lactobacilli [127–130]. The major protective nutrient/functional food direct effects of prebiotics include improved bowel functions (e.g., as treatment of irritable bowel syndrome and constipation), increased mineral absorption [131–133], altered lipid metabolism, and possibly a reduced risk of colon cancer [134, 135].

Clinical trials have been more limited. In abstract form, 2 studies have evaluated prebiotic-supplemented infant cereal. A study among young children attending day care showed that prebiotic-supplemented cereal was associated with fewer episodes of diarrhea with fever than control cereal, although the overall rate of diarrhea episodes was not different in the groups [136]. A study in which Peruvian children were similarly supplemented did not show a reduction in diarrhea, other infections, or change in serum IgE [137].

Prebiotics therefore require significantly more clinical study before they can be widely accepted as important gut-protective nutrients. Long-term trials with valid and important health outcomes are needed.

Conclusions

A number of GI protective nutrients exist, and it is likely that future studies will uncover important roles for a variety of additional such nutrients. As we have pointed out, gaps and deficiencies exist in the published literature, including significant problems in some studies with design, enrollment and data analysis. Other have noted similar shortcomings in the design and implementation of these and similar nutrition studies [138–140]. We [19] and others [141] have also previously noted that the unique way in which dietary supplements are regulated in many countries may contribute to this state of affairs. The future of nutritional science is certainly promising with respect to the ability of the practitioners of tomorrow to individualize nutrient mixes for the promotion of optimal health. As newer products come to market with advertised health benefits, the practitioner of today would be well-served to appreciate both the promise and limitations of the data supporting the use of these nutrients.

References

1 Roesler TA, Barry PC, Bock SA: Factitious food allergy and failure to thrive. Arch Pediatr Adolesc Med 1994;148:1150–1155.
2 Carvalho NF, Kenney RD, Carrington PH, Hall DE: Severe nutritional deficiencies in toddlers resulting from health food milk alternatives. Pediatrics 2001;107:E46.
3 Kennedy KI: Effects of breastfeeding on women's health. Int J Gynaecol Obstet 1994; 47(suppl):S11–S21.
4 Fomon S: Nutrition of Normal Infants. St Louis, Mosby, 1993.
5 Host A: Cow's milk protein allergy and intolerance in infancy. Some clinical, epidemiological and immunological aspects. Pediatr Allergy Immunol 1994;5(suppl):1–36.
6 Hidvégi E, Arató A, Cserháti E, et al: Slight decrease in bone mineralization in cow milk-sensitive children. J Pediatr Gastroenterol Nutr 2003;36:44–49.
7 Kalkwarf HJ, Khoury JC, Lanphear BP: Milk intake during childhood and adolescence, adult bone density, and osteoporotic fractures in US women. Am J Clin Nutr 2003;77:257–265.
8 Rigo J, Salle BL, Picaud JC, et al: Nutritional evaluation of protein hydrolysate formulas. Eur J Clin Nutr 1995;49(suppl 1):S26–S38.
9 Isolauri E, Sutas Y, Makinen-Kiljunen S, et al: Efficacy and safety of hydrolyzed cow milk and amino acid-derived formulas in infants with cow milk allergy. J Pediatr 1995;127:550–557.
10 Rigo J, Senterre J: Metabolic balance studies and plasma amino acid concentrations in preterm infants fed experimental protein hydrolysate preterm formulas. Acta Paediatr Suppl 1994;405:98–104.
11 Abrams SA, Griffin IJ, Davila PM: Calcium and zinc absorption from lactose-containing and lactose-free infant formulas. Am J Clin Nutr 2002;76:442–446.

12 Strom BL, Schinnar R, Ziegler EE, et al: Exposure to soy-based formula in infancy and endocrinological and reproductive outcomes in young adulthood. JAMA 2001;286:807–814.
13 de Boissieu D, Matarazzo P, Dupont C: Allergy to extensively hydrolyzed cow milk proteins in infants: Identification and treatment with an amino acid-based formula. J Pediatr 1997;131:744–747.
14 Jones M, Campbell KA, Duggan C, et al: Multiple micronutrient deficiencies in a child fed an elemental formula. J Pediatr Gastroenterol Nutr 2001;33:602–605.
15 Yuwono M, Claxton N, Tjota A, Rossi T: Presentation of scurvy on complete enteral feeding: A case report. Gastroenterology 1999;116:A588.
16 Piccoli R, Gelio S, Fratucello A, Valletta E: Risk of low micronutrient intake in neurologically disabled children artificially fed. J Pediatr Gastroenterol Nutr 2002;35:583–584.
17 Roberfroid MB: Functional effects of food components and the gastrointestinal system: Chicory fructooligosaccharides. Nutr Rev 1996;54:S38–S42.
18 Koletzko B, Aggett PJ, Bindels JG, et al: Growth, development and differentiation: A functional food science approach. Br J Nutr 1998;80(suppl 1):S5–S45.
19 Duggan C, Gannon J, Walker WA: Protective nutrients and functional foods for the gastrointestinal tract. Am J Clin Nutr 2002;75:789–808.
20 Bulus N, Cersosimo E, Ghishan F, Abumrad N: Physiologic importance of glutamine. Metabolism 1989;38(suppl 1):1–5.
21 Tamada H, Nezu R, Imamura I, et al: The dipeptide alanyl-glutamine prevents intestinal mucosal atrophy in parenterally fed rats. JPEN J Parenter Enteral Nutr 1992;16:110–116.
22 Burrin DG, Shulman RJ, Langston C, Storm MC: Supplemental alanylglutamine, organ growth, and nitrogen metabolism in neonatal pigs fed by total parenteral nutrition. JPEN J Parenter Enteral Nutr 1994;18:313–319.
23 Li J, Langkamp-Henken B, Suzuki K, Stahlgren LH: Glutamine prevents parenteral nutrition-induced increases in intestinal permeability. JPEN J Parenter Enteral Nutr 1994;18:303–307.
24 Harward TR, Coe D, Souba WW, et al: Glutamine preserves gut glutathione levels during intestinal ischemia/reperfusion. J Surg Res 1994;56:351–355.
25 Tamada H, Nezu R, Matsuo Y, et al: Alanyl glutamine-enriched total parenteral nutrition restores intestinal adaptation after either proximal or distal massive resection in rats. JPEN J Parenter Enteral Nutr 1993;17:236–242.
26 Gouttebel M, Astre C, Briand D, et al: Influence of N-acetylglutamine or glutamine infusion on plasma amino acid concentrations during the early phase of small-bowel adaptation in the dog. JPEN J Parenter Enteral Nutr 1992;16:117–121.
27 Vanderhoof JA, Blackwood DJ, Mohammadpour H, Park JH: Effects of oral supplementation of glutamine on small intestinal mucosal mass following resection. J Am Coll Nutr 1992;11:223–227.
28 Van der Hulst R, van Kreel B, von Meyenfeldt M, et al: Glutamine and the preservation of gut integrity. Lancet 1993;334:1363–1365.
29 Tremel H, Kienle B, Weilemann L, et al: Glutamine dipeptide-supplemented parenteral nutrition maintains intestinal function in the critically ill. Gastroenterology 1994;107:1595–1601.
30 O'Dwyer S, Smith R, Hwang T, Wilmore D: Maintenance of small bowel mucosa with glutamine-enriched parenteral nutrition. JPEN J Parenter Enteral Nutr 1989;13:579–585.
31 Klimberg V, Souba W, Dolson D, et al: Prophylactic glutamine protects the intestinal mucosa from radiation injury. Cancer 1990;66:62–68.
32 Burke D, Alverdy J, Aoys E, Moss G: Glutamine-supplemented total parenteral nutrition improves gut immune function. Arch Surg 1989;124:1396–1369.
33 Alverdy J: Effects of glutamine-supplemented diets on immunology of the gut. JPEN J Parenter Enteral Nutr 1990;14:109S–113S.
34 O'Riordain M, Fearon K, Ross J, et al: Glutamine-supplemented total parenteral nutrition enhances T-lymphocyte response in surgical patients undergoing colorectal resection. Ann Surg 1994;220:212–221.
35 Byrne T, Persinger R, Young L, et al: A new treatment for patients with short-bowel syndrome. Growth hormone, glutamine, and a modified diet. Ann Surg 1995;222:243–254.
36 Gianotti L, Alexander J, Gennari R, et al: Oral glutamine decreases bacterial translocation and improves survival in experimental gut-origin sepsis. JPEN J Parenter Enteral Nutr 1995;19:69–74.

37 Zhang W, Frankel WL, Bain A, et al: Glutamine reduces bacterial translocation after small bowel transplantation in cyclosporine-treated rats. J Surg Res 1995;58:159–164.
38 Ziegler TR, Young LS, Benfell K, et al: Clinical and metabolic efficacy of glutamine-supplemented parenteral nutrition after bone marrow transplantation. A randomized, double-blind, controlled study. Ann Intern Med 1992;116:821–828.
39 Neu J, Roig J, Meetze W, et al: Enteral glutamine supplementation for very low birth weight infants decreases morbidity. J Pediatr 1997;131:691–699.
40 Bhan MK, Mahalanabis D, Fontaine O, Pierce NF: Clinical trials of improved oral rehydration salt formulations: A review. Bull WHO 1994;72:945–955.
41 Beaugerie L, Carbonnel F, Hecketsweiler B, et al: Effects of an isotonic oral rehydration solution, enriched with glutamine, on fluid and sodium absorption in patients with a short-bowel. Aliment Pharmacol Ther 1997;11:741–746.
42 Poindexter B, Ehrenkranz R, Stoll B, et al: Parenteral glutamine supplementation in ELBW infants: A multicenter randomized clinical trial. Pediatr Res 2002;51:317A.
43 Novak F, Heyland DK, Avenell A, et al: Glutamine supplementation in serious illness: a systematic review of the evidence. Crit Care Med 2002;30:2022–2029.
44 Barbul A: Arginine: Biochemistry, physiology, and therapeutic implications. JPEN J Parenter Enteral Nutr 1986;10:227–238.
45 Moncada S, Higgs A: The *L*-arginine-nitric oxide pathway. N Engl J Med 1993;329: 2002–2012.
46 Barbul A, Rettura G, Levenson S: Arginine: Thymotropic and wound healing promoting agent. Surg Forum 1977;28:101–103.
47 Leon P, Redmond HP, Stein TP, et al: Arginine supplementation improves histone and acute-phase protein synthesis during gram-negative sepsis in the rat. JPEN J Parenter Enteral Nutr 1991;15:503–508.
48 Ye SL, Istfan NW, Driscoll DF, Bistrian BR: Tumor and host response to arginine and branched chain amino acid-enriched total parenteral nutrition. A study involving Walker 256 carcinosarcoma-bearing rats. Cancer 1992;69:261–270.
49 Oka T, Ohwada K, Nagao M, et al: Arginine-enriched solution induces a marked increase in muscle glutamine concentration and enhances muscle protein synthesis in tumor-bearing rats. JPEN J Parenter Enteral Nutr 1994;18:491–496.
50 Alican I, Kubes P: A critical role for nitric oxide in intestinal barrier function and dysfunction. Am J Physiol 1996;270:G225–G237.
51 Kanwar S, Wallace JL, Befus D, Kubes P: Nitric oxide synthesis inhibition increases epithelial permeability via mast cells. Am J Physiol 1994;266:G222–G229.
52 Mourad FH, O'Donnell LJ, Andre EA, et al: *L*-Arginine, nitric oxide, and intestinal secretion: Studies in rat jejunum in vivo. Gut 1996;39:539–544.
53 Mueller AR, Platz KP, Heckert C, et al: *L*-Arginine application improves mucosal structure after small bowel transplantation. Transplant Proc 1998;30:2336–2338.
54 Mueller AR, Platz KP, Schirmeier A, et al: *L*-Arginine application improves graft morphology and mucosal barrier function after small bowel transplantation. Transplant Proc 2000;32: 1275–1277.
55 Welters CF, Dejong CH, Deutz NE, Heineman E: Effects of parenteral arginine supplementation on the intestinal adaptive response after massive small bowel resection in the rat. J Surg Res 1999;85:259–266.
56 Gurbuz AT, Kunzelman J, Ratzer EE: Supplemental dietary arginine accelerates intestinal mucosal regeneration and enhances bacterial clearance following radiation enteritis in rats. J Surg Res 1998;74:149–154.
57 Kharitonov SA, Lubec G, Lubec B, et al: *L*-Arginine increases exhaled nitric oxide in normal human subjects. Clin Sci 1995;88:135–139.
58 Becker RM, Wu G, Galanko JA, et al: Reduced serum amino acid concentrations in infants with necrotizing enterocolitis. J Pediatr 2000;137:785–793.
59 Zamora SA, Amin HJ, McMillan DD, et al: Plasma *L*-arginine concentrations in premature infants with necrotizing enterocolitis. J Pediatr 1997;131:226–232.
60 Amin H, Zamora S, McMillan D, et al: Arginine supplementation prevents necrotizing enterocolitis in the premature infant. J Pediatr 2002;140:425–431.
61 Heyland DK, Novak F, Drover JW, et al: Should immunonutrition become routine in critically ill patients? A systematic review of the evidence. JAMA 2001;286:944–953.

62 Filipe PM, Fernandes AC, Manso CF: Effects of zinc on copper-induced and spontaneous lipid peroxidation. Biol Trace Elem Res 1995;47:51–56.
63 Shankar AH, Prasad AS: Zinc and immune function: the biological basis of altered resistance to infection. Am J Clin Nutr 1998;68(suppl):447S–463S.
64 Follis R, Day H, McCollum E: Histologic studies of the tissues of rats fed a diet extremely low in zinc. J Nutr 1941;22:223–235.
65 Koo SI, Turk DE: Effect of zinc deficiency on the ultrastructure of the pancreatic acinar cell and intestinal epithelium in the rat. J Nutr 1977;107:896–908.
66 Virgili F, Canali R, Figus E, et al: Intestinal damage induced by zinc deficiency is associated with enhanced CuZn superoxide dismutase activity in rats: Effect of dexamethasone or thyroxine treatment. Free Radic Biol Med 1999;26:1194–1201.
67 Nobili F, Vignolini F, Figus E, Mengheri E: Treatment of rats with dexamethasone or thyroxine reverses zinc deficiency-induced intestinal damage. J Nutr 1997;127:1807–1813.
68 Ghishan FK: Transport of electrolytes, water, and glucose in zinc deficiency. J Pediatr Gastroenterol Nutr 1984;3:608–612.
69 Wapnir RA: Zinc deficiency, malnutrition and the gastrointestinal tract. J Nutr 2000; 130(suppl): 1388S–1392S.
70 Moynahan E: Acrodermatitis enteropathica: a lethal inherited human zinc deficiency disorder. Lancet 1974;i:399–400.
71 Hambidge K: Zinc and diarrhea. Acta Paediatr Suppl 1992;381:82–86.
72 Castillo-Duran C, Vial P, Uauy R: Trace mineral balance during acute diarrhea in infants. J Pediatr 1988;113:452–457.
73 Castillo-Duran C, Vial P, Uauy R: Oral copper supplementation: Effect on copper and zinc balance during acute gastroenteritis in infants. Am J Clin Nutr 1990;51:1088–1092.
74 Roy S, Behrens R, Haider R, et al: Impact of zinc supplementation on intestinal permeability in Bangladeshi children with acute diarrhoea and persistent diarrhoea syndrome. J Pediatr Gastroenterol 1992;15:289–296.
75 Bhutta ZA, Bird SM, Black RE, et al: Therapeutic effects of oral zinc in acute and persistent diarrhea in children in developing countries: Pooled analysis of randomized controlled trials. Am J Clin Nutr 2000;72:1516–1522.
76 Bhutta ZA, Black RE, Brown KH, et al: Prevention of diarrhea and pneumonia by zinc supplementation in children in developing countries: Pooled analysis of randomized controlled trials. Zinc Investigators' Collaborative Group. J Pediatr 1999;135:689–697.
77 Baqui AH, Black RE, Arifeen SE, et al: Effect of zinc supplementation started during diarrhoea on morbidity and mortality in Bangladeshi children: Community randomised trial. BMJ 2002; 325:1059.
78 Bahl R, Bhandari N, Saksena M, et al: Efficacy of zinc-fortified oral rehydration solution in 6- to 35-month-old children with acute diarrhea. J Pediatr 2002;141:677–682.
79 Bhandari N, Bahl R, Taneja S, et al: Substantial reduction in severe diarrheal morbidity by daily zinc supplementation in young north Indian children. Pediatrics 2002;109:e86.
80 Osendarp SJ, Santosham M, Black RE, et al: Effect of zinc supplementation between 1 and 6 mo of life on growth and morbidity of Bangladeshi infants in urban slums. Am J Clin Nutr 2002;76:1401–1408.
81 Strand TA, Chandyo RK, Bahl R, et al: Effectiveness and efficacy of zinc for the treatment of acute diarrhea in young children. Pediatrics 2002;109:898–903.
82 Rojanapo W, Lamb AJ, Olson JA: The prevalence, metabolism and migration of goblet cells in rat intestine following the induction of rapid, synchronous vitamin A deficiency. J Nutr 1980; 110:178–188.
83 Warden RA, Strazzari MJ, Dunkley PR, O'Loughlin EV: Vitamin A-deficient rats have only mild changes in jejunal structure and function. J Nutr 1996;126:1817–1826.
84 Ahmed F, Jones DB, Jackson AA: The interaction of vitamin A deficiency and rotavirus infection in the mouse. Br J Nutr 1990;63:363–373.
85 Warden RA, Noltorp RS, Francis JL, et al: Vitamin A deficiency exacerbates methotrexate-induced jejunal injury in rats. J Nutr 1997;127:770–776.
86 Fawzi W, Chalmers T, Herrera M, Mosteller F: Vitamin A supplementation and child mortality: A meta-analysis. JAMA 1993;269:898–903.
87 Ghana VAST Study Team: Vitamin A supplementation in northern Ghana: Effects on clinic attendances, hospital admissions, and child mortality. Lancet 1993;342:7–12.

88 Hossain S, Biswas R, Kabir I, et al: Single dose vitamin A treatment in acute shigellosis in Bangladesh children: Randomised double blind controlled trial. BMJ 1998;316:422–426.
89 Barreto M, Santos L, Assis A, et al: Effect of vitamin A supplementation on diarrhoea and acute lower respiratory tract infections in young children in Brazil. Lancet 1994;344:228–231.
90 Bhandari N, Bhan M, Sazawal S: Impact of massive dose of vitamin A given to preschool children with acute diarrhoea on subsequent respiratory and diarrhoeal morbidity. BMJ 1994; 309:1404–1407.
91 Bhandari N, Bahl R, Sazawal S, Bhan MK: Breast-feeding status alters the effect of vitamin A treatment during acute diarrhea in children. J Nutr 1997;127:59–63.
92 Fawzi WW, Mbise RL, Spiegelman D, et al: Vitamin A supplements and diarrheal and respiratory infections among children in Dar es Salaam, Tanzania. J Pediatr 2000;137:660–667.
93 Fawzi WW, Mbise RL, Hertzmark E, et al: A randomized trial of vitamin A supplements in relation to mortality among human immunodeficiency virus-infected and uninfected children in Tanzania. Pediatr Infect Dis J 1999;18:127–133.
94 Gibson GR, Roberfroid MB: Dietary modulation of the human colonic microbiota: Introducing the concept of prebiotics. J Nutr 1995;125:1401–1412.
95 Isolauri E, Majamaa H, Arvola T, et al: *Lactobacillus casei* strain GG reverses increased intestinal permeability induced by cow milk in suckling rats. Gastroenterology 1993;105: 1643–1650.
96 Lu L, Walker WA: Pathologic and physiologic interactions of bacteria with the gastrointestinal epithelium. Am J Clin Nutr 2001;73:1124S–1130S.
97 Walker WA: Role of nutrients and bacterial colonization in the development of intestinal host defense. J Pediatr Gastroenterol Nutr 2000;30(suppl 2):S2–S7.
98 Vanderhoof JA: Probiotics: Future directions. Am J Clin Nutr 2001;73:1152S–1155S.
99 Fonder R, Mogensen G, Tanka R, et al: Effect of fermented dairy products on intestinal microflora, human nutrition, and health: Current knowledge and future perspectives. Brussels, International Dairy Federation Publications, 1999.
100 Bengmark S: Econutrition and health maintenance: A new concept to prevent inflammation, ulceration and sepsis. Clin Nutr 1996;15:1–10.
101 Madsen KL, Doyle JS, Jewell LD, et al: Lactobacillus species prevents colitis in interleukin 10 gene-deficient mice. Gastroenterology 1999;116:1107–1114.
102 Steidler L, Hans W, Schotte L, et al: Treatment of murine colitis by *Lactococcus lactis* secreting interleukin-10. Science 2000;289:1352–1355.
103 Caplan MS, Miller-Catchpole R, Kaup S, et al: Bifidobacterial supplementation reduces the incidence of necrotizing enterocolitis in a neonatal rat model. Gastroenterology 1999; 117:577–583.
104 Brady LJ, Gallaher DD, Busta FF: The role of probiotic cultures in the prevention of colon cancer. J Nutr 2000;130(suppl 2):410S–414S.
105 Langhendries JP, Detry J, Van Hees J, et al: Effect of a fermented infant formula containing viable bifidobacteria on the fecal flora composition and pH of healthy full-term infants. J Pediatr Gastroenterol Nutr 1995;21:177–181.
106 Saavedra JM, Bauman NA, Oung I, et al: Feeding of *Bifidobacterium bifidum* and *Streptococcus thermophilus* to infants in hospital for prevention of diarrhoea and shedding of rotavirus. Lancet 1994;344:1046–1049.
107 Majamaa H, Isolauri E, Saxelin M, Vesikari T: Lactic acid bacteria in the treatment of acute rotavirus gastroenteritis. J Pediatr Gastroenterol Nutr 1995;20:333–338.
108 Shornikova AV, Casas IA, Mykkanen H, et al: Bacteriotherapy with *Lactobacillus reuteri* in rotavirus gastroenteritis. Pediatr Infect Dis J 1997;16:1103–1107.
109 Guarino A, Canani RB, Spagnuolo MI, et al: Oral bacterial therapy reduces the duration of symptoms and of viral excretion in children with mild diarrhea. J Pediatr Gastroenterol Nutr 1997;25:516–519.
110 Oberhelman RA, Gilman RH, Sheen P, et al: A placebo-controlled trial of lactobacillus GG to prevent diarrhea in undernourished Peruvian children. J Pediatr 1999;134:15–20.
111 Szajewska H, Kotowska M, Mrukowicz JZ, et al: Efficacy of lactobacillus GG in prevention of nosocomial diarrhea in infants. J Pediatr 2001;138:361–365.
112 Surawicz CM, McFarland LV, Greenberg RN, et al: The search for a better treatment for recurrent *Clostridium difficile* disease: Use of high-dose vancomycin combined with *Saccharomyces boulardii*. Clin Infect Dis 2000;31:1012–1017.

113 Gorbach SL, Chang TW, Goldin B: Successful treatment of relapsing *Clostridium difficile* colitis with lactobacillus GG. Lancet 1987;2:1519.
114 Biller JA, Katz AJ, Flores AF, et al: Treatment of recurrent *Clostridium difficile* colitis with lactobacillus GG. J Pediatr Gastroenterol Nutr 1995;21:224–226.
115 Vanderhoof JA, Whitney DB, Antonson DL, et al: Lactobacillus GG in the prevention of antibiotic-associated diarrhea in children. J Pediatr 1999;135:564–568.
116 D'Souza AL, Rajkumar C, Cooke J, Bulpitt CJ: Probiotics in prevention of antibiotic associated diarrhoea: Meta-analysis. BMJ 2002;324:1361.
117 Isolauri E, Kaila M, Arvola T, et al: Diet during rotavirus enteritis affects jejunal permeability to macromolecules in suckling rats. Pediatr Res 1993;33:548–553.
118 Isolauri E, Juntunen M, Rautanen T, et al: A human lactobacillus strain (*Lactobacillus casei* sp strain GG) promotes recovery from acute diarrhea in children. Pediatrics 1991;88: 90–97.
119 Majamaa H, Isolauri E: Probiotics: A novel approach in the management of food allergy. J Allergy Clin Immunol 1997;99:179–185.
120 Isolauri E, Arvola T, Sutas Y, et al: Probiotics in the management of atopic eczema. Clin Exp Allergy 2000;30:1604–1610.
121 Kalliomaki M, Salminen S, Arvilommi H, et al: Probiotics in primary prevention of atopic disease: A randomised placebo-controlled trial. Lancet 2001;357:1076–1079.
122 Kirjavainen PV, Arvola T, Salminen SJ, Isolauri E: Aberrant composition of gut microbiota of allergic infants: A target of bifidobacterial therapy at weaning? Gut 2002;51:51–55.
123 Gionchetti P, Rizzello F, Venturi A, Campieri M: Probiotics in infective diarrhoea and inflammatory bowel diseases. J Gastroenterol Hepatol 2000;15:489–493.
124 Rotimi VO, Duerden BI: The development of the bacterial flora in normal neonates. J Med Microbiol 1981;14:51–62.
125 Gnoth MJ, Kunz C, Kinne-Saffran E, Rudloff S: Human milk oligosaccharides are minimally digested in vitro. J Nutr 2000;130:3014–3020.
126 Dai D, Walker WA: Protective nutrients and bacterial colonization in the immature human gut. Adv Pediatr 1999;46:353–382.
127 Gibson GR, Beatty ER, Wang X, Cummings JH: Selective stimulation of bifidobacteria in the human colon by oligofructose and inulin. Gastroenterology 1995;108:975–982.
128 Roberfroid MB: Prebiotics and synbiotics: Concepts and nutritional properties. Br J Nutr 1998;80:S197–S202.
129 Gibson GR, Wang X: Enrichment of bifidobacteria from human gut contents by oligofructose using continuous culture. FEMS Microbiol Lett 1994;118:121–127.
130 Kleessen B, Sykura B, Zunft HJ, Blaut M: Effects of inulin and lactose on fecal microflora, microbial activity, and bowel habit in elderly constipated persons. Am J Clin Nutr 1997;65: 1397–1402.
131 Scholz-Ahrens KE, Schaafsma G, van den Heuvel EG, Schrezenmeir J: Effects of prebiotics on mineral metabolism. Am J Clin Nutr 2001;73(suppl):459S–464S.
132 Ohta A, Ohtsuki M, Baba S, et al: Calcium and magnesium absorption from the colon and rectum are increased in rats fed fructooligosaccharides. J Nutr 1995;125:2417–2424.
133 Delzenne N, Aertssens J, Verplaetse H, et al: Effect of fermentable fructo-oligosaccharides on mineral, nitrogen and energy digestive balance in the rat. Life Sci 1995;57:1579–1587.
134 Reddy BS, Hamid R, Rao CV: Effect of dietary oligofructose and inulin on colonic preneoplastic aberrant crypt foci inhibition. Carcinogenesis 1997;18:1371–1374.
135 Hughes R, Rowland IR: Stimulation of apoptosis by two prebiotic chicory fructans in the rat colon. Carcinogenesis 2001;22:43–47.
136 Saavedra J, Tschernia A, Moore N, et al: Gastrointestinal function in infants consuming a weaning food supplemented with oligo-fructose, a prebiotic. J Pediatr Gastroenterol Nutr 1999;29:513.
137 Duggan C, Penny M, Hibberd P, et al: The effects of infant cereal supplemented with oligofructose in Peruvian infants: A randomized, double blind trial. Am J Clin Nutr 2001; 75(suppl):348S.
138 Heyland DK: In search of the magic nutraceutical: Problems with current approaches. J Nutr 2001;131:2591S–2595S.
139 Buchman AL: Glutamine: Commercially essential or conditionally essential? A critical appraisal of the human data. Am J Clin Nutr 2001;74:25–32.

140 de Roos NM, Katan MB: Effects of probiotic bacteria on diarrhea, lipid metabolism, and carcinogenesis: A review of papers published between 1988 and 1998. Am J Clin Nutr 2000; 71:405–411.
141 Falk M: Model for a third-party review of the evidence substantiating food and dietary supplement claims. J Nutr 2001;131:2219–2223.
142 Scheltinga MR, Young LS, Benfell K, et al: Glutamine-enriched intravenous feedings attenuate extracellular fluid expansion after a standard stress. Ann Surg 1991;214:385–395.
143 MacBurney M, Young L, Ziegler T, Wilmore D: A cost-evaluation of glutamine-supplemented parenteral nutrition in adult bone marrow transplant patients. J Am Diet Assoc 1994;94: 1263–1266.
144 Ziegler TR, Bye RL, Persinger RL, et al: Effects of glutamine supplementation on circulating lymphocytes after bone marrow transplantation: A pilot study. Am J Med Sci 1998;315: 4–10.
145 Schloerb PR, Amare M: Total parenteral nutrition with glutamine in bone marrow transplantation and other clinical applications (a randomized, double-blind study). JPEN J Parenter Enteral Nutr 1993;17:407–413.
146 Jensen GL, Miller RH, Talabiska DG, et al: A double-blind, prospective, randomized study of glutamine-enriched compared with standard peptide-based feeding in critically ill patients. Am J Clin Nutr 1996;64:615–621.
147 Bozzetti F, Biganzoli L, Gavazzi C, et al: Glutamine supplementation in cancer patients receiving chemotherapy: A double-blind randomized study. Nutrition 1997;13:748–751.
148 Griffiths RD, Jones C, Palmer TE: Six-month outcome of critically ill patients given glutamine-supplemented parenteral nutrition. Nutrition 1997;13:295–302.
149 Anderson PM, Ramsay NK, Shu XO, et al: Effect of low-dose oral glutamine on painful stomatitis during bone marrow transplantation. Bone Marrow Transplant 1998;22:339–344.
150 Brown SA, Goringe A, Fegan C, et al: Parenteral glutamine protects hepatic function during bone marrow transplantation. Bone Marrow Transplant 1998;22:281–284.
151 de Beaux AC, O'Riordain MG, Ross JA, et al: Glutamine-supplemented total parenteral nutrition reduces blood mononuclear cell interleukin-8 release in severe acute pancreatitis. Nutrition 1998;14:261–265.
152 Houdijk AP, Rijnsburger ER, Jansen J, et al: Randomised trial of glutamine-enriched enteral nutrition on infectious morbidity in patients with multiple trauma. Lancet 1998;352:772–776.
153 Morlion BJ, Stehle P, Wachtler P, et al: Total parenteral nutrition with glutamine dipeptide after major abdominal surgery: A randomized, double-blind, controlled study. Ann Surg 1998; 227:302–308.
154 Noyer CM, Simon D, Borczuk A, et al: A double-blind placebo-controlled pilot study of glutamine therapy for abnormal intestinal permeability in patients with AIDS. Am J Gastroenterol 1998; 93:972–975.
155 Yoshida S, Matsui M, Shirouzu Y, et al: Effects of glutamine supplements and radiochemotherapy on systemic immune and gut barrier function in patients with advanced esophageal cancer. Ann Surg 1998;227:485–491.
156 Barbosa E, Moreira EA, Goes JE, Faintuch J: Pilot study with a glutamine-supplemented enteral formula in critically ill infants. Rev Hosp Clin Fac Med Sao Paulo 1999;54:21–4.
157 Decker-Baumann C, Buhl K, Frohmuller S, et al: Reduction of chemotherapy-induced side-effects by parenteral glutamine supplementation in patients with metastatic colorectal cancer. Eur J Cancer 1999;35:202–207.
158 Den Hond E, Hiele M, Peeters M, et al: Effect of long-term oral glutamine supplements on small intestinal permeability in patients with Crohn's disease. JPEN J Parenter Enteral Nutr 1999;23:7–11.
159 Jones C, Palmer TE, Griffiths RD: Randomized clinical outcome study of critically ill patients given glutamine-supplemented enteral nutrition. Nutrition 1999;15:108–115.
160 Okuno SH, Woodhouse CO, Loprinzi CL, et al: Phase III controlled evaluation of glutamine for decreasing stomatitis in patients receiving fluorouracil (5-FU)-based chemotherapy. Am J Clin Oncol 1999;22:258–261.
161 Powell-Tuck J, Jamieson CP, Bettany GE, et al: A double blind, randomised, controlled trial of glutamine supplementation in parenteral nutrition. Gut 1999;45:82–88.
162 Schloerb PR, Skikne BS: Oral and parenteral glutamine in bone marrow transplantation: A randomized, double-blind study. JPEN J Parenter Enteral Nutr 1999;23:117–122.

163 Shabert JK, Winslow C, Lacey JM, Wilmore DW: Glutamine-antioxidant supplementation increases body cell mass in AIDS patients with weight loss: A randomized, double-blind controlled trial. Nutrition 1999;15:860–864.
164 Akobeng AK, Miller V, Stanton J, et al: Double-blind randomized controlled trial of glutamine-enriched polymeric diet in the treatment of active Crohn's disease. J Pediatr Gastroenterol Nutr 2000;30:78–84.
165 Coghlin Dickson T, Wong R, et al: Effect of oral glutamine supplementation during bone marrow transplantation. JPEN J Parenter Enteral Nutr 2000;24:61–66.
166 Cerra FB, Lehman S, Konstantinides N, et al: Effect of enteral nutrient on in vitro tests of immune function in ICU patients: A preliminary report. Nutrition 1990;6:84–88.
167 Gottschlich MM, Jenkins M, Warden GD, et al: Differential effects of three enteral dietary regimens on selected outcome variables in burn patients. JPEN J Parenter Enteral Nutr 1990;14:225–236.
168 Daly JM, Lieberman MD, Goldfine J, et al: Enteral nutrition with supplemental arginine, RNA, and omega-3 fatty acids in patients after operation: Immunologic, metabolic, and clinical outcome. Surgery 1992;112:56–67.
169 Sigal RK, Shou J, Daly JM: Parenteral arginine infusion in humans: Nutrient substrate or pharmacologic agent? JPEN J Parenter Enteral Nutr 1992;16:423–428.
170 Moore FA, Moore EE, Kudsk KA, et al: Clinical benefits of an immune-enhancing diet for early postinjury enteral feeding. J Trauma Injury Infect Crit Care 1994;37:607–615.
171 Bower R, Cerra F, Bershadsky B, et al: Early enteral administration of a formula (Impact) supplemented with arginine, nucleotides, and fish oil in intensive care unit patients: Results of a multicenter, prospective, randomized, clinical trial. Crit Care Med 1995;23:436–449.
172 Daly JM, Weintraub FN, Shou J, et al: Enteral nutrition during multimodality therapy in upper gastrointestinal cancer patients. Ann Surg 1995;221:327–338.
173 Kemen M, Senkal M, Homann HH, et al: Early postoperative enteral nutrition with arginine-omega-3 fatty acids and ribonucleic acid-supplemented diet versus placebo in cancer patients: An immunologic evaluation of Impact. Crit Care Med 1995;23:652–659.
174 Senkal M, Kemen M, Homann HH, et al: Modulation of postoperative immune response by enteral nutrition with a diet enriched with arginine, RNA, and omega-3 fatty acids in patients with upper gastrointestinal cancer. Eur J Surg 1995;161:115–122.
175 Braga M, Gianotti L, Cestari A, et al: Gut function and immune and inflammatory responses in patients perioperatively fed with supplemented enteral formulas. Arch Surg 1996;131:1257–1265.
176 Braga M, Vignali A, Gianotti L, et al: Immune and nutritional effects of early enteral nutrition after major abdominal operations. Eur J Surg 1996;162:105–112.
177 Kudsk KA, Minard G, Croce MA, et al: A randomized trial of isonitrogenous enteral diets after severe trauma. An immune-enhancing diet reduces septic complications. Ann Surg 1996;224:531–543.
178 Schilling J, Vranjes N, Fierz W, et al: Clinical outcome and immunology of postoperative arginine, omega-3 fatty acids, and nucleotide-enriched enteral feeding: A randomized prospective comparison with standard enteral and low calorie/low fat i.v. solutions. Nutrition 1996;12:423–429.
179 Gianotti L, Braga M, Vignali A, et al: Effect of route of delivery and formulation of postoperative nutritional support in patients undergoing major operations for malignant neoplasms. Arch Surg 1997;132:1222–1230.
180 Heslin MJ, Latkany L, Leung D, et al: A prospective, randomized trial of early enteral feeding after resection of upper gastrointestinal malignancy. Ann Surg 1997;226:567–580.
181 Heys SD, Segar A, Payne S, et al: Dietary supplementation with *L*-arginine: Modulation of tumour-infiltrating lymphocytes in patients with colorectal cancer. Br J Surg 1997;84:238–241.
182 Mendez C, Jurkovich GJ, Garcia I, et al: Effects of an immune-enhancing diet in critically injured patients. J Trauma Injury Infect Crit Care 1997;42:933–941.
183 Saffle JR, Wiebke G, Jennings K, et al: Randomized trial of immune-enhancing enteral nutrition in burn patients. J Trauma Injury Infect Crit Care 1997;42:793–802.
184 Senkal M, Mumme A, Eickhoff U, et al: Early postoperative enteral immunonutrition: Clinical outcome and cost-comparison analysis in surgical patients. Crit Care Med 1997;25:1489–1496.

185 Atkinson S, Sieffert E, Bihari D: A prospective, randomized, double-blind, controlled clinical trial of enteral immunonutrition in the critically ill. Guy's Hospital Intensive Care Group. Crit Care Med 1998;26:1164–1172.
186 Braga M, Gianotti L, Vignali A, et al: Artificial nutrition after major abdominal surgery: Impact of route of administration and composition of the diet. Crit Care Med 1998;26:24–30.
187 Braga M, Gianotti L, Vignali A, Di Carlo V: Immunonutrition in gastric cancer surgical patients. Nutrition 1998;14:831–835.
188 Weimann A, Bastian L, Bischoff WE, et al: Influence of arginine, omega-3 fatty acids and nucleotide-supplemented enteral support on systemic inflammatory response syndrome and multiple organ failure in patients after severe trauma. Nutrition 1998;14:165–172.
189 Braga M, Gianotti L, Radaelli G, et al: Perioperative immunonutrition in patients undergoing cancer surgery: Results of a randomized double-blind phase 3 trial. Arch Surg 1999;134:428–433.
190 Buchman AL, O'Brien W, Ou CN, et al: The effect of arginine or glycine supplementation on gastrointestinal function, muscle injury, serum amino acid concentrations and performance during a marathon run. Int J Sports Med 1999;20:315–321.
191 Gianotti L, Braga M, Fortis C, et al: A prospective, randomized clinical trial on perioperative feeding with an arginine-, omega-3 fatty acid-, and RNA-enriched enteral diet: Effect on host response and nutritional status. JPEN J Parenter Enteral Nutr 1999;23:314–320.
192 Senkal M, Zumtobel V, Bauer KH, et al: Outcome and cost-effectiveness of perioperative enteral immunonutrition in patients undergoing elective upper gastrointestinal tract surgery: A prospective randomized study. Arch Surg 1999;134:1309–1316.
193 Galban C, Montejo JC, Mesejo A, et al: An immune-enhancing enteral diet reduces mortality rate and episodes of bacteremia in septic intensive care unit patients. Crit Care Med 2000;28:643–648.
194 Berard MP, Zazzo JF, Condat P, et al: Total parenteral nutrition enriched with arginine and glutamate generates glutamine and limits protein catabolism in surgical patients hospitalized in intensive care units. Crit Care Med 2000;28:3637–3644.
195 Gianotti L, Braga M, Gentilini O, et al: Artificial nutrition after pancreaticoduodenectomy. Pancreas 2000;21:344–351.
196 Riso S, Aluffi P, Brugnani M, et al: Postoperative enteral immunonutrition in head and neck cancer patients. Clin Nutr 2000;19:407–412.
197 van Bokhorst-de van der Schueren MA, Quak JJ, von Blomberg-van der Flier BME, et al: Effect of perioperative nutrition, with and without arginine supplementation, on nutritional status, immune function, postoperative morbidity, and survival in severely malnourished head and neck cancer patients. Am J Clin Nutr 2001;73:323–332.

Discussion

Dr. Isolauri: Just a brief question on the last comment you made about the treatment of acute diarrhea: 'If the feeding practices were standardized'. What specifically do you mean by that?

Dr. Duggan: I know ESPGAN has been very aggressively encouraging early feeding after rehydration, but there have been a number of studies in oral rehydration therapy that have not standardized early resumption of enteral nutrition and that can have an effect on diarrheal disease outcomes.

Dr. Isolauri: I just want to make a correction because half of the studies you were quoting were our studies, and more than 10 years ago we studied rapid refeeding including milk and milk products after 6 h of oral rehydration, and that is the standard practice. Gradual feeding, starving and any other things are no longer accepted by our ethics committee. In all those studies the feeding was standardized beginning after 6 h of rehydration.

Dr. Walker: In your review of the topic would protective nutrients be considered earlier as a preventive process? It is important that they have an optimum nutritional environment for the gut to develop properly which is thought to be the basis for not developing an adverse reaction such as allergy. Although not used as a primary therapy, could protective nutrients be used as an adjunctive therapy or, as you suggested earlier, should they be used in conjunction with some other primary therapies?

Dr. Duggan: To answer your first question, there are no clinical data to look at the time of introduction of these nutrients, unless we go back to Dr. Bergmann's presentation and say what is the most commonly used protective nutrient and that would be breast milk. So the timing of breast-feeding obviously would be the way to do that. And again, the idea that some of these nutrients might be helpful in an adjunctive response to anti-inflammatory medications in the case of inflammatory bowel disease, is an open question.

Dr. Guesry: One of the major differences between breast milk and most infant formula of the past is an imbalance between n-6 and n-3 fatty acids. Do you have any direct, more scientific studies comparing the role of n-3, which is an anti-inflammatory nutriment, in relationship with allergy?

Dr. Duggan: Many such studies exist but time constraints limited my ability to include them in this talk.

Dr. Endres: You mentioned under special diets and protein hydrolysates that nitrogen accretion is suboptimal or not optimal in preterm infants. In the context of the topic of our workshop, what do you mean by 'I am not aware of studies showing that here is an inadequate nitrogen accretion by giving protein hydrolysates', i.e. in preterm, not in term infants?

Dr. Duggan: There are at least 3 studies that I know of, 2 were published by Rigo [1, 2] that looked at serum amino acid profiles as well as nitrogen accretion with balance studies, and I believe Dr. Isolauri had a publication in the 1990s looking at the same topic [3]. Looking at nitrogen economy in intact protein formulas versus protein hydrolysate formulas, I believe serum threonine was higher and in the patients given hydrolysate formulas serum histidine was lower.

Dr. Vandenplas: The study that you quoted from Rigo is from Belgium. As far I remember these formulas were never commercialized because they were test formulas in which problems could happen. I don't think he has ever shown that this also happens in commercialized products.

Dr. Lack: You mentioned the increased alkaline phosphatase and decreased mineralization in children with cow's milk and soy allergies. Were these children on formula supplementation or were they on breast milk?

Dr. Duggan: I believe most of them were on protein hydrolysate formulas.

Dr. Lack: Is there anything known about children who are on prolonged breast-feeding perhaps because of atopy and eczema in the family. We are seeing increasing numbers of children presenting with nutritional rickets after prolonged exclusive breast-feeding because of food allergies or eczema. Is there anything known biochemically about this group of children who are on prolonged breast-feeding?

Dr. Duggan: Breast milk has a relatively low concentration of vitamin D, and in the US that fact is often ignored by pediatricians and these children are just not supplemented with vitamin D as they should be.

Dr. Saavedra: Just one more comment with regard to a few of the reports that occasionally come out with specialized diets or avoidance diets. Unfortunately there is always the difficulty of separating what might be the actual problem of the individuals and of course all their potential problems with absorption or digestion. So it is hard to subscribe that to a particular diet as being responsible for the problem rather than the individual in whom that diet is being given who probably needed something different than what he was getting to avoid the problem. Certainly it would not apply to healthy babies.

Dr. Vandenplas: Regarding the negative nutritional effects of those special diets. How long were these patients followed with that special diet? You could imagine that they have nutritional inadequacy because of the disease, and that your special diet would just, if you follow them, correct the malnutrition. What we did with partial and with extensive hydrolysates was put healthy babies from birth on these special diets and then follow them over 3 months. The nutritional parameters measured at the age of 3 months, and we could not find any deficiency.

Dr. Duggan: Clearly I think there is a strong track record for the safety of soy formulas and protein hydrolysate formulas in terms of short-term outcomes and perhaps long-term outcomes if you consider 12-months growth a long-term outcome. My point is that not all nutritional outcomes can be measured with a scale and a measuring tape. Bone health is a good example of that: (a) you need a special machine, and (b) sometimes you have to wait 50 years for fractures to develop. I just used these anecdotes to illustrate these points that altering diets might have long-term consequences that may not be easy to see or measure.

Dr. Guesry: I would like to come back to what you showed on glutamine because although the theory of the nutrition aspect is very challenging, there is a big technological problem that glutamine solution is highly unstable, and most of the people who thought they were injecting or giving orally glutamine were in fact giving glutamic acid.

Dr. Duggan: There are a number of problems with glutamine studies. In fact the studies that have looked at higher doses of parenteral glutamine supplementation actually seem to show more of an effect than enteral supplementation.

Dr. Hill: My question relates to your assessment regarding bone demineralization in those who have food allergy. It is a considerable concern for us. Many of these infants who are on hydrolysate amino acid preparations don't in fact take adequate nutrition. Do you get a sense of when it is reasonable to commence screening for bone mineral density in terms of identifying the child who is at most risk for these long-term problems?

Dr. Duggan: It is an excellent question because those children in the study by Hidvégi et al. [4] were studied not with DEXA scanning but with single photon absorbtiometry. This calls into question standards, how good the reference data are, and whether it makes sense to screen. At least in our center, we don't generally perform DEXA until the age of 8 years because good normative data don't exist at this time.

Dr. Hourihane: The other secular trend we have seen in Europe over the last 20 years is vegetarianism. What is the effect of elective meat exclusion from maternal diets on the quality or micronutrient composition of breast milk? Are there any extensive data?

Dr. Duggan: I am sure there are changes but I know throughout the world many people are vegetarian and they breast-feed successfully.

Dr. Hourihane: But throughout the rest of the world there are vegetarian populations but not highly atopic populations.

Dr. Salminen: I would like to ask you about your prebiotic study because you reported that there were no effects in Peruvian children. What exactly were your prebiotics? What was the composition of whatever you were giving the children?

Dr. Duggan: It was oligofructose and it was administered with an infant cereal, rice or oat cereal.

Dr. Ham Pong: There has been an association reported between a diet high in red meat and the increased frequency of asthma. Do you have any explanation for this association? There have been epidemiological studies that suggest this.

Dr. Duggan: I can't explain why that would be.

Dr. Endres: What was the daily amount of fructo-oligosaccharides in these cereals?

Dr. Duggan: The average intake was 18 g of cereals/day and the cereals were supplemented with 0.55 g/15 g cereal.

Dr. Walker: With regard to beef allergy, the allergic response is frequently a function of age. There was a conference several years ago in which fish fed early on as a weaning food caused fish allergy, when beef was fed early it was beef allergy. So it is a matter not so much of beef being a highly allergenic substance as timing of the exposure.

References

1 Rigo J, Salle BL, Picaud JC, et al: Nutritional evaluation of protein hydrolysate formulas. Eur J Clin Nutr 1995;49(suppl 1):S26–S38.
2 Rigo J, Senterre J: Metabolic balance studies and plasma amino acid concentrations in preterm infants fed experimental protein hydrolysate preterm formulas. Acta Paediatr Suppl 994;405: 98–104.
3 Isolauri E, Suta Y, Makinen-Kiljunen S, et al: Efficacy and safety of hydrolyzed cow milk and amino acid-derived formulas in infants with cow milk allergy. J Pediatr 1995;127:550–557.
4 Hidvégi E, Arató A, Cserháti E, et al: Slight decrease in bone mineralization in cow milk-sensitive children. J Pediatr Gastroenterol Nutr 2003;36:44–49.

Isolauri E, Walker WA (eds): Allergic Diseases and the Environment.
Nestlé Nutrition Workshop Series Pediatric Program, Vol. 53, pp. 251–265,
Nestec Ltd.; Vevey/S. Karger AG, Basel, © 2004.

Identification of Probiotics and Prebiotics with Antiallergenic Properties[1]

S. Salminen and E. Isolauri

Department of Biochemistry and Food Chemistry and Department of Pediatrics,
University of Turku, Turku, Finland

Introduction

Probiotics have been defined as bacterial preparations which impart clinically verified beneficial health effects on the host when consumed orally. Prebiotics are nonabsorbable carbohydrates which act by promoting beneficial members of intestinal microbiota in a manner that provides demonstrated health benefits to humans [1]. Most probiotics are currently either lactic acid bacteria or bifidobacteria, but new species and genera are being assessed for probiotic use. Common prebiotics are based on fructo-oligosaccharides from plant sources or lactose-based galacto-oligosaccharides resembling those found in breast milk [1].

Current knowledge of probiotics and prebiotics shows that mechanisms of probiotic action are multi-facetted and each probiotic or prebiotic may have specific functions affecting the host. The criteria for effective probiotics were defined based on the general properties of probiotics. It may be necessary to redefine these criteria and acquire new standards to allow the development of probiotics for specific functions and targets [2]. The same is required for prebiotics as most of them were developed as substrates for intestinal bifidobacteria in general without understanding their role in microbiota–host interactions. The focus on here is to characterize probiotics and prebiotics in

[1] A Nutrition, Allergy, Mucosal Immunology and Intestinal Microbiota (NAMI) Research Group report.

general and define the steps needed to develop probiotics and potentially also prebiotics with antiallergenic efficacy.

Intestinal Microbiota: Basis of Probiotic and Prebiotic Development

The generation of immunophysiological regulation in the gut depends on the establishment of indigenous microbiota. The microbiota of a newborn develops rapidly after birth and it is initially strongly dependent on the mother's microbiota, mode of birth and birth environment, and subsequently influenced by feeding practices and the environment of the child. Most microbiota succession studies have been based on culture method studies. Recent molecular studies have indicated that the microbiota in infants develops rapidly during the first week and remains unstable for the first year of life. We know that lactic acid bacteria account for <1% of the total microbiota in infants but bifidobacteria can range from 60 to 90% of the total fecal microbiota in breast-fed infants [3, 4]. The composition of bifidobacteria microbiota in infants was first clarified by Benno and Mitsuoka [5]. Usually bifidobacteria appear after birth and within a week they have been reported to be the dominant bacterial group with *Bifidobacterium breve* and *Bifidobacterium bifidum* as the most common species present in healthy infants. Comparing breast-fed and formula-fed infants the greatest differences appear to be in lactic acid bacteria colonization and species of bifidobacteria present. In breast-fed infants *Lactobacillus gasseri* and *B. breve* are the most common species present in culture method studies [5]. Similar results have been reported with more detailed information on the distribution of bifidobacterial species using 16S rRNA primers and modern taxonomy [6]. *B. breve, Bifidobacterium infantis* and *Bifidobacterium longum* are frequently found in fecal samples from infants. Using molecular methods, the most common lactobacilli in breast-fed and formula-fed infant feces were *Lactobacillus acidophilus* (*sensu lacto*) group organisms [3, 7].

The development of intestinal microbiota has to be characterized in a manner defining the composition that assists the infant to remain healthy. Specific aberrancies in intestinal microbiota may predispose the infant to allergic disease. Such aberrancies include decreased numbers of bifidobacteria and an atypical composition of bifidobacterial microbiota [8]. Also aberrancies in the clostridium content and composition have been reported to be important [8–11]. Compositional differences among clostridia and their relation to bifiobacterial composition and concentration need to be assessed carefully as they may predispose the infant to allergic diseases. Similar predisposing factors may also exist in terms of microbiota and risk for rotavirus diarrhea [12]. Thorough knowledge of intestinal microbiota composition offers a basis for future probiotic development and the search of antiallergenic strains.

Optimal Characteristics for Probiotics

Tolerance to Upper Gastrointestinal Environment

The effects of gastrointestinal (GI) conditions, such as pH, bile, and digestive enzymes on the survival [13] and adhesion properties [14] of probiotic bacteria have been documented. Various bacteria show different levels of tolerance to the GI conditions. For example, the adhesion of *Lactobacillus rhamnosus* GG on mucus was reduced to 1/10, while the adhesion of *Lactobacillus johnsonii* La1 was also reduced after pretreatment with amylase, pepsin, bile and pancreatin [14]. Such properties have to be clarified for all candidate probiotics.

Adhesion

Adhesion on the intestinal surface lengthens the retention time of a probiotic, and it is particularly important for the small intestine. The resident time of intestinal material in the small intestine is relatively short.

L. rhamnosus GG, which has been reported to adhere and also colonize also the small intestine, was found to be effective in shortening rotavirus diarrhea in infants [15, 16]. *Lactobacillus bulgaricus*, which could not adhere to and colonize the intestine, had no effect on infant diarrhea. Similarly, a highly adhesive strain *Bifidobacterium lactis* Bb12 has been proved to be effective in preventing and treating acute diarrhea in infants [17]. Recent information on the genome of *B. longum* indicates that the strain has specific gene sequences that assist in the adherence to intestinal mucosa especially in the colon [18]. The genetic coding may predispose some strains and species to inhabit specific target sites in the intestinal tract of infants and these properties should be carefully characterized for each strain.

The ability of probiotics to adhere to intestinal mucous glycoprotein is likely to reflect the persistence of a probiotic to intestinal contents, but it may not necessarily be related to their capacity to successfully adhere to intestinal tissue [19]. A probiotic bacterium that binds strongly on mucin glycoprotein would compete with pathogens for adhesion on the mucous surface, but may have a high turnover rate on the mucosal surface, due to their continuous dislodgement from the intestinal surface together with mucus that they bind to. Conversely, a probiotic bacterium that penetrates the mucous layer may adhere to the epithelial surface [19, 20].

Specificity to Target Sites

Orally consumed probiotics pass along the entire GI tract and, therefore, selecting new candidate probiotics from members of the normal microbiota, the candidate strains are likely to have prerequisite survival and specificity depending on isolation location. An effective probiotic should reside sufficiently long at desirable target sites and at sufficient concentrations to elicit probiotic effects. Moreover, adhesion and even temporary multiplication of probiotic bacteria at the target sites would result in enhanced concentrations of probiotics at the optimal places of action, achieving the desirable responses even at a lower dosage [19, 21, 22].

Growth and Metabolic Activity

Without adhesion to the intestinal mucosa, the concentration of probiotic bacteria would be diluted to an insignificant level following a meal or drink. It is not clear whether all probiotics could grow in an intestinal environment. No commercial probiotics have been reported to be able to establish permanently in the human intestine, which suggests that even if there is cell division the specific growth rates are not fast enough to replenish detached probiotic cells on the intestinal surface [1].

Growth in the intestinal tract increases population size and the metabolic products of probiotics, and their ability to alter GI bacterial activities. We have yet to see evidence demonstrating the growth of probiotics in the GI tract. Some probiotics attach to the intestinal mucosa and can be recovered in biopsies much longer than reported by Alander et al. [23] and Zoetendal et al. [24]. Thus, adherence studies need to complement fecal recovery assessment, preferably in biopsies. The importance of viability is underscored in reports in which immune-enhancing effects during probiotic treatment of rotavirus diarrhea were only observed with viable probiotics [25]. Another aspect of viability concerns metabolite production. Acid and peroxide production by bacteria are linked to growth, but secondary metabolites are non-growth linked and produced when cells are not multiplying. These metabolites may play an important role in locally modulating GI microbiota.

Prebiotic Characteristics

Bifidogenicity

The basis for prebiotics is the selective stimulation of bifidobacteria observed in the assessment of fecal or intestinal contents [1]. This is the major characteristic for each candidate prebiotic. Rather than the current requirement for enhanced bifidobacterial concentrations in feces, one key factor for antiallergenic properties may be the influence on the bifidobacterial composition in the intestinal tract. We have reported that different bifidobacterial species and strains may be involved when antiallergenic properties are considered. Infants that later develop allergies or are allergic are more often colonized by adult type of bifidobacteria, *Bifidobacterium adolescentis*, whilst children that remain healthy have a different bifidobacterial composition [10]. Thus, future prebiotics for antiallergenic properties may need to be formulated to promote specific species and strains of bifidobacteria, not just the *Bifidobacterium* ssp in general.

Microbiota Effects of Prebiotics

Most studies on the prebiotic effects on intestinal microbiota have concentrated on bifidobacteria and little is know about the effects of many prebiotics on other intestinal microbiota compositions. One of the oldest prebiotics is lactulose, which has been extensively studied and used in adults and infants. It has the required bifidogenic effects reported and lactulose resembling lacto-oligosaccharides are also found in breast milk. Lactulose also has a long history of safe use in intestinal microbiota management in adults and children [26, 27]. The potential antiallergenic properties of lactulose have not been assessed. This requires work on intestinal microbiota composition and long-term effects in human subjects. Fructo-oligosaccharides have mainly been assessed in adults, but recently also applications in infant formula have been introduced. The long-term microbiota effects of early fructo-oligosaccharide administration in infancy are not yet known.

Future prebiotic assessment needs to focus on intestinal microbiota as a whole and the search for prebiotics or prebiotic mixes with antiallergenic properties. Assessment of beneficial as well as potentially harmful components are needed in a qualitative and quantitative manner. The same targets apply as indicated for probiotics.

Characterizing Antiallergenic Probiotic and Prebiotics

It is clear that new selection criteria are needed in addition to the traditional ones if antiallergenic efficacy is to be obtained. One proposed scheme that requires a relatively long time and interaction by multidisciplinary research groups is presented in figure 1. It is based on characterizing the normal microbiota for infants who remain healthy for several years. Healthy infants are compared to infants who later develop allergic diseases and the microbiota aberrancies need to be monitored. At the same time, bifidobacteria and lactobacilli in healthy infants are characterized and assessed for their influence on normalizing microbiota aberrancies. Within the proposed scheme it will take several years to identify new probiotic candidates for future clinical trials. Such strains should be carefully characterized prior to application in human studies (table 1). Investigations needed for this assessment are presented in table 2.

Probiotics, Prebiotics and Intestinal Microbiota and Immunity

One of the main selection criteria for probiotics has been competitive exclusion of pathogens. Probiotics compete directly or hinder the adhesion of pathogens on stereo-specific receptors on the GI surface [28]. They can also

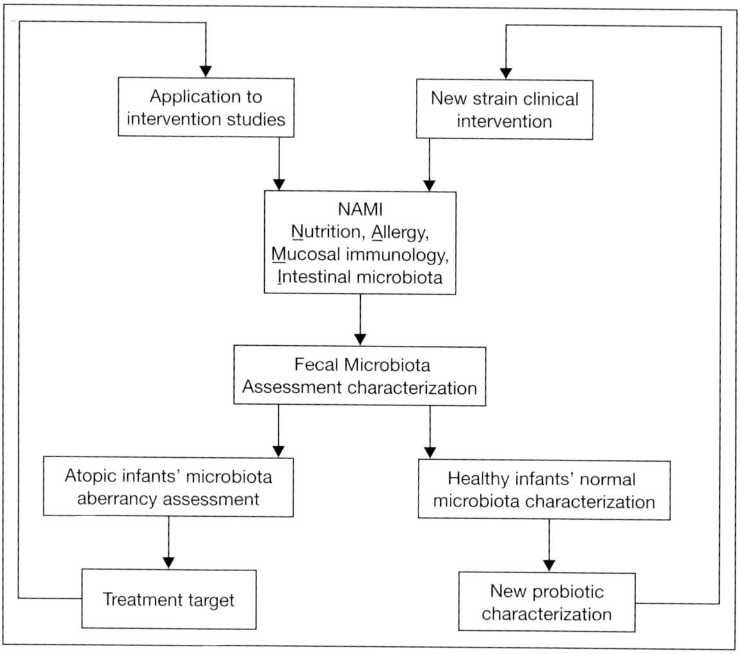

Fig. 1. Proposed approach for isolating and characterizing new probiotic strains with antiallergenic properties. NAMI = University of Turku combined research program on Nutrition, Allergy, Mucosal Immunology and Intestinal Microbiota.

influence the development of intestinal microbiota in infants. The outcome of the competition would depend on the specificity of the bacteria adhesins for the receptors and the relative concentration of the two competing bacteria. The effective dosage of a probiotic is thus determined by the relative affinity for the receptor sites.

Probiotic bacteria have been shown to modulate the intestinal and systemic immune responses [2, 29–31]. Activation of immunological cells and tissues likely requires close contact of probiotics with the immune cells and tissue on the intestinal surface [32]. Interestingly, both lactobacilli and bifidobacteria, which mainly colonize the small and large intestine, respectively, given as probiotic supplements, were able to modify immunological reactions related to allergic inflammation, but lactobacilli were ineffective in protection against cow's milk allergy [2, 32–34]. In this respect, preferential binding of probiotics to the specific antigen-processing cells (macrophages, dendritic and epithelial cells) [35, 36] may be even more important than the location of adhesion. We have also shown that the cytokine stimulation profiles of different bifidobacterium strains vary and strains isolated from healthy infants mainly stimulate noninflammatory cytokines. Probiotic properties also vary in

Table 1. Properties of probiotics to be assessed during the development of new strains and new probiotic functional foods

Property	Target and method
Specificity to species and target	Source or origin to be assessed, gut commensals as a source, target defined
Resistance to pH	Model systems for gastric and bile effects
Adhesion and colonization	Several model systems to be used for adhesion (e.g. cell cultures, mucus, intestinal segments)
Competitive exclusion	Colonization in human studies adhesion and competitive exclusion of pathogens in in vitro and in vivo model systems
Immune regulation	In vitro and human studies – Cytokine profile – Contact with immune cells – Adhesion related to immune effects – Improvement of gut barrier and permeability disorders
Function specificity	Adhesion Immune function Competitive exclusion
Safety	Safety clearance and post-market monitoring
Technological properties	Stability and activity throughout the processes
Sensory assessment	Acceptance of probiotic and prebiotic products
Efficacy assessment	Human clinical intervention studies with final product formulations, at least two independent studies to show efficacy in target populations and safety in all consumer groups

Table 2. Examples of target-specific searches for optimal probiotics

Target for probiotic action	Selection criteria
Alleviation of lactose maldigestion symptoms	High lactase producing strongly site specific adhesion LAB
Intestinal inflammation	Site specific adhesion properties, anti-inflammatory cytokine expression, mucosal properties to alleviate permeability disorder and gut microbiota aberrancy
Alleviation or food allergy symptoms, reducing the risk of atopic diseases	Adherence to small intestine, induction of local TGF-β production, proteolytic properties
Reducing the risk of colon cancer	Target-specific adhesion to distal and or proximal colon, mucosal butyric acid production, competitive exclusion of inflammatory bacteria, toxin binding and promotion of nontoxigenic mucosal microbiota

Table 3. Future challenges for the health-promoting probiotics

- Preclinical testing of probiotics: efficacy and safety
- Different and often opposite immunological effects of the specific strains of gut microbiota
- Different role of gut microbiota and the effects of probiotics and prebiotics in the healthy versus inflamed mucosa
- Identification of specific strain in prevention and management of infectious and inflammatory diseases
- Identification and mechanisms of effective dietary components
- Development of novel functional foods with specific probiotics, prebiotics and supporting dietary compounds

this respect. *Lactobacillus casei* has been reported to induce IL-12 and transforming growth factor-α from murine dendritic cells while *Lactobacillus reuteri* causes IL-10 production and downregulates the effects of *L. casei*. The gut microbiota provides crucial maturational signals for the immune system in infancy and interferes and also actively controls gut-associated immunological homeostasis later in life. Indeed, it is not because of food antigens but because of the antigens of the microbiota that fully matured gut-associated lymphoid tissue is the largest immunological organ containing greater numbers of T cells than the rest of the body combined. Duchmann et al. [37] have demonstrated that healthy individuals are tolerant to their own microbiota. Specific strains of the gut microbiota have also been shown to contribute to a T-helper cell population that maintains a disease-free state of the gut. These interactions should be taken into account when selecting the candidate probiotics (table 3).

Conclusions

It is clear that intestinal microbiota development is of major importance to the health of the newborn. It appears that due to their concentration and composition bifidobacteria are more important than lactic acid bacteria during early intestinal colonization. These factors form the basis for selecting probiotics from the currently available ones, suggesting bifidobacteria as the first option, and specific lactic acid bacteria that may stimulate intestinal bifidobacteria as the second option. The qualitative effects of current probiotics and prebiotics on intestinal microbiota should be understood prior to being used in infant foods.

The knowledge of intestinal microbiota development, nutrition, immunity and allergic diseases should be carefully combined in the search for new probiotics and prebiotics with antiallergenic properties.

References

1 Salminen S, Bouley MC, Boutron-Rualt MC, et al: Functional food science and gastrointestinal physiology and function. Br J Nutr 1998;80(suppl 1):S147–S171.
2 Isolauri E, Rautava S, Kalliomaki M, et al: Role of probiotics in food hypersensitivity. Curr Opin Allergy Clin Immunol 2002;2:263–271.
3 Vaughan E, de Vries M, Zoetendal E, et al: The intestinal LABs. Antonie Van Leeuwenhoek 2002;82:341–352.
4 Favier C, Vaughan E, de Vos W, Akkermans A: Molecular monitoring of succession of bacterial communities in human neonates. Appl Environ Microbiol 2002;68:219–226.
5 Benno Y, Mitsuoka T: Development of intestinal microflora in humans and animals. Bifidobacteria Microflora 1986;5:13–25.
6 Matsuki T, Watanabe K, Tanaka R, et al: Distribution of Bifidobacterial species in human intestinal microflora examined with 16S rRNA-gene-targeted species-specific primers. Appl Environ Microbiol 1999;65;4506–4512.
7 Satokari RM, Vaughan EE, Akkermans AD, et al: Bifidobacterial diversity in human feces detected by genus-specific PCR and denaturing gradient gel electrophoresis. Appl Environ Microbiol 2001;67:504–513.
8 Kalliomäki M, Kirjavainen P, Eerola E, et al: Distinct patterns of neonatal gut microflora in infants developing or not developing atopy. J Allergy Clin Immunol 2001;107:129–134.
9 Björkstén B, Sepp E, Julge K, et al: Allergy development and the intestinal microflora during the first year of life. J Allergy Clin Immunol 2001;108:516–520.
10 He F, Ouwehand A, Isolauri E, et al: Comparison of mucosal adhesion and species identification of bifidobacteria isolated from healthy and allergic infants. FEMS Immunol Med Microbiol 2000;1285:43–47.
11 He F, Morita H, Hashimoto H, et al: Intestinal bifidobacterium species induce varying cytokine production. J Allergy Clin Immunol 2002;109:1035–1036.
12 Juntunen M: Treatment and Prevention of Childhood Diarrhoea with Probiotics and Early Refeeding; PhD thesis, University of Turku, 2001.
13 Havenaar, R, Huis in't Veld JHJ: Selection of strains for probiotic use; in Fuller R (ed): Probiotics, the Scientific Basis. London, Chapman & Hall, 1992, pp 209–224.
14 Ouwehand AC, Tolkko S, Salminen S: The effect of digestive enzymes on the adhesion of probiotic bacteria in vitro. J Food Sci 2001;66:856–859.
15 Isolauri E, Juntunen M, Rautanen T, et al: A human lactobacillus strain (*Lactobacillus casei* sp strain GG) promotes recovery from acute diarrhea in children. Pediatrics 1991;88:90–97.
16 Guandalini S, Pensabene L, Zikri M, et al: Lactobacillus GG administered in an oral rehydration solution to children with acute diarrhea: A multicenter European trial. J Pediatr Gastroenterol Nutr 2000;30:54–60.
17 Saavedra J, Bauman N, Oung I, et al: Feeding of *Bifidobacterium bifidum* and *Streptococcus thermophilus* to infants in hospital for prevention of diarrhea and shedding of rotavirus. Lancet 1994;344:1046–1049.
18 Schell MA, Karmirantzou M, Snel B, et al: The genome sequence of *Bifidobacteium longum* reflects its adaptation to the human gastrointestinal tract. Proc Natl Acad Sci USA 2002;99: 14422–14427.
19 Ouwehand AC, Salminen S, Tölkkö S, et al: Resected human colonic tissue: New model for characterizing adhesion of lactic acid bacteria. Clin Diagn Lab Immunol 2002;9:184–186.
20 Apostolou, E, Pelto L, Kirjavainen PV, et al: Differences in the gut bacterial flora of healthy and milk-hypersensitive adults, as measured by fluorescence in situ hybridization. FEMS Immunol Med Microbiol 2001;30:217–221.
21 Lee YK, Lim CY, Teng WL, et al: Qualitative approach in the study of adhesion of lactic acid bacteria on intestinal cells and their competition with enterobacteria. Appl Environ Microbiol 2000;66:3692–3697.
22 Ouwehand AC, Tuomola EM, Lee YK, Salminen S: Microbial interactions to intestinal mucosal models. Methods Enzymol 2001;337:200–12.
23 Alander M, Satokari R, Korpela R, et al: Persistence of colonization of human colonic mucosa by a probiotic strain, *Lactobacillus rhamnosus* GG, after oral consumption. Appl Environ Microbiol 1999;65:351–354.

24 Zoetendal E, Wright A, Vilpponen-Salmela T, et al: Mucosa associated bacteria in the human gastrointestinal tract are uniformly distributed along the colon and differ from the community recovered from the faeces. Appl Environ Microbiol 2002;68:3401–3407.
25 Majamaa H, Isolauri E, Saxelin M, Vesikari T: Lactic acid bacteria in the treatment of acute rotavirus gastroenteritis. J Pediatr Gastroenterol Nutr 1995;20:333–338.
26 Ballongue J, Schumann C, Quignon P: Effects of lactulose and lactitol on colonic microflora and enzymatic activity. Scand J Gastroenterol Suppl 1997;222:41–44.
27 Schumann C: Medical, nutritional and technological properties of lactulose. An update. Eur J Nutr 2002;41(suppl 1):I17–I25.
28 Lee YK, Puong KY: Competition for adhesion between probiotics and human gastrointestinal pathogens in the presence of carbohydrate. Br J Nutr 2002;88(suppl 1):S101–S108.
29 Miettinen M, Lehtonen A, Julkunen I, Matikainen S: Lactobacilli and streptococci activate NF-kappa B and STAT signalling pathways in human macrophages. J Immunol 2000;164:3733–3740.
30 Isolauri E, Arvola T, Sutas Y, et al: Probiotics in the management of atopic eczema. Clin Exp Allergy 2000;30:1604–1610.
31 Neish AS, Gewirtz, AT, Zeng H, et al: Prokaryotic regulation of epithelia responses by inhibition of IkappaB-alpha ubiquitination. Science 2000;289:1560–1563.
32 Schiffrin E.J, Brassart D, Servin AL, et al: Immune modulation of blood leukocytes in humans by lactic acid bacteria: criteria for strain selection. Am J Clin Nutr 1997;66:155S–520S.
33 Kalliomäki M, Salminen S, Arvilommi H, et al: Probiotics in the prevention of atopic diseases: A randomised placebo-controlled trial. Lancet 2001;357:1076–1079.
34 Kirjavainen PV, Arvola T, Salminen SJ, Isolauri E: Aberrant composition of gut microbiota of allergic infants: A target of bifidobacterial therapy at weaning? Gut 2002;51:51–55.
35 Hemmi H, Takeuchi O, Kawai T: A Toll-like receptor recognizes bacterial DNA. Nature 2000;408:740–745.
36 Cario E, Rosenberg IM, Brandwein SL: Lipopolysaccharide activates distinct signaling pathways in intestinal epithelial cell lines expressing Toll-like receptors. J Immunol 2000;164:966–972.
37 Duchmann R, Kaiser I, Hermann E, et al: Tolerance exists towards resident intestinal flora but is broken in active inflammatory bowel disease (IBD). Clin Exp Immunol 1995;102:448–455.

Discussion

Dr. Endres: You mentioned that lactobacilli are able to enhance the growth of bifidobacteria. As we all have a similar definition of prebiotics in mind, we could say that lactobacilli have a prebiotic effect on bifidobacteria, but I think this is not the right conclusion because it is another mechanism. I think that the prebiotics create the right environment and are in a certain way food for probiotic bacteria, aren't they?

Dr. Salminen: I quite agree with you. I was trying to point out that the probiotic effect can be similar to the prebiotic effect, but of course by definition you are absolutely right, it could not go that way. But we have been lucky in a way because many of the current lactobacillus strains used actually may have that effect.

Dr. Walker: This was an excellent overview because this is an important area of investigation that needs to be carefully analyzed. My concern is that when you put in a procaryotic against the eucaryotic, the procaryotic usually wins the battle because it can adapt so much more easily to the environment than can a whole organism, so a problem develops. One of the concerns is that prebiotics modulate the environment. As a result of their modulation you get increased bifidobacteria but, because you have other bacteria, they can adapt and the prebiotic effect is a short-term rather than a long-term effect. The other concern that I would like to have you comment on is: there was a really excellent article in *Science* [1] where they genetically engineered lactobacillus to produce IL-10 that could be delivered directly to the mucosal surface and showed in an experimental model of inflammatory bowel disease that they could downregulate the inflammation. This is an area that we really need to be looking at in the future because we might be able to use probiotics not only themselves, but genetically engineer them to deliver medications/factors directly to the gut.

Dr. Salminen: I really appreciate the last comment, it is a very important area. I left it out because we are actually discussing infant nutrition and at the moment the genetic engineering question is such that it is very controversial even in adults. But I quite agree, I know the study presented in *Science* and it certainly actually offers some mechanisms that we should consider. From the discussions that we have in Europe today, I would say that it certainly has great potential in the pharmaceutical field, but perhaps we are a bit off in infant foods. We are trying to understand the genome and perhaps, for infant food purposes, select strains or species that are natural and naturally adapted to the infant gut, such as *B. longum*, and the more we know about the genome, the more choices and the more possibilities we will have. But I take your other point also as a very valuable addition to the discussion. Of course we know the genome in the bifidobacteria but we need to know a little bit more about what the bacteria do to our intestinal cells and their gene expression. So we are only starting to know the first part of a cross-talk, what kinds of signals there are perhaps in the bifidobacteria. However, we know very little about how those signals affect our intestinal cells. So in those terms I think that you are absolutely right, we need to know more and we need to understand them, but still I think that perhaps we would use the genetically modified organisms more in the pharmaceutical area.

Dr. Walker: My other concern is that we are being artificial when we introduce the single organism into a gut to do a major job like prevent allergy or produce inflammation. This is a strong case for the use of cocktails of bacteria that can work in concert to produce a potentially stronger effect than a single organism, particularly if you chose the wrong organism.

Dr. Salminen: I agree with that comment also, but before we go into the cocktails we have to know the safety properties of each single strain and component in the cocktail, and I think we should understand the steps that the infant has in acquiring its microbiota a little bit more. Because if we start very early it may be one or two species of bifidobacteria that form 90% of the microbiota but how they then influence the next step is not known.

Dr. Guesry: To prolong the question of Dr. Endres on the potential prebiotic role of a certain type of probiotic bacteria, I think we should enlarge the discussion to the point of what is the role of dead probiotic bacteria compared to living probiotic bacteria, because we have some indication that there are sometimes synergies between dead and living bacteria. Do you have a comment on that?

Dr. Salminen: I think you have touched upon a very important area both in terms of intestinal microbiota research and in terms of probiotics. Most of the genetic methods that are used today in assessing microbiota include all, both viable and nonviable bacteria, and if we compare the viable bifidobacteria counts, for instance, usually the counts in gut samples are lower than the genetic methods for the total number of bifidobacteria. In a recent review that we wrote with Dr. Isolauri [2] we suggested that one should also consider nonviable bacteria because even though the bacterial cells are not presently alive in the gut, they are probably present in the mucosa and possibly influence a local effect. So I think you are absolutely right, but we also have to do studies on nonviable bacteria. Again I would refer to Dr. Isolauri because she has done diarrhea studies with viable and nonviable bacteria, and if I recall well I think the clinical effects were similar but the immune effects were not the same [2]. So they may be efficacious in some aspects and we should look at that.

Dr. Guesry: In that case it is another dogma that we have put down this morning since the living bacteria is part of the definition.

Dr. Salminen: Let me just point out that I use the commonly accepted definition of probiotics. We have proposed another one that will also take into account nonviable bacteria.

Dr. Sorensen: Thank you for a very nice review of a topic I know nothing about, which I think explains why I am going to ask you this question. Why do you exclude non-pathogenic *Escherichia coli* from your list of useful bacteria? There is plenty of evidence that infants by 1 year of age have developed antibodies and isoagglutinins. I understand there are antibodies against galactosamines on the surface of *E. coli*, so they clearly have an effect on infant immunity and a normal child may never have had diarrhea but plenty of evidence of having many *E. coli*. Why do you ignore them?

Dr. Salminen: I do not discriminate against them at all. I was only trying to point out that there is no straightforward categorization of harmful or not so harmful. I think clostridia are another example. If we lose all the clostridia in our gut, we might be in trouble and it is probably the same with the *E. coli*. Again, the early colonization of the gut is so much dependent on the environment in which we are born that we cannot say that one bacteria, one species, not even some genera, are really strictly harmful, but we should rather find a way not to kill them, not to eradicate them, but to live together with them. That comes back to the composition: how do we understand the composition? The European Union has been investing a lot of money in defining healthy European gut microbiota, but we are giving up because there is no such thing. There are individual healthy gut microbiota that between us will probably be dramatically different. I would not eradicate, but would try to coexist happily with the microbes we are born with and only start eradicating when there is serious disease.

Dr. Szajewska: We know from the recent meta-analysis [3] that there is a dose-related effect, at least in diarrheal diseases. Can you please comment on the minimum dose, to summarize data, and also do you think that we have to be worried about too much bacteria being given to an infant?

Dr. Salminen: These are two very excellent questions that all of us should consider. The first question I think the clinicians should answer. From the microbiological point of view I think the dose that is used currently for most probiotics is 10^9 colony forming units/day/person. It is some kind of average of many studies and I would say that it comes back to the unique individual strain properties. I think most of the studies have used that dose to be sure to guarantee enough exposure. How much lower you can go, I don't think anybody knows. We can probably go lower but how much lower. There are no dose-response studies that go to 10^6–10^5, the lowest effects are usually seen in 10^8, in some studies 10^8 is not enough. But then I think it comes to the other question, viability, how important is survival, what is a strain-specific property, survival in the gastric acid conditions, survival and adherence to the gut, local effects? So I think 10^9 is a rule of thumb, but when we learn the mechanisms in more detail we could probably use lower doses with some strains. However, if you were running a clinical study, would you risk going lower without knowing?

Dr. Saavedra: I agree completely with what you just said. But from the point of view of dose, I think a lot will also depend on what the use of the probiotic is. Because a good part of what is currently presented relates to therapeutic effects of probiotics, that is to treat a particular condition once the condition has been initiated, whether it is allergy or for treatment of diarrhea, versus the application of probiotics for what we would consider an adjuvant in terms of gut health or modifications of gut function on a chronic basis. These are completely different approaches incorporating it on a long-term and chronic basis, and of course even then it is even harder to know what the minimal doses are going to be. Can you comment on what an overdose of probiotics is? But I think it is almost impossible.

Dr. Salminen: I am sorry, by discussing the dose I forgot to discuss your second question. As long as we have been conducting safety assessment of different specific probiotic strains, there doesn't seem to be an achievable toxic dose. However, we know from the use of lactobacilli that one has always to remember that when you have viable living bacteria, and that is another question concerning viability, under some circumstances it is viable bacteria that can cause a problem. However, I would say that with lactobacilli the problems are extremely rare as far as we know, with bifidobacteria they are almost unreported. I would almost think that bifidobacteria are even onefold safer than lactic acid bacteria. We know for instance for the *Lactobacillus bulgaricus* or *Streptococcus thermophilus* that, if I recall correctly, no problems have ever been reported for these two common yogurt strains in the literature.

Dr. Lack: We tend to think now of certain probiotics and prebiotics as being beneficial perhaps for allergy, and antibiotics as being harmful or evil. As someone who knows very little about the field I just wanted to ask, could antibiotics have a beneficial role, could they have a prebiotic effect in the sense of allowing you to then come in with the good guys (the probiotics)?

Dr. Salminen: If you really take a bright look into the future, why would one not be able to develop an antibiotic that would perhaps very specifically decrease some components of the microbiota and enhance some other microbiota parts. I think the lactobacillus question is stimulatory in a way, but the more wide-spectrum things you use, the more important microbes and indifferent ones you are wiping out, and again from the microbiological point of view it is a similar thing to your hygiene hypothesis. Most of us working with food have always been told how to kill every single bacteria in the food before moving it to the consumer. Recent studies from the US, for instance, have shown that cheese produced under very hygienic conditions is also more prone to spoilage because there is no natural bacteria to fight against, so there is no competitive exclusion against the spoilages causing bacteria. Perhaps also in the food industry we have gone one step too far, and now people, again with the European Union funding, are trying to look at selective ways of pasteurizing or sterilizing food so that you don't kill everything, but you kill the predominant problem causing organisms and let the indifferent ones live perhaps to better preserve the food in the long-term.

Dr. Lack: You distinguish between looking at probiotics as a group and perhaps focusing rather than on genus, on species and strains with their very specific immunological effects. Do you think different host immune responses may come into play as well? I think you show differences between atopic and nonatopic responses in terms of IL-10 production. Could we explain the differences in the colonization of the gut in relation to the host immune response as a reverse causal effect?

Dr. Salminen: It could be part of it but I would leave it to the clinicians to look at the effects. I can only assess what happens in the microbiota.

Dr. Isolauri: I think you missed a slide because it was not an immune response producing more IL-10 in atopic infants, but it was the bifidobacteria isolated from atopic infants which were producing less IL-10, while in healthy infants bifidobacteria caused the high IL-10. So it was the bifidobacteria isolated from the fecal samples of the patients [4].

Dr. Saavedra: I think the question on antibiotics was a very provocative one, but at the same time from that point of view, I think one of the criteria that we chose, in particular probiotics, is that they don't have the ability to transfer antibiotic resistance, for example, which would make things very complicated. It is again another reason why we need to go stepwise and very slowly with these strains.

Dr. Manjra: Are there any studies with regard to the duration of therapy with probiotics?

Dr. Salminen: There are studies but again I would leave that to the clinical specialists in the audience.

Dr. Neijens: How much documentation do we have on the effect of probiotics on different cell populations like coli bacteria and rotavirus because this interaction might be very important? *E. coli*, for instance, produce a lot of IL-12. My second question is what do we know of the effects of antibiotics given to the child on the different strains? Should we advise not to give antibiotics or to be very restrictive, or should we follow that up? My third question is what is the documentation as far as the exchange of genetic material between different strains? What do we know about the exchange of genetic material like DNA or plasmids, etc.?

Dr. Salminen: I think you are presenting excellent questions but we need a regulatory authority to answer. I can try to give you a couple of points. First of all the documentation between strains varies tremendously. There are very well-documented strains, there are strains that have practically no documentation behind them. So there is very wide use of the term 'probiotic', and there is no good single answer to that. All the probiotics that have been used by the food and clinical nutrition industry are actually very well documented for nontransfer of antibiotic resistance, whether by plasmids or by other means, so that has been one of our selection criteria. I did not define the selection criteria that we used on safety studies. So most are lactic acid bacteria, lactobacilli or bifidobacteria, and you can be sure that there is no transfer of genetic material. However, there are still some enterococci which are known to transfer antibiotic resistance, but at least the producers of such strains claim that their particular strain does not do the transfer. Now how good or bad the documentation is, I don't know. I think we should really address the regulatory people for this.

Dr. Szajewska: From a microbiological point of view, could you please comment on why probiotics or lactobacillus GG, for example, are effective in rotavirus gastroenteritis, but are not shown to be effective in bacterial gastroenteritis? What is your explanation?

Dr. Salminen: I think there are simple explanations that are related to the clinical studies. Looking at the microbiota, at the duration of diarrhea, they may sometimes change from viral to microbial, and you may be able to alter the outcome of the microbial phase. It has also been suggested that it could be related to the absorption of rotavirus particles. Now I don't have any evidence on that, but it has been suggested that it may be just a physical barrier between the virus and the intestinal epithelium. But I think the clinical effects are for others to relate to the bacteria.

Dr. Endres: I would like to ask Dr. Szajewska, in your study, the ESPGAN study, it has been shown that viral diarrhea responded better to an oral rehydration solution with lactobacillus GG, whereas in the case of other kinds of diarrhea there has been a less pronounced effect, hasn't there?

Dr. Szajewska: No, as a matter of fact in the ESPGHAN study [5] we confirmed the inefficiency of lactobacillus GG in proven bacterial infectious diarrhea. That is why I was asking my question: why do you think that lactobacillus GG was ineffective? I could not find good data in the literature.

Dr. Guesry: Yes, but your study was not prophylactic since the GG bacteria were given with oral rehydration salt or solution, it was on babies who already had diarrhea, and that is for me a main difference. In our study with Dr. Saavedra, we make it prophylactic and it works. As a treatment it is another question.

Dr. Szajewska: But my question was regarding treatment, I was not asking about prophylaxis.

Dr. Isolauri: I think that question needs to be studied especially in target groups. There are very little data to say that there is no effect or there is an effect. An additional reason is that we are not thinking about why we see an effect in some populations and no effect in another. It could be that even though we use the same strain with the same name on the label, we might finally have a different kind of product, it having been handled differently. We have looked at this in some in vitro systems and finally there might be different products.

Dr. Salminen: Perhaps a comment for the industry people, the quality control for probiotics is very important. One has to be sure that it is similar to the original strain properties because especially in the dairy industry, when butter milk, yogurt or other dairy products are continuously cultured, the properties perhaps decrease and the bile acid's tolerance also decreases. There is absolutely no published study on the strain properties. So it is important for quality control purposes to make sure that the strain remains similar to the original.

Dr. Rijntjes: Children who are allergic have another gut flora and after birth the gut flora of the mother is important for colonization. Can you tell me if there is any literature on the colonization from the gut of the father to the child, because in modern society the father is looking after the child more and more?

Dr. Salminen: I am sure that there is some exchange of bacteria as was said earlier for the real father, and I am quite sure that some of those bacteria are transmitted to the infant, but to my knowledge there are no studies looking at that aspect. But when you have contact you exchange bacteria even if you kiss, and if you have more intensive contact then you exchange more bacteria. It is quite likely that the father has some bacteria that might be affiliated to both parents.

Dr. Rijntjes: There could also be a genetic predisposition to have the gut flora of the father, when he is the real father of course.

Dr. Al-Malik: I understand from your talk that prebiotics are used to treat gut infections and also to reduce food hypersensitivity. Has there been any attempt to use these to treat respiratory allergy or respiratory infections?

Dr. Salminen: To my knowledge there are not many studies with great success. There have been quite a few studies even on the infection or the viral side and, as we heard in the morning, they have not produced any effect. So I think it comes back to defining what is your real prebiotic and is it the right prebiotic for the target.

References

1 Steidler L, Hans W, Schotte L, et al: Treatment of murine colitis by *Lactococcus lactis* secreting interleukin-10. Science 2000;289:1352–1355.

2 Isolauri E, Rautava S, Kalliomaki M, et al: Role of probiotics in food hypersensitivity. Curr Opin Allergy Clin Imunol 2002;2:263–271.

3 Van Niel C, Freudtner C, Garrison MM, et al: Lactobacillus therapy for acute infectious diarrhea in children: A meta-analysis. Pediatrics 2002;109:678–684.

4 He F, Morita H, Hashimoto H, et al: Intestinal bifidobacterium species induce varying cytokine production. J Allergy Clin Immunol 2002;109:1035–1036.

5 Guandalini S, Pensabene L Abu Zikri M, et al: Lactobacillus GG administered in oral rehydration solution to children with acute diarrhea: A multicenter European trial. J Pediatr Gastroenterol Nutr 2000;30:54–60.

Isolauri E, Walker WA (eds): Allergic Diseases and the Environment.
Nestlé Nutrition Workshop Series Pediatric Program, Vol. 53, pp. 267–284,
Nestec Ltd.; Vevey/S. Karger AG, Basel, © 2004.

Can We Prevent the Allergic Child from Becoming a Chronic Asthmatic Adult?

Andrew H. Liu

Division of Allergy and Immunology, Department of Pediatrics,
National Jewish Medical and Research Center, and
University of Colorado Health Sciences Center, Denver, Colo., USA

A rich body of evidence provides the basis for paradigms of asthma development, intervention strategies, and studies to test prevention hypotheses (fig. 1). Longitudinal prospective studies of asthma provide the strongest epidemiological evidence for supporting causal relationships in asthma development and prevention. These studies suggest an 'allergic march' in childhood, of food allergies and atopic dermatitis (AD) in infancy progressing to allergic airways disease and persistent, allergy-associated asthma. Allergy-associated asthma appears to be the most common asthma phenotype in locales where this has been studied. Pathogenically, a combination of environmental, lifestyle and genetic factors are believed to influence immune development in early life, providing an immunologic milieu that can lead to allergic diseases and asthma. Respiratory infections, inhaled allergens, and airway toxicants can injure and inflame the lower airways, targeting immune pathogenic processes to the lungs. Aberrant repair of persistent and/or recurrent airways injury are believed to underlie the many abnormalities found in asthmatic airways.

Prevalence studies reveal that most asthma begins in early life – ~80% of asthmatics are first diagnosed by 6 years of age. However, most young children who experience lower respiratory tract infections with coughing and/or wheezing do not develop persistent asthma. Therefore, in early life, persistent asthmatics coexist within a larger group of transient early wheezers. In preschool-age children with recurrent wheezing, atopy manifestations comprise the majority of risk factors for persistent asthma (table 1). However, it is important to note that many atopic children will not develop persistent asthma; also, asthma can develop and persist in nonallergic children.

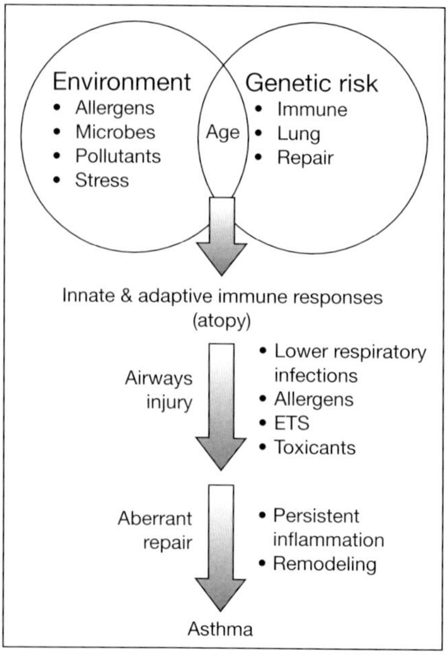

Fig. 1. A pathogenesis schema for asthma. A combination of genetic and environmental factors in early life shape how the immune system develops and responds to microbes and allergens. Atopic immune responses are an indication of pro-asthmatic immune development. Respiratory microbes and inhaled allergens and toxicants that can injure the lower airways target the disease process to the lungs. Aberrant immune and repair responses to airways injury lead to persistent disease.

Table 1. Asthma Predictive Index for children (Tucson Children's Respiratory Study; Tucson, Ariz., USA) [13]

Major criteria	Minor criteria
Parental asthma	Allergic rhinitis
Eczema	Wheezing apart from colds
	Eosinophils >4%
Inhalant allergen sensitization*	Food allergen sensitization*

Through a statistically optimized model for 2- to 3-year-old children with frequent wheezing in the past year, 1 major criterion or 2 minor criteria provided a 77% positive predictive value and 97% specificity for asthma in later childhood (i.e. at 6, 8, 11 and/or 13 years of age).

* Other studies implicate inhalant and food allergen sensitization in early childhood as additional risk factors for persistent asthma.

Strategies to prevent asthma can be conceptualized as targeting different stages of asthma development: (1) early intervention in the early years of asthma development; (2) secondary prevention in at-risk (e.g., allergic) children prior to pulmonary disease manifestations, and (3) primary prevention in infancy and early childhood. The preschool years may be a critical period for such interventions to be effective, during the period of greatest immune maturation and lung growth. Naturally occurring exposures and lifestyle differences in early childhood that have been associated with less subsequent allergy and asthma include prolonged breast-feeding (e.g., >4 months), infections (e.g., common colds, hepatitis A, ascaris), endotoxin, and domestic animals and pet ownership. Randomized controlled interventions in children to prevent allergy and/or asthma have studied the effects of allergenic food avoidance, indoor inhalant allergen reduction, environmental tobacco smoke (ETS) reduction, pharmacologic intervention with antihistamine (cetirizine), inhaled corticosteroid (budesonide), nedocromil, Calmette-Guérin bacillus (BCG), and lactobacillus. These studies provide important clues in the search for effective and safe interventions.

The Natural History of Asthma

Introducing the Allergic March

Natural history studies provide a rich resource for etiologic hypotheses and risk factor assessments of the development and persistence of asthma. Three prospective, longitudinal, birth cohort studies exemplify optimized natural history studies from birth trough early childhood: (1) the Tucson Children's Respiratory Study (CRS) in Tucson, Ariz., USA (begun in 1980); (2) the German Multicenter Allergy Study (MAS) in Germany (begun in 1990), and (3) a Kaiser-based study in San Diego, Calif., USA (begun in 1981). The major findings of these studies have been consistent and reveal a common pattern of allergy and asthma development that begins in infancy.

(1) The highest incidence of AD and food allergies is in the first 2 years of life [1–3]. It is generally believed that infants rarely manifest allergic symptoms in the first month of life. By 3 months of age, however, AD, food allergies, and wheezing problems are common.

(2) This is paralleled by a high prevalence of food allergen sensitization in the first 2 years of life [4]. Early food allergen sensitization is an important risk factor for food allergies, AD, and asthma.

(3) Allergic airways diseases generally begin slightly later in childhood. Most persistent asthma begins before 12 years of age [5]. Childhood asthma often initially manifests with a lower respiratory tract infection or bronchiolitis episode in the first few years of life.

(4) The development of persistent asthma is paralleled by a rise in inhalant allergen sensitization [4]. Perennial inhalant allergen sensitization (i.e. cat dander, dust mites) emerges between 2 and 5 years of age. Seasonal inhalant allergen sensitization becomes apparent slightly later in life (ages 3–5 years).

These observations introduce a link and possibly a progression of atopic immunity to allergic manifestations, and often to asthma – the so-called 'allergic march' of childhood.

When Does Asthma Begin?

Approximately 80% of asthmatics have disease onset prior to 6 years of age [6]. However, of all young children who experience recurrent wheezing, only a minority will go on to have persistent asthma in later life. The most common form of recurrent wheezing in preschool children occurs primarily with viral infections. These 'transient wheezers' or 'wheezy bronchitics' are not at an increased risk of having asthma in later life. This is demonstrated in a large birth cohort study in Tucson, Ariz. – the CRS. In the first 6 years of life, 49% of their birth cohort reported wheezing symptoms [7]. These early childhood wheezers were further subdivided into: (1) 'transient early wheezers', with wheezing only <3 years of life; (2) 'persistent wheezers', with manifestations both <3 years and between 3–6 years, and (3) 'late onset wheezers', with manifestations only between 3 and 6 years. Transient wheezers comprised the largest proportion of the group at 20%. Persistent wheezers and late onset wheezers made up slightly smaller proportions, 14 and 15%, respectively. Of these 3 groups, persistent wheezers had the greatest likelihood of persistent asthma in later childhood (i.e. age 11 years; Martinez FD, personal commun.). Late onset wheezers also had an increased likelihood of persistent childhood asthma. In contrast, the likelihood of persistent asthma in the transient wheezer group was not different from non-wheezers.

Lung function in the Tucson CRS was measured in the first year of life (prior to the occurrence of lower respiratory tract infections) and at 6 years of age. Interestingly, transient wheezers had the lowest airflow measures in infancy, suggesting that they had the narrowest airways and/or the smallest lungs at birth [7]. Their reduced lung function improved significantly by 6 years of age. In comparison, persistent wheezers demonstrated normal lung function in the first few months of life, but a significant decline in airflow measures by 6 years of age. Therefore, alterations in lung function were consistent with clinical disease manifestations in the first 6 years of life.

Asthma from Childhood to Adulthood

A cohort of asthmatic 7-year-olds living in Melbourne, Australia, were re-studied for persistence and severity of asthma at 10, 14, 21, 28 and 35 years of age. At 35 years of age, 70% of the asthmatics and 90% of the severe asthmatics continued to have asthma symptoms; 75% of the severe asthmatics reported frequent or persistent asthma [8]. In comparison, 24% of 'wheezy bronchitics' (i.e. wheezing only with colds at 7 years of age) reported frequent or persistent asthma. These observations – that many asthmatic children experience disease remission or improvement in early adulthood, but that severe asthma persists with age – are remarkably similar to those of several other natural history studies of childhood asthma into adulthood: i.e. Aberdeen, Scotland [9], Tasmania, Australia [10], and a national British study [11].

Objective measures of lung function both validate and bring further insights to these natural history studies. Spirometric measures of lung function of the Melbourne study children initially revealed that asthmatics (especially severe asthmatics) had lung function impairment, while wheezy bronchitics (i.e. 'transient' wheezers) had lung function that was not different from nonasthmatics. Over the ensuing years, these differences in lung function impairment between groups persisted in parallel, without a greater rate of decline in lung function in any group [12]. In the Aberdeen study, greater lung function impairment in asthmatics vs. wheezy bronchitics or controls was complemented by a greater proportion of asthmatic subjects with bronchial hyperresponsiveness (BHR) when compared with the wheezy bronchitis or control groups [9]. These findings support the importance of the early childhood years in asthma development – the establishment of chronic disease and lung function impairment in school-age children appears to predict persistent asthma well into adulthood.

Allergic Risk Factors for Persistent Asthma

Essentially all of the current natural history studies have found that allergic disease or evidence of pro-allergic immune development are significant risk factors for persistent asthma. In the Tucson CRS, early AD, allergic rhinitis (AR), elevated serum IgE levels in the first year of life, and peripheral blood eosinophilia were all significant risk factors for persistent asthma [7, 13]. In the Berlin MAS study, additional risk factors for asthma and BHR at age 7 years included persistent sensitization to foods (i.e. hen's egg, cow's milk, wheat and/or soy) and perennial inhalant allergens (i.e. dust mite, cat), especially in early life [14, 15]. At age 7 years, food allergen sensitization was not associated with asthma; however, the combination of food allergen sensitization by age 2 years and inhalant allergen sensitization by age 7 years ('persistent sensitization') was associated with a significantly higher prevalence of asthma and BHR [16]. In the Kaiser San Diego study, milk or peanut allergen sensitization were risk factors for asthma [2].

Natural history studies of asthma that have extended into adulthood continue to find allergy to be a risk factor for persistent asthma [8, 10, 11]. Two studies found that food allergen sensitization in the first 2 years of life was associated with asthma at ages 7 [16] and 22 years [17]. For allergen sensitization to egg and/or milk in the first year of life, sensitivity and specificity for asthma at age 22 years was 57 and 89%, respectively [18].

Severe AD in early childhood is associated with a high prevalence of allergen sensitization and airways allergic disease in later childhood (i.e. 4 years later) [19]. In young patients with severe AD, 100% developed inhalant allergen sensitization, and 75% developed an allergic respiratory disease (mostly asthma) over 4 years. In contrast to severe AD, mild-to-moderate AD patients were not as likely to develop allergen sensitization (36%) or an allergic respiratory disease (26%).

Natural history studies of asthma have also identified other biologic, genetic, and environmental risk factors for persistent asthma. These include male gender, parental asthma, and ETS exposure. Certain respiratory viral infections in early life have been associated with persistent wheezing problems in children, especially respiratory syncytial virus, parainfluenza virus, adenovirus, and metapneumovirus. It is not known if persistent airways abnormalities are primarily the result of virus-induced damage, or of vulnerable individuals revealing their airways' susceptibility to virus-induced airflow obstruction, or injury with aberrant repair. From the Tucson CRS, a statistical optimization of the major risk factors for persistent asthma was recently published [13]. In 2- to 3-year-old children with recurrent wheezing in the past year, risk factor assessment provided 97% specificity and 77% positive-predictive value for persistent asthma in later childhood (table 1) [13].

Asthma Pathogenesis

Briefly, the pathogenic hallmarks of asthma, in addition to atopic inflammation, include: (1) fibrotic changes that occur in the tissues surrounding the airway lumen; (2) smooth muscle hypertrophy/hyperplasia; (3) mucous gland hypertrophy/hyperplasia, and (4) damaged respiratory epithelium. Hypothetically, these 'remodeling' abnormalities might result from aberrant repair processes following airways injury and inflammation. Alternatively, sustained inflammation may not allow for optimal repair processes to heal airways injury.

An immune paradigm for asthma development asserts that pro-allergic type-2 T-helper (Th2) cells are: (1) differentiated to produce cytokines that direct allergic responses and inflammation (e.g., IL-4, IL-5, IL-9, IL-13), and (2) opposed by Th1 cells that produce counterregulatory cytokines that inhibit Th2 differentiation (i.e. IL-12, IFN-γ). Th2 cell-derived IL-4, IL-5, and granulocyte-macrophage colony-stimulating factor support eosinophil and mast cell development and differentiation in allergic inflammation. The development of allergen-specific IgE antibodies is an indication of allergen-specific Th2 lymphocytes that are guiding B lymphocytes to differentiate and produce allergen-specific IgE.

Recent studies on the influence of IFN-γ and IL-4 on airways tissues broaden the scope of potential influence of these Th1/Th2 cytokines on asthma pathogenesis and airway healing. Intriguingly, Th2 cytokines (IL-4, IL-13) induce fibroblasts to proliferate and produce collagen in vitro [20–22]. Therefore, IFN-γ's downregulatory influence on IL-4 production would be expected to provide a milieu for airway repair without fibrosis. IFN-γ also directly inhibits the proliferation of lung fibroblasts, their differentiation into myofibroblasts, and collagen synthesis [23–26]. The potential for IFN-γ immune responses to augment other aspects of airway repair after injury is less clear, but still considerable. Murine models of asthma have recently revealed that Th2-type cytokines (i.e. IL-4, IL-9, IL-13) are strongly linked to mucous gland hypertrophy, hyperplasia, and hypersecretion [27–31] and that IFN-γ-producing T cells are essential to the regulation and prevention of this pathologic process [27, 32]. Greater numbers of mast cells are typically found in asthmatic airways [33, 34], especially in the late-phase asthmatic response to allergen [35, 36]. While the in vivo mechanisms leading to mast cell accumulation in the airways are unclear, IFN-γ directly inhibits the proliferation of human mast cells in vitro [37, 38]. IFN-γ also protects the airways by inhibiting viral replication in epithelial cells through several well-defined cell molecular mechanisms. Since viral replication in airway epithelial cells is strongly linked to epithelial proinflammatory cytokine production and damage in response to viral infections, a vigorous IFN-γ response to viruses may protect the epithelium by containing virus-mediated damage and inflammation.

Infants with diminished Th1 responses may be more susceptible to developing asthma due to: (1) poor containment of viral infections with tropism for respiratory epithelium, and (2) aberrant repair responses to infection-induced airways injury. Bronchiolitic infants who continued to have persistent wheezing and airflow obstruction produce less IFN-γ [39]. This suggests that infants who produce less IFN-γ to ubiquitous allergens and to airway viral infections are susceptible to chronic allergic diseases and asthma because: (1) they are less able to impede the development of allergen-specific T cells and IgE, and (2) they are more likely to manifest persistent airways abnormalities following respiratory viral infections.

Asthma- and Allergy-Protective Influences

Some naturally occurring lifestyle differences may impart asthma- and/or allergy-protective effects.

Breast-Feeding

Numerous studies have investigated the potential of early breast-feeding as a protective influence against the development of allergy and asthma. Meta-analyses of prospective studies of exclusive breast-feeding for 4 or more months from birth have been associated with less AD and asthma (summary odds ratios of 0.68 and 0.70, respectively) [40, 41]. In the Tucson CRS, breast-feeding generally reduced the risk of recurrent wheezing up to 2 years of age (odds ratio 0.45); however, in a subgroup of atopic children who were exclusively breast-fed for 4 months by asthmatic mothers, the risk of persistent asthma between 6–13 years of age was increased (odds ratio 8.7) [42]. These conflicting findings have been further corroborated by recently published studies. A prospective birth cohort study of ~2,600 Australian children found that exclusive breast-feeding for longer than 4 months was associated with less MD-diagnosed asthma at age 6 years, regardless of maternal asthma history [43]. However, a longitudinal study of ~1,000 New Zealand children to age 26 years found that infants breast-fed for ≥4 weeks had a higher prevalence of allergen sensitization and asthma that was independent of maternal asthma or hay fever history [44].

The Hygiene Hypothesis

Numerous epidemiologic studies have found that a variety of microbial exposures are associated with a lower likelihood of allergen sensitization, allergic disease, and asthma. This has led to a 'hygiene' hypothesis which proposes that the reduction in childhood microbial exposures in modernized countries has led to the rise in allergy and asthma. To address this hypothesis, natural history studies and detailed population studies have begun to explore the causal relationships between infections and microbial exposures and the subsequent development of allergies and asthma.

Common Colds. In the Tucson CRS, children raised in larger families or in day care from an early age (i.e. <6 months old) were less likely to have asthma symptoms in later childhood [45]. Children placed in day care in the first 2 years of life experience more infections, generally common colds. In the German MAS, more runny nose colds in the first 3 years of life were associated with a lower likelihood of allergen sensitization, asthma, and BHR at 7 years of age [46]. A dose-dependent effect was observed, such that children who experienced ≥8 colds by age 3 years had an adjusted odds ratio of 0.16 for asthma at age 7 years.

Gastrointestinal Infections and Flora. In a large US cohort, serologic antibody evidence of previous hepatitis A, *Toxoplasma gondii*, and herpes simplex virus 1 infections (but not hepatitis B or C) were associated with less asthma, hay fever, and allergen sensitization, mirroring previous similar studies of Italian military cadets [47]. Recent evidence in a mouse model of asthma of a new asthma-susceptibility gene for T-cell membrane proteins that is homologous to the human hepatitis A receptor, implicates hepatitis A and its receptor as a gene–environment interaction in the development of asthma and allergy [48].

In two birth cohort studies of infants followed through the first year of life, allergic infants (i.e. with allergic disease or allergen sensitization) had less gastrointestinal tract colonization with enterococci and bifidobacteria, and more colonization with clostridia and *Staphylococcus aureus* [16, 17]. Such alterations in the gut flora of infants from dietary differences (i.e. breast vs. formula feeding, semi-sterile food, antibiotic use) may have an allergy-protective effect on the developing immune system.

Meanwhile, in rural Africa, parasitic infestations with schistosomiasis [18] or ascaris/hookworm [49] have been associated with less allergen sensitization and asthma. The paradox of less atopy in Th2-inducing parasite-infested children has excited interest in the potential disease-mitigating role of IL-10-producing cells [50]. For example, in a study of Gabonese schoolchildren in which schistosome infestation was common, peripheral blood cells from non-allergic patients demonstrated greater schistosome-specific IL-10 production in vitro [18]. Mechanistically, IL-10 can differentially regulate IL-4-stimulated B cells to produce IgG4 instead of IgE, block mast cell degranulation, and downregulate IL-4 and IL-5 production. 'Regulatory' IL-10-producing CD4+ CD25+ T lymphocytes, capable of abrogating autoimmunity and transplant rejection in some animal models, may also play a role in alleviating and preventing atopic inflammatory diseases.

Endotoxin. In infants with a history of recurrent wheezing, greater exposure levels of naturally occurring bacterial endotoxin were associated with a lack of early allergen sensitization, and correlated with increased proportions of Th1-type lymphocytes [51]. In a different German birth cohort study ('LISA'), early childhood endotoxin exposure was associated with a lower likelihood of AD in the first 6 months of life [52].

European investigators of several farm/non-farm communities have reported some important associations between greater endotoxin exposure and asthma and allergy outcomes in school-age children: (1) farm children are exposed to more endotoxin (as measured in house dust, barn dust, and mattress dust) [53, 54]; (2) greater endotoxin exposure is associated with less allergen sensitization, hay fever symptoms, and atopic asthma, in a dose-dependent manner [53]; (3) the blood cells of farmer's children expressed higher amounts of CD14 and Toll-like receptor 2, which are innate immune receptors for microbial compounds that include endotoxin [55]; (4) recollection of early life exposures to farm barns and unpasteurized milk had the strongest associations with low asthma and allergy prevalences [56], and (5) high levels of endotoxin exposure were associated with an increased prevalence of non-atopic wheeze [53].

Therefore, natural endotoxin exposure may promote early Th1-type immune development, thereby preventing the development of allergen sensitization, allergic airways conditions, and asthma.

Pet and Animal Exposure. Two recent longitudinal, prospective birth cohort studies in US metropolitan communities have found less asthma in children raised with pet dogs [57], and less allergen sensitization with increasing numbers of pet cats and/or dogs in early life [58]. Similarly, in farming and rural locales, a lower likelihood of allergy and asthma has been associated with animal contact or the keeping of domestic animals in the home [59]. Although the mechanism(s) for this potentially protective influence are unclear, one possibility is that greater bacterial endotoxin exposure occurs with animal contact and/or animal/pet-keeping in the home. Recent studies have reported that indoor pets are a major factor associated with higher indoor endotoxin levels in metropolitan homes [59].

Early Intervention and Prevention Studies

Early intervention studies to prevent the development of allergic disease and asthma have had limited success so far. Nevertheless, because of their prospective design, such studies can add valuable insights to the natural history of asthma, and the potential for disease prevention. Although difficult to accomplish in early childhood, investigators have attempted to modify some of the risk factors described above.

Lifestyle and Home Environment Interventions

Avoidance of Allergenic Foods in Infancy. Perhaps the best-studied 'environmental' intervention so far has been a 7-year follow-up of a randomized controlled intervention study performed at Kaiser Permanente in San Diego, Calif., in which the common allergenic foods (cow's milk, peanut, egg, fish) were eliminated from the diets of at-risk infants (i.e. with 1 parent with an atopic disorder and allergen sensitization), from the third trimester of pregnancy to 24 months of life [3]. Although this intervention significantly reduced the prevalence of food allergen sensitization, AD and urticarial rash in the first year of life [3], a lower prevalence of allergic disease did not persist at either age 4 or 7 years (table 1) [2]. Furthermore, no effect was observed on inhalant allergen sensitization or asthma.

Indoor Inhalant Allergen Elimination/Reduction. Addition of thorough dust mite reduction measures to food allergen avoidance for 1 year reduced the likelihood of AD from 1 to 4 years of age, and also reduced the incidence of allergen sensitization at age 4 years [60–62]. Decreased asthma was observed in the first year of life, but not at ages 2 or 4 years. Randomized controlled studies of the influence of indoor allergen reduction alone on the development of allergies and asthma have generally not shown any benefit. One challenge of such studies has been the difficulty of substantially lowering perennial allergen exposure through home mitigation, although recent improvements in this area (i.e. de-humidification) now make such studies feasible [63]. The recent controversial studies of the link between pets and animal exposure in early life and less subsequent allergen sensitization and asthma are discussed above.

Breast-Feeding. This has been best addressed in the prospective, controlled studies, discussed above.

Environmental Tobacco Smoke Elimination/Reduction. The acquisition of definitive proof of the preventive value of reducing or eliminating ETS exposure in infancy and childhood has been hindered by the difficulties in achieving long-term smoking cessation in randomized controlled studies. ETS exposure at all ages, from prenatal exposure of mothers to smoking in asthmatic adults, is associated with more wheezing problems and more severe disease. When considered with other health benefits of ETS exposure avoidance, this is strongly recommended.

Pharmacologic Interventions

Several studies represent first attempts to determine if conventional therapy for allergy and asthma may be able to alter the natural course of the allergic march, or to prevent persistent allergic disease and chronic asthma.

Antihistamines. In the Early Treatment of the Atopic Child (ETAC) study, the antihistamine cetirizine was administered for 18 months to young children at high risk for asthma because of a history of AD and/or a family history of asthma. Of subjects receiving cetirizine, only young children with early allergen sensitization to mites or grass pollen were less likely to develop asthma symptoms during the treatment period [64]. Eighteen months after cetirizine discontinuation, a slightly lower incidence of asthma symptoms continued for the cetirizine-treated, grass-allergic subjects only [65].

Conventional 'Controller' Pharmacotherapy for Asthma. In the CAMP study, 5- to 12-year-old children were treated with either daily inhaled corticosteroid (budesonide), daily inhaled nonsteroidal anti-inflammatory medication (nedocromil), or placebo for more than 4 years [66]. Study medication was then discontinued. The budesonide-treated subjects demonstrated significant improvement in most of the clinical outcomes and lung function measures of asthma, including BHR to methacholine. After discontinuation of budesonide; however, the mean BHR of the budesonide-treated group regressed to that of the placebo group. Nedocromil-treated subjects did not improve BHR when compared with placebo. This suggests that, although long-term administration of inhaled corticosteroids in school-age asthmatic children significantly improves asthma severity, it might not increase the likelihood of asthma remission in later childhood or adulthood. To qualify this observation, the outcome of asthma remission was not the intent of the CAMP study and, therefore, forthcoming studies designed to determine the influence of asthma pharmacotherapy on asthma persistence or remittance in childhood will be valuable.

Allergen-Specific Immunotherapy (AIT). AIT has been studied to determine if it can reduce the likelihood of asthma development in children with AR. A recently published randomized controlled study found that a 3-year AIT course administered to children with birch and/or grass pollen AR reduced the likelihood of asthma symptom development, and was associated with less BHR to methacholine [67]. Moreover, the clinical benefit and immune-modifying effects of AIT can persist for years after its administration. For example, completion of a 3-year AIT course can induce sustained clinical improvement in AR and asthma for at least 3 additional years [68]. AIT has also been associated with a lack of progression of inhalant allergen sensitization in asthmatic children. This prevention of new sensitization to inhalant allergens has persisted for several years after AIT discontinuation [69, 70]. These studies suggest that AIT may alter the allergic march of inhalant allergen sensitization and asthma, but the difficulties and risks of conventional AIT in children warrants careful consideration.

BCG and Mycobacterium vaccae. Derived from *Mycobacterium bovis*, BCG has been used for many years as a childhood vaccination for tuberculosis. A study of Japanese schoolchildren (who all received up to 3 BCG immunizations in childhood) revealed that those who had a positive tuberculin response were less likely to develop atopy, allergic disease, or asthma [71]. BCG 'responders' had more IFN-γ and less Th2-type cytokines in their serum. There is debate over the meaning of this provocative finding. Was the lower prevalence of atopy and asthma in BCG responders due to: (1) tuberculosis, leading to a larger tuberculin response and the association with less atopy and asthma; (2) the BCG vaccine itself, or (3) the tuberculin skin test response to vaccine serving to identify Th1-biased children less likely to develop allergy and asthma? Other studies have not consistently confirmed this original observation [72]. However, in children in Guinea-Bissau, West Africa, BCG vaccination, especially in the first week of life, was associated with less allergen sensitization [73]. BCG vaccination induces memory Th1-type immune response in newborns [74], and also improves antibody and cellular responses to other early childhood immunizations (i.e. hepatitis B, oral polio vaccine) [75]. In a randomized controlled trial of BCG re-administration to asthmatic adults, BCG treatment was followed by a reduction in asthma medication use and significant lung function improvement [76].

M. vaccae has been developed as an immune modulator similar to BCG, but without antigenic cross-reactivity to *M. tuberculosis*. In a randomized, controlled trial, one intradermal injection of killed *M. vaccae* improved AD in children for 3 months [77]. Interestingly, clinical trials with *M. vaccae* for psoriasis have also demonstrated sustained improvement similar to that seen for AD. Since psoriasis is considered to be a Th1-mediated disease, this suggests that *M. vaccae* primarily works through neither Th1 nor Th2 immune mechanisms (perhaps through regulatory T cells). Preliminary clinical studies with *M. vaccae* have also been published for cancer therapy (i.e. inoperable lung cancer, mesothelioma), multiple sclerosis therapy, and for pulmonary tuberculosis in several clinical settings: new-onset cases, multidrug-resistant cases, and for prevention of HIV-associated tuberculosis.

Lactobacillus. Some studies suggest that lactobacillus supplementation may also prevent allergies and asthma by promoting Th1-type and/or regulatory T lymphocyte (i.e. anti-inflammatory) immune development [78]. A randomized controlled trial of daily lactobacillus given to at-risk infants (i.e. of mothers with at least 1 first-degree relative or partner with AD, AR, or asthma) for the first 6 months of life was recently reported [78]. At age 2 years, a lower AD incidence was observed in the treated group. Interestingly, in breast-feeding mothers who received lactobacillus supplementation, their breast milk had higher concentrations of the anti-inflammatory cytokine TGF-β, and their infants had a reduced relative risk of AD of 0.32 [79]. This observation did not extend, however, to other allergic conditions or measures of allergen sensitization at this young age. Mechanistically, lactobacillus ingestion has been associated with increased peripheral blood IL-10 production and serum IL-10 levels. Oral lactobacillus supplementation is currently US FDA-approved for the prevention of antibiotic-associated diarrhea in children and adults. Randomized controlled trials with oral lactobacillus have also demonstrated preventive efficacy for necrotizing enterocolitis in the neonatal intensive care unit, nosocomial diarrhea in hospitalized young children, and therapeutic efficacy for irritable bowel syndrome and acute infectious diarrhea in infants and children. Other published clinical studies with lactobacillus suggest its therapeutic potential in inflammatory bowel diseases (e.g. Crohn's disease) and to reduce significant respiratory infection manifestations in young children.

Conclusions

Allergic diseases and asthma commonly develop in the early childhood years. Current paradigms of immune development and lung growth shape our understanding of disease pathogenesis. The cumulative evidence does not establish whether asthma in adulthood can be prevented through interventions in childhood. A rich body of data provides substantive paradigms upon which interventions for asthma prevention can be targeted. Current experience also provides many tools and the know-how to rigorously study and prove the effectiveness and determine the safety of preventive interventions for asthma.

References

1 Wahn U: Review Series VI: The immunology of fetuses and infants. What drives the allergic march? Allergy 2000;55:591–599.
2 Zeiger RS, Heller S: The development and prediction of atopy in high-risk children: Follow-up at age seven years in a prospective randomized study of combined maternal and infant food allergen avoidance. J Allergy Clin Immunol 1995;95:1179–1190.
3 Zeiger RS, Heller S, Mellon MH, et al: Effect of combined maternal and infant food-allergen avoidance on development of atopy in early infancy: A randomized study. J Allergy Clin Immunol 1989;84:72–89.
4 Kulig M, Bergmann R, Klettke U, et al: Natural course of sensitization to food and inhalant allergens during the first 6 years of life. J Allergy Clin Immunol 1999;103:1173–1179.
5 Rhodes HL, Thomas P, Sporik R, et al: A birth cohort study of subjects at risk of atopy. Am J Respir Crit Care Med 2002;165:176–180.
6 Yunginger JW, Reed CE, O'Connell, et al: A community-based study of the epidemiology of asthma. Incidence rates, 1964–1983. Am Rev Respir Dis 1992;146:888–894.
7 Martinez FD, Wright AL, Taussig LM, et al: Asthma and wheezing in the first six years of life. N Engl J Med 1995;332:133–138.
8 Oswald H, Phelan PD, Lanigan A, et al: Outcome of childhood asthma in mid-adult life. BMJ 1994;309:95–96.
9 Godden DJ, Ross S, Abdalla M, et al: Outcome of wheeze in childhood. Am J Respir Crit Care Med 1994;149:106–112.
10 Jenkins MA, Hopper JL, Bowes G, et al: Factors in childhood as predictors of asthma in adult life. BMJ 1994;309:90–93.

11 Strachan DP, Butland BK, Anderson HR: Incidence and prognosis of asthma and wheezing illness from early childhood to age 33 in a national British cohort. BMJ 1996;312:1195–1199.
12 Oswald H, Phelan PD, Lanigan A, et al: Childhood asthma and lung function in mid-adult life. Pediatr Pulmonol 1997;23:14–20.
13 Castro-Rodriguez JA, Holberg CJ, Wright AL, Martinez FD: A clinical index to define risk of asthma in young children with recurrent wheezing. Am J Respir Crit Care Med 2000;162: 1403–1406.
14 Kulig M, Bergmann R, Tacke U, et al: Long-lasting sensitization to food during the first two years precedes allergic airway disease. The MAS Study Group, Germany. Pediatr Allergy Immunol 1998;9:61–67.
15 Lau S, Illi S, Sommerfeld C, et al: Early exposure to house-dust mite and cat allergens and development of childhood asthma: A cohort study. Multicentre Allergy Study Group. Lancet 2000;356:1392–1397.
16 Bjorksten B, Sepp E, Julge K, et al: Allergy development and the intestinal microflora during the first year of life. J Allergy Clin Immunol 2001;108:516–520.
17 Kalliomaki M, Kirjavainen P, Eerola E, et al: Distinct patterns of neonatal gut microflora in infants in whom atopy was and was not developing. J Allergy Clin Immunol 2001;107:129–134.
18 van den Biggelaar AH, van Ree R, Rodrigues LC, et al: Decreased atopy in children infected with *Schistosoma haematobium*: A role for parasite-induced interleukin-10. Lancet 2000; 356:1723–1727.
19 Patrizi A, Guerrini V, Ricci G, et al: The natural history of sensitizations to food and aeroallergens in atopic dermatitis: A 4-year follow-up. Pediatr Dermatol 2000;17:261–265.
20 Postlethwaite AE, Holness MA, Katai H, Raghow R: Human fibroblasts synthesize elevated levels of extracellular matrix proteins in response to interleukin 4. J Clin Invest 1992;90: 1479–1485.
21 Gillery P, Fertin C, Nicolas JF, et al: Interleukin-4 stimulates collagen gene expression in human fibroblast monolayer cultures. Potential role in fibrosis. FEBS Lett 1992;302:231–234.
22 Sempowski GD, Beckmann MP, Derdak S, Phipps RP: Subsets of murine lung fibroblasts express membrane-bound and soluble IL-4 receptors. Role of IL-4 in enhancing fibroblast proliferation and collagen synthesis. J Immunol 1994;152:3606–3614.
23 Diaz A, Jimenez SA: Interferon-gamma regulates collagen and fibronectin gene expression by transcriptional and post-transcriptional mechanisms. Int J Biochem Cell Biol 1997;29: 251–260.
24 Duncan MR, Berman B: Gamma interferon is the lymphokine and beta interferon the monokine responsible for inhibition of fibroblast collagen production and late but not early fibroblast proliferation. J Exp Med 1985;162:516–527.
25 Goldring MD, Sandell LJ, Stephenson ML, Krane SM: Immune interferon suppresses levels of procollagen mRNA and type II collagen synthesis in cultured human articular and costal chondrocytes. J Biol Chem 1986;261:9049–9055.
26 Jimenez SA, Freundlich B, Rosenbloom J: Selective inhibition of human diploid fibroblast collagen synthesis by interferons. J Clin Invest 1984;74:1112–1116.
27 Cohn L, Homer RJ, Niu N, Bottomly K: T helper 1 cells and interferon gamma regulate allergic airway inflammation and mucus production. J Exp Med 1999;190:1309–1318.
28 Cohn L, Homer RJ, MacLeod H, et al: Th2-induced airway mucus production is dependent on IL-4R alpha, but not on eosinophils. J Immunol 1999;162:6178–6183.
29 Longphre M, Li D, Gallup M, et al: Allergen-induced IL-9 directly stimulates mucin transcription in respiratory epithelial cells. J Clin Invest 1999;104:1375–1382.
30 Louahed J, Toda M, Jen J, et al: Interleukin-9 upregulates mucus expression in the airways. Am J Respir Cell Mol Biol 2000;22:637–639.
31 Zhu Z, Homer RJ, Wang Z, et al: Pulmonary expression of interleukin-13 causes inflammation, mucus hypersecretion, subepithelial fibrosis, physiologic abnormalities, and eotaxin production. J Clin Invest 1999;103:779–788.
32 Schmitt E, Germann T, Goedert S, et al: IL-9 production of naive CD4+T cells depends on IL-2, is synergistically enhanced by a combination of TGF-beta and IL-4, and is inhibited by IFN-gamma. J Immunol 1994;153:3989–3996.
33 Ollerenshaw SL, Woolcock AJ: Characteristics of the inflammation in biopsies from large airways of subjects with asthma and subjects with chronic airflow limitation. Am Rev Respir Dis 1992;145:922–927.

34 Laitinen LA, Laitinen A, Haahtela T: Airway mucosal inflammation even in patients with newly diagnosed asthma. Am Rev Respir Dis 1993;147:697–704.
35 Crimi E, Chiaramondia M, Milanese M, et al: Increased numbers of mast cells in bronchial mucosa after the late-phase asthmatic response to allergen. Am Rev Respir Dis 1991;144: 1282–1286.
36 Kassel O, de Blay F, Duvernelle C, et al: Local increase in the number of mast cells and expression of nerve growth factor in the bronchus of asthmatic patients after repeated inhalation of allergen at low-dose. Clin Exp Allergy 2001;31:1432–1440.
37 Kirshenbaum AS, Worobec AS, Davis TA, et al: Inhibition of human mast cell growth and differentiation by interferon gamma-1b. Exp Hematol 1998;26:245–251.
38 Ochi H, Hirani WM, Yuan Q, et al: T helper cell type 2 cytokine-mediated comitogenic responses and CCR3 expression during differentiation of human mast cells in vitro. J Exp Med 1999;190:267–280.
39 Renzi PM, Turgeon JP, Marcotte JE, et al: Reduced interferon-γ production in infants with bronchiolitis and asthma. Am J Respir Crit Care Med 1999;159:1417–1422.
40 Gdalevich M, Mimouni D, David M, Mimouni M: Breast-feeding and the onset of atopic dermatitis in childhood: A systematic review and meta-analysis of prospective studies. J Am Acad Dermatol 2001;45:520–527.
41 Gdalevich M, Mimouni D, Mimouni M: Breast-feeding and the risk of bronchial asthma in childhood: A systematic review with meta-analysis of prospective studies. J Pediatr 2001;139: 261–266.
42 Wright AL, Holberg CJ, Taussig LM, Martinez FD: Factors influencing the relation of infant feeding to asthma and recurrent wheeze in childhood. Thorax 2001;56:192–197.
43 Oddy WH, Peat JK, de Klerk NH: Maternal asthma, infant feeding, and the risk of asthma in childhood. J Allergy Clin Immunol 2002;110:65–67.
44 Sears MR, Greene JM, Willan AR, et al: Long-term relation between breastfeeding and development of atopy and asthma in children and young adults: A longitudinal study. Lancet 2002;360:887–888.
45 Ball TM, Castro-Rodriguez JA, Griffith KA, et al: Siblings, day-care attendance, and the risk of asthma and wheezing during childhood. N Engl J Med 2000;343:538–543.
46 Illi S, von Mutius E, Lau S, et al: Early childhood infectious diseases and the development of asthma up to school age: A birth cohort study. BMJ 2001;322:390–395.
47 Matricardi PM, Rosmini F, Panetta V, et al: Hay fever and asthma in relation to markers of infection in the United States. J Allergy Clin Immunol 2002;110:381–387.
48 McIntire JJ, Umetsu SE, Akbari O, et al: Identification of Tapr (an airway hyperreactivity regulatory locus) and the linked Tim gene family. Nat Immunol 2001;2:1095–1096.
49 Scrivener S, Yemaneberhan H, Zebenigus M, et al: Independent effects of intestinal parasite infection and domestic allergen exposure on risk of wheeze in Ethiopia: A nested case-control study. Lancet 2001;358:1493–1499.
50 Yazdanbakhsh M, Kremsner PG, van Ree R: Allergy, parasites, and the hygiene hypothesis. Science 2002;296:490–494.
51 Gereda JE, Leung DYM, Thatayatikom A, et al: Relation between house-dust endotoxin exposure, type 1 T-cell development, and allergen sensitization in infants at high risk of asthma. Lancet 2000;355:1680–1683.
52 Gehring U, Bolte G, Borte M, et al: Exposure to endotoxin decreases the risk of atopic eczema in infancy: A cohort study. J Allergy Clin Immunol 2001;108:847–854.
53 Braun-Fahrlander C, Riedler J, Herz U, et al: Environmental exposure to endotoxin and its relation to asthma in school-age children. N Engl J Med 2002;347:869–877.
54 Gereda JE, Leung DYM, Liu AH: House-dust endotoxin is higher in rural homes in developing countries and farm homes, where asthma is less prevalent. JAMA 2000;284:1652–1653.
55 Lauener RP, Birchler T, Adamski J, et al: Expression of CD14 and Toll-like receptor 2 in farmers' and non-farmers' children. Lancet 2002;360:465–466.
56 Riedler J, Braun-Fahrlander C, Eder W, et al: Exposure to farming in early life and development of asthma and allergy: A cross-sectional survey. Lancet 2001;358:1129–1133.
57 Remes ST, Castro-Rodriguez JA, Holberg CJ, et al: Dog exposure in infancy decreases the subsequent risk of frequent wheeze but not of atopy. J Allergy Clin Immunol 2001;108:509–515.
58 Ownby DR, Johnson CC, Peterson EL: Exposure to dogs and cats in the first year of life and risk of allergic sensitization at 6 to 7 years of age. JAMA 2002;288:963–972.

59 Liu AH: Endotoxin exposure in allergy and asthma: Reconciling a paradox. J Allergy Clin Immunol 2002;109:379–392.

60 Arshad SH, Matthews S, Gant C, Hide DW: Effect of allergen avoidance on development of allergic disorders in infancy. Lancet 1992;339:1493–1497.

61 Hide DW, Matthews S, Matthews L, et al: Effect of allergen avoidance in infancy on allergic manifestations at age two years. J Allergy Clin Immunol 1994;93:842–846.

62 Hide DW, Matthews S, Tariq S, Arshad SH: Allergen avoidance in infancy and allergy at 4 years of age. Allergy 1996;51:89–93.

63 Arlian LG, Neal JS, Morgan MS, et al: Reducing relative humidity is a practical way to control dust mites and their allergens in homes in temperate climates. J Allergy Clin Immunol 2001;107:99–104.

64 ETAC Study Group: Allergic factors associated with the development of asthma and the influence of cetirizine in a double-blind, randomized, placebo-controlled trial: First results of ETAC. Early treatment of the atopic child. Pediatr Allergy Immunol 1998;9:116–124.

65 Warner JO: A double-blinded, randomized, placebo-controlled trial of cetirizine in preventing the onset of asthma in children with atopic dermatitis: 18 months' treatment and 18 months' posttreatment follow-up. J Allergy Clin Immunol 2001;108:929–937.

66 The Childhood Asthma Management Program Research Group: Long-term effects of budesonide or nedocromil in children with asthma. N Engl J Med 2000;343:1054–1063.

67 Moller C, Dreborg S, Ferdousi HA, et al: Pollen immunotherapy reduces the development of asthma in children with seasonal rhinoconjunctivitis (the PAT-study). J Allergy Clin Immunol 2002;109:251–256.

68 Durham SR, Walker SM, Varga EM, et al: Long-term clinical efficacy of grass-pollen immunotherapy. N Engl J Med 1999;341:468–475.

69 Purello-D' Ambrosio F, Gangemi S, et al: Prevention of new sensitizations in monosensitized subjects submitted to specific immunotherapy or not. A retrospective study. Clin Exp Allergy 2001;31:1295–1302.

70 Des Roches A, Paradis L, Menardo JL, et al: Immunotherapy with a standardized *Dermatophagoides pteronyssinus* extract. VI. Specific immunotherapy prevents the onset of new sensitizations in children. J Allergy Clin Immunol 1997;99:450–453.

71 Shirakawa T, Enomoto T, Shimazu S, Hopkin JM: The inverse association between tuberculin responses and atopic disorder. Science 1997;275:77–79.

72 Alm JS, Lilja G, Pershagen G, Scheynius A: Early BCG vaccination and development of atopy. Lancet 1997;350:400–403.

73 Aaby P, Shaheen SO, Heyes CB, et al: Early BCG vaccination and reduction in atopy in Guinea-Bissau. Clin Exp Allergy 2000;30:644–650.

74 Marchant A, Goetghebuer T, Ota MO, et al: Newborns develop a Th1-type immune response to *Mycobacterium bovis* bacillus Calmette-Guérin vaccination. J Immunol 1999;163:2249–2255.

75 Ota MO, Vekemans J, Schlegel-Haueter SE, et al: Influence of *Mycobacterium bovis* bacillus Calmette-Guérin on antibody and cytokine responses to human neonatal vaccination. J Immunol 2002;168:919–925.

76 Choi IS, Koh YI: Therapeutic effects of BCG vaccination in adult asthmatic patients: A randomized, controlled trial. Ann Allergy Asthma Immunol 2002;88:584–591.

77 Arkwright PD, David TJ: Intradermal administration of a killed *Mycobacterium vaccae* suspension (SRL 172) is associated with improvement in atopic dermatitis in children with moderate-to-severe disease. J Allergy Clin Immunol 2001;107:531–534.

78 Kalliomaki M, Salminen S, Arvilommi H, et al: Probiotics in primary prevention of atopic disease: A randomized placebo-controlled trial. Lancet 2001;357:1076–1079.

79 Rautava S, Kalliomaki M, Isolauri E: Probiotics during pregnancy and breast-feeding might confer immunomodulatory protection against atopic disease in the infant. J Allergy Clin Immunol 2002;109:119–121.

Discussion

As the author of this paper was unable to join the workshop, the presentation and the discussion were conducted by R. Sorensen, USA.

Dr. Hill: I am from the Royal Children's Hospital in Melbourne that was the home of the Melbourne asthma study in which the oldest reported subject now has a 42-year follow-up. I want to make a comment regarding the data you quoted from Martinez, the data I presented on Monday, and also severe egg asthma in adulthood. Basically, the children are 14 years old when we do the lung function test and they have been followed since the age of 7. In my first report in the *British Medical Journal*, the interesting thing was that at that stage the children with severe problems had severe atopic dermatitis. They were recalled, and when we looked at the skin test reactivity at that stage the allergen skin-testing extracts were very poorly characterized. But the thing that came through, even though a very crude method of assigning reactivity was used, was that the rate of sensitization was much higher and those children had severe disease at that stage and maintained that phenomenon right through into adulthood. So frequently positive sensitization to egg was evident at the 7-year follow-up. It is a very unusual finding. Most children with egg sensitization in infancy lose their sensitization. How is it relevant to what I was talking about? Remember I said that at 12 months of age in our study there are 600 babies, the infants who had severe atopic dermatitis had IgE food allergy. If you look at those children at the age of 5, the risk of asthma was in fact increased 7-fold compared to the atopic group who had no evidence of eczema or sensitization to food. So clearly we are seeing the potentially severe asthmatic. The final point was that when we looked at the sensitization inhalants at 12 months of age, already the children who had severe atopic dermatitis were sensitized particularly to house dust mite and cat dander. Now by contrast, I think Martinez started his skin testing at the age of 3 years and in fact the risk for asthma, he assigned a minor scoring for the presence of food sensitization at 3, and of course by 3 years of age a lot of food sensitization would have come into remission.

Dr. Sorensen: Thank you very much for that comment. Indeed Dr. Martinez gets in trouble regularly when he presents to immunologists because they criticize his choice of the age at which he did the skin testing and also his choice of allergens. I don't think he included mites, he concentrated on molds, so he may have missed sensitization to other allergens. For your reassurance I think that Dr. Liu in his presentation quotes your studies too; obviously it should be used to modify the criteria that were presented here because I think that we should refine the tools for early detection of infants at risk.

Dr. Guesry: The title of the presentation is 'Can we prevent the allergic child from becoming a chronic asthmatic adult'. I would like to share with you the results of an epidemiological survey, conducted in Switzerland, as part of a European survey on 14-year-old children during 3 periods over the last 15 years. You can see that, in Switzerland for the first time in the last 30 years, there has been a decrease in the frequency of asthma and not by a small margin: a reduction of 50% in the prevalence of asthma, and a stabilization of the other manifestations of allergy. This is true for all countries in Europe that participated in the study, which means Germany, France, Belgium and Italy, except the UK. The author of this report [1] wonders why there was no such improvement in the UK. My interpretation, which may not be right, is that 17 years ago in Germany, France, Switzerland and Belgium the hypoallergenic infant formula was launched, but not in the UK.

Dr. R. Bergmann: It would be helpful to show what primary prevention would mean. In our study we were looking at what it would look like if we could project our results on atopic diseases in the first 2 years onto the population. This was the distribution of risks, the atopic history in parents, therefore in Germany 5% of all infants had both parents with some kind of allergic disease, and 31% just 1 parent, and 64% neither. When we looked at the association, of course there was a highly significant association of allergy in the first 2 years compared to the parents' allergy. But if you count you find that in numbers most children come from this part. So if we are aiming at primary prevention we should address the whole population instead of children at risk.

Dr. Lack: Just relating to that comment and to the previous comment by Dr. Hill. Yes, family histories aren't good enough, but I do agree that the presence of eczema and sensitization to foods early on, particularly egg, is a very good way of identifying the children who will go onto develop asthma. So we don't need necessarily to invoke a family history. Similarly in line with what Dr. Hill was suggesting, we just published a study on children with severe life-threatening asthma, a case-control study, who have all been ventilated for their asthma, compared to mild asthmatic controls [2]. The strongest risk factor that emerged was actually the presence of persistent food allergy so that more than 50% of our severe life-threatening asthmatics were either egg or peanut allergic. So food allergies may be both a good early predictor of the tendency to develop asthma and also a marker of asthma severity.

Dr. Lack: We all know about the progression of allergic symptoms which we call the allergic march, and which we spoke of a few days ago. What we don't know is at the secondary prevention level whether preventing or treating eczema well will decrease the follow-on in terms of food allergies and whether treating food allergies well will prevent allergic rhinitis. We don't know whether treating allergic rhinitis well will actually prevent the subsequent development of asthma. There are some data showing that treating allergic rhinitis may improve asthma when they coexist. If we are going to target an intervention we have got to know what the links are between the individual steps before we can just do something very early on in the first 6 months of life and expect to see an outcome 7 years down the line in terms of asthma.

Dr. K. Bergmann: Renate, my wife, has just completed a longitudinal control study on the efficacy of anticipatory guidance. She enrolled newborn infants, and as far as I know she has looked at eczema and obesity. Renate, would you like to comment on that?

Dr. R. Bergmann: We observed the children for 2 years so we can't say very much about obesity, but what we could see is that infants in the intervention group program were more often breast-fed and had late introduction of solid foods. Then we tried to get the parents to stop smoking. We had a smoking intervention study. At 2 years of age the children had a normal skin fold thickness in the intervention group. It is a small group, only 200 children without a special risk. There was less eczema.

Dr. Sorensen: I think that the whole issue of obesity is very important because many of our children are obese, if you ask them how they are doing, they say: I am fine, I don't have asthma, I don't wheeze, I don't do anything. Then you ask them if they participate in any sport and the answer is no. Then you do a pulmonary function test and they have deeply abnormal pulmonary function. They have adapted to less oxygen by being very sedentary and being sedentary increases the problem of obesity. So to me it is essential that any prospective program needs to include the early recognition and management of the children who are going into obesity too. As we understand it today obesity is an inflammatory disease, and it is a contributing factor to the severity of asthma.

References

1 Grize L, Gassner M, Heiniger U, et al: No further increase in asthma, hayfever and atopic sensitisation rates in Swiss adolescents (abstract). European Respiratory Society Congress, Stockholm, 2002.

2 Roberts G, Patel N, Levi-Schaffer F, et al: Food allergy as a risk factor for life-threatening asthma in childhood: A case controlled study. J Allergy Clin Immunol 2003;112:168–174.

Isolauri E, Walker WA (eds): Allergic Diseases and the Environment.
Nestlé Nutrition Workshop Series Pediatric Program, Vol. 53, pp. 285–300,
Nestec Ltd.; Vevey/S. Karger AG, Basel, © 2004.

The German Infant Nutritional Intervention Study[1] (GINI): A Model for Allergy Prevention

Andrea von Berg

Department of Pediatrics, Marien Hospital Wesel, Wesel, Germany

Introduction

It is widely accepted that the early contact of the neonatal immune system with food antigens plays an important role in the complex process of allergy development, especially in children with an atopic genotype. The immune response of fetuses/newborns with an atopic genotype is influenced by the T-helper type-2 (Th2) milieu of pregnancy from the normal T-helper type-1 (Th1) response towards a Th2 response with the production of IgE [1, 2].

The mechanism is probably a reduced downregulation of IgE production by B cells within the lymphoid follicles of the gastrointestinal tract and reduced facilitation of switch from a Th2 to a Th1 response in the gut.

---

[1] The GINI study group is a cooperation of one epidemiological and three clinical centers in Germany, represented by:

Andrea von Berg, MD (Department of Pediatrics, Marien Hospital Wesel), Sibylle Koletzko, MD (Department of Pediatrics, Ludwig Maximilian University, Munich), Armin Grübl, MD (Department of Pediatrics, Technical University of Munich), Birgit Filipiak-Pittroff, MSc (GSF-National Research Center for Environment and Health, Institute of Epidemiology, Neuherberg), H.-Erich Wichmann, PhD, MD (GSF_National Research Center for Environment and Health, Institute of Epidemiology, Neuherberg), Carl Peter Bauer, MD (Department of Pediatrics, Technical University of Munich), Dietrich Reinhardt, MD (Department of Pediatrics, Ludwig Maximilian University, Munich), and Dietrich Berdel, MD (Department of Pediatrics, Marien Hospital Wesel).

The study was supported by the Federal Ministry for Education, Science, Research and Technology, grant No.01 EE 9401–4.

The companies Nestlé, Hipp, Milupa, Numico, and Mead Johnson provided the study formula and SHS provided the formula for elimination diet. The Child Health Foundation, Munich, Germany, gave financial support.

In contrast, the immunological development of a nonatopic child is a Th1-skewed immune response which goes along with the production of IgG antibodies and clinical tolerance.

The aim of reduced antigen exposure by feeding an elimination diet, such as hydrolysates, in the postnatal period to children at risk of atopy is therefore to induce a normal, Th1/Th2-balanced immune response, and thereby to reduce IgE production and allergic reactions. However, it remains unclear to what extend exposure to antigens should be reduced in order to avoid allergic reactions and at the same time actively induce oral tolerance.

The current feeding recommendations for infants with a hereditary risk of allergy include: breast milk for 4–6 months; in the case of insufficient breast milk, hypoallergenic infant formula as the only substitute or supplement for at least 4 months, and the introduction of solid foods not before 4–6 months of age [3]. Although several studies have been performed to investigate the allergy-preventive effect of partially hydrolyzed formula (pHF) [4, 5] and extensively hydrolyzed formula (eHF) [6, 7], no definite conclusions with regard to the preferability of one or the other type of hypoallergenic formula could be drawn [8]. Most of the studies are not comparable, even though they were performed according to rather strict quality criteria, because of differences in inclusion criteria, co-interventions, control of compliance and confounders, and most important, because of differences in the definition of endpoints [8]. Although two studies that directly compared the effect of pHF and eHF observed a trend towards a superior effect of eHF [9, 10], the ESPGHAN and ESPAACI recommended more studies to help answer unresolved questions as to the effectiveness of allergy prevention by nutritional intervention with hydrolysates of different degrees of antigenicity in newborns and infants at high risk of atopy [3].

The German Infant Nutritional Intervention Program (GINI) was initiated to prospectively compare, in a randomized and double-blind design, the allergy-preventive effect of three differently hydrolyzed infant formulas with a conventional cow's milk-based formula (CMF) in a cohort of infants at high risk of atopy [11].

Methods

The design of the study has recently been described in detail [11]. Briefly, 2,252 infants were recruited for the study between September 1995 and June 1998 in obstetric units throughout two areas in Germany (Wesel, North Rhine Westphalia, and Munich, Bavaria). Only healthy newborns with at least 1 family member (mother, father, or biological sibling) with an allergic disease according to a questionnaire, administered to the parents, containing 18 items on past or present asthma, allergic rhinitis, atopic dermatitis (AD), allergic urticaria or food allergy (symptoms, doctor diagnosed or relevant treatment), were enrolled when written informed consent was obtained from both parents. Exclusion criteria were: severe acquired or congenital diseases; gestational age <37 weeks; birth weight $<2{,}500$ g; age >14 days; intake of any CMF prior to inclusion, or inability of the parents to comply with the study protocol. The study protocol was approved by the ethic committees of each of the study centers.

At inclusion infants were randomized by a computer-generated list to one of the study formulas, stratified by an independent person for single (1 parent and/or sibling) or double (biparental only) heredity of atopy and study region. Blinding of parents and the study team was guaranteed by using identically labeled tins for the study formula, coded with 4 different letters for each of the 4 formulas.

The following 3 hydrolyzed formulas, differing in terms of the nitrogen source and the molecular weight profile, were used for intervention and compared with standard CMF (Nutrilon premium, Nutricia/Numico, Zoetermeer Netherlands): (1) a partially hydrolyzed whey formula (pHF-W: Beba HA, Nestlé, Vevey, Switzerland); (2) an extensively hydrolyzed whey formula (eHF-W: Hipp HA/, Hipp, Pfaffenhofen, Germany, until 1999 on the German market and identical to Nutrilon Pepti, Nutricia/ Numico, Zoetermeer Netherlands), and (3) an extensively hydrolyzed, lactose-free casein formula (eHF-C: Nutramigen, Mead Johnson, Diezenbach, Germany).

At inclusion all mothers received the same nutritional recommendations on feeding the child during the first year of life. They were encouraged to exclusively breastfeed for at least 4 months (strict intervention period), preferably 6 months. No dietary restrictions for the lactating mother were recommended. The timing of weaning and introduction of study formula was left exclusively to the mother. The randomized study formulas were applied only if exclusive breast-feeding for the first 6 months was not feasible. In addition, mothers were advised to withhold solid food during the strict intervention period. Thereafter no more than one new food per week should be added, but milk and dairy products, hen's egg, soy products, fish, nuts, tomatoes and citrus fruits should be avoided during the first year.

From weekly diaries during the first 6 months information was gathered on the kind of milk the infant was fed (breast milk, study formula, brand of non-study formula if fed), time of first introduction of study formula, kind of new solid foods, and any health problems. These diaries together with structured interviews served to assess parental compliance with the feeding recommendations [12]. Children were excluded from the protocol analysis, if the diaries during the intervention period showed noncompliance with the milk-feeding recommendations or if one of the weekly diaries was missing.

Follow-up visits with structured interviews and physical examination in the clinical centers by a study physician were scheduled at 1, 4, 8 and 12 months of age, and symptoms related to AD, allergic urticaria and food allergy with manifestations in the gastrointestinal tract (FA-GIT) were recorded. Information on sociodemographic factors, family and living conditions, and smoking habits were documented. Unscheduled visits were made when symptoms suggestive of allergy appeared.

Definition of Endpoints

Allergic manifestation (AM) was defined when at least one of the following allergic diseases were documented during the first 12 months: AD, allergic urticaria or FA-GIT.

AD was defined using a computer algorithm based on the following modified criteria [13]: (1) typical morphology and distribution of skin lesions (face, neck and scalp, flexural folds, hands and extensor sides of the extremities, assessed by the study physician); (2) pruritus (signs of scratching) or treatment with steroids/oral antihistamines, and (3) duration of at least 14 days without treatment and/or chronically relapsing. The final morphologic diagnosis of AD was based on skin examination by a second physician specially trained in pediatric allergology, who was not aware of the infant's feeding history. Case definition required all three criteria. Only definite diagnoses were included as cases in the statistical analysis.

The severity of AD was rated using the SCORAD method [14].

Allergic urticaria was diagnosed if at least two episodes of itching eruptions or swelling with typical appearance, observed by the parents or a physician, were caused by the same allergen. In case of a single episode, immunological evidence (skin-prick test with the suspected undiluted native allergen, wheal size ≥3 mm, or allergen-specific IgE ≥0.35 KU/l, CAP, Pharmacia) or a positive provocation with the suspected allergen was needed for definite diagnosis.

For the diagnosis of FA-GIT we considered both IgE- and non-IgE-mediated immunological reactions [15]. The causal relation of the suspected formula or food with symptoms such as blood-stained stools, diarrhea, vomiting or frequent regurgitation, colicky behavior, and/or failure to thrive not explained by any other condition, had to be proven by an elimination and challenge procedure. In symptomatic breast-fed infants the mothers were advised not to eat cow's milk products, eggs, fish, nuts and peanuts. In case of severe continuous symptoms discontinuation of breast-feeding and supplementation with an amino acid-derived infant formula (Neocate®, SHS, Heilbronn, Germany) was recommended. Only definite cases were included in the analysis. FA-GIT was defined as definite if a standardized elimination/challenge procedure was performed and positive under supervision of the GINI team in the clinic (for early reactions) or at home (for late reactions). Double-blind placebo-controlled food challenge (DBPCFC) was performed in cases of uncertain reactions.

Statistical Methods

The sample size calculation was based on: (1) an expected loss due to drop out and exclusively breast-feeding of about 50% [7, 9]; (2) an estimated prevalence of allergic diseases in the CMF group of 30% [4, 5], and (3) an expected reduction in prevalence with the hydrolyzed formula of 30% (which corresponds to an expected incidence of 20%) [6]. We calculated with a significance error of 5% (two-tailed) and power of 80% in a sample size of at least 313 infants for each formula (reaching a total of 2,400 children included).

Frequencies in baseline characteristics were compared with Pearson's χ^2 test, and for comparison of means analyses of variance for unbalanced data were used. The 1-year incidences of AMs and the odds ratio (OR) for the hydrolysate groups with the CMF group as reference were calculated. For control of potential confounders, multiple logistic regression models were used. Factors without influence on the exposure or outcome variables were excluded from the model in a back-stepping procedure. For the final model, adjusted ORs with 95% confidence interval (CI) are given.

In addition to the adherence to protocol analysis the final multiple regression model was repeated in the intention-to-treat population with and without the exclusively breast-fed infants. All calculations were performed using the Statistical Analysis System (SAS), release 6.12.

Results

Baseline Characteristics

Follow-up data at age 1 year were available for 945 infants who received study formula and were compliant with the milk-feeding regime and the study protocol. 304/2,252 (13.5%) of the infants had left the study by their first birthday, 6.1% were considered noncompliant with the milk-feeding regime and the 865 remaining children were exclusively breast-fed during the first 4 months of life [11].

The 4 study formula groups did not differ significantly with reference to feeding and baseline characteristics, family history of allergies and sociodemographic data. The mean age at first exposure to study formula was 2 weeks and the mean duration of feeding the study formula was 12 weeks. The mean percentage of children fed exclusively with study formula was 9%, with no significant differences between the groups. Also, children who had received study formula, but dropped out in the first 12 months, did not differ significantly between groups. The main reasons for dropouts (personal problems within families, nutritional problems of the infant, change of permanent residence, refusal to use blinded study formula, death unrelated to study formula or design) were equally distributed between the groups [11].

By the age of 12 months 119/945 (13%) infants had developed at least one of the 3 AMs. 106 (11%) children had developed AD, 5 (0.5%) infants were diagnosed with allergic urticaria, and 12 (1.3%) with FA-GIT. More than 1 allergic disorder was diagnosed in 4 children [11].

Significant risk factors for the development of AM in the first year were found to be male gender (boys 15%, girls 10%; $p = 0.018$), and the presence of AD in a family member (children with AD in the family 18%, without AD in the family 10%; $p \leq 0.001$). A biparental family history of atopy compared with a single family history of atopy increased the incidence of AM in the offspring, though not significantly ($p = 0.087$). Neither parental education, nationality and siblings in the family nor study center influenced the incidence of AM [11].

The incidence of AM was significantly lower in infants fed eHF-C compared to the CMF-fed group ($p = 0.036$), whereas the reduction in incidence in both groups fed whey hydrolysates did not reach significance (pHF-W, $p = 0.114$, and eHF-W, $p = 0.677$; table 1). This effect was unaffected after adjusting for risk factors and confounders in a multiple logistic regression model [11].

Because AD was the predominant AM in the first year, the analysis was repeated for AD alone. We observed a significant reduction for eHF-C, but also for pHF-W on the incidence of AD (table 2). In addition, because AD in the core family was shown to be the main risk factor for an AM in the first year, and AD was the predominant allergic disease, the data were reanalyzed and stratified with respect to this risk factor. 342 children had AD in the core family, while 603 had not. In the children without AD in the family, the 1-year incidence of AD was lower in all 4 study groups, and compared with the CMF-fed group, the risk was reduced by 54% (pHF-W), 42% (eHF-W) and 58% (eHF-C; table 2). In contrast, in infants with a positive family history of AD, only eHF-C reduced the risk of AD by 57%, whereas pHF-W led only to a reduction of 28%, and eHF-W had no preventive effect (table 2).

Intention-to-treat analyses confirmed the results of the adherence to protocol analysis regardless of whether the data of all children with a follow-up of at least 4 weeks or the data of all infants exposed to a study formula were included.

Table 1. First-year incidence of atopic dermatitis (AD), allergic urticaria, gastrointestinal food allergy (FA-GIT) and allergic manifestation (AM) with crude odds ratio from logistic regression dependent on the feeding regime

		CMF (n = 256)	pHF-W (n = 241)	eHF-W (n = 238)	eHF-C (n = 210)
AD	n	38	22	31	15
	%	14.8	9.1	13.0	7.1
Urticaria	n	1	0	1	3
	%	0.4	0.0	0.4	1.4
FA-GIT	n	1	5	2	4
	%	0.4	2.1	0.8	1.9
AM	n	40	26	34	19
	%	15.6	10.8	14.3	9.1
Crude OR		1	0.65	0.90	0.54
95% CI			0.39–1.1	0.55–1.5	0.30–0.96
p value			0.114	0.677	0.036

Adapted from von Berg et al. [11].

Table 2. Adjusted odds ratio[1] for atopic dermatitis (AD) dependent on the feeding regime and stratified by AD in family history (FH)

AD	CMF	pHF-W	eHF-W	eHF-C
All				
Incidence, n/N	38/256 (15%)	22/241 (9%)	31/238 (13%)	15/210 (7%)
Adj. OR[1] (95% CI)	1	0.56 (0.32–0.99)	0.81 (0.48–1.4)	0.42(0.22–0.79)
p value		0.048	0.44	0.007
No AD in FH (n = 603)				
Incidence, n/N	21/165 (13%)	10/162 (6%)	11/142 (8%)	8/134 (6%)
Adj. OR[2] (95% CI)	1	0.46 (0.21–1.02)	0.58 (0.27–1.3)	0.42 (0.18–1.00)
p value		0.055	0.173	0.050
AD in FH (n = 342)				
Incidence, n/N	17/91 (19%)	12/79 (15%)	20/96 (21%)	7/76 (9%)
Adj. OR[2] (95% CI)	1	0.75 (0.33–1.7)	1.1 (0.54–2.3)	0.43 (0.17–1.1)
p value		0.494	0.757	0.077

Results of the multivariable models, adapted and modified from von Berg et al. [11].
[1] Adjusted for AD in FH, gender and maternal smoking after birth.
[2] Adjusted for gender and maternal smoking after birth.

Discussion

The aim of the GINI study was to answer three main questions: (1) are hydrolyzed infant formulas able to reduce the incidence of allergic diseases in children at high risk of atopy; (2) are there differences in the magnitude of the allergy-preventive effect of the hydrolysates compared with CMF, and (3) is the preventive effect of a hydrolysate dependent on the degree of hydrolyzation (partially or extensively hydrolyzed) or on the nitrogen source (whey or casein).

Our results confirm that prevention of AM in the first year of life of infants with at least 1 first-degree atopic family member is feasible by feeding hydrolyzed formulas as a supplement or substitute for the first 4 months of life, if breast-feeding is insufficient. It could be shown that the 1-year incidence of AM as defined here (AD and/or allergic urticaria and/or FA-GIT) was 15.6% in the CMF group, 10.8% in the group fed pHF-W, 14.3% in the eHF-W fed group, and 9.1% in the eHF-C fed group. The reduction of 30% which was anticipated to be of clinical relevance, could be observed only in the eHF-C group (table 1). However, if only AD was considered, a significant and, according to our definition, clinically relevant preventive effect was observed in the pHF-W and the eHF-C group compared with the CMF group (table 2).

The number of cases of allergic urticaria and of FA-GIT were too few to test for differences between the groups. Allergic urticaria is generally very rare in this age group. FA-GIT was probably underestimated in our study because many parents refused the standardized elimination and provocation procedure, which is necessary for a definite diagnosis.

In the current dietary prevention guidelines for children with a genetically determined risk of developing allergies, extensively hydrolyzed formulas are recommended as being more potent in preventing allergies. However, from previous cohort studies with hydrolysates in atopy-prone infants, it remains inconclusive whether eHF or pHF is preferable for allergy prevention. Both, eHF and pHF have been shown to prevent allergies, mainly food allergy and AD, when compared with regular CMF [4, 6]. In our study, AM was significantly prevented by eHF-C, and as the predominant allergic disease during infancy AD was also prevented by pHF-W but not by eHF-W. These results are difficult to compare to the findings of the 2 Scandinavian studies that investigated the allergy-preventive effect of pHF and eHF [9, 10]. Halken et al. [9] used the same eHF-C and pHF-W as we did, but a different brand of eHF-W and no CMF group for comparison. They did not find significant differences regarding the incidence of AD between the groups, and both eHF-W and eHF-C were equally effective [9]. Oldaeus et al. [10] compared the same eHF-C as we did with CMF, but used a partially hydrolyzed whey/casein formula which is not commercially available. They also recommended a hypoallergenic diet to the pregnant and lactating mother as co-intervention. The cumulative incidence of AD was significantly reduced at 9 months (17% in eHF-C vs. 44% in the pHF and 41% in CMF), but not at 12 and 18 months of age [10].

The different preventive effects of the two extensively hydrolyzed formulas, eHF-C and eHF-W, in our study are struggling, and together with the good effect of the pHF-W unexpected. Clearly these findings suggest that neither the molecular weight profile nor the nitrogen source alone is responsible for the effect. An explanation for the lack of effect of the eHF-W is difficult. It can only be speculated that the enzymatic processing of hydrolyzation influences the remaining epitopes and the residual antigenicity [16], or causes a loss of tolerogenic epitopes. However, this result has clinical implications because it clearly shows that the effect of formulas aiming for allergy prevention needs to be proven in clinical trials.

From several previous studies it is well known that hereditary factors are important risk factors for allergic diseases like atopy in the family [17], especially maternal atopy [18]. Eczema or perennial rhinitis in the mother are associated with elevated cord blood IgE [19, 20], and maternal AD, asthma and sensitization are associated with AD and recurrent wheezing during the first 2 years of life [21]. In a recent epidemiological study the genetic trait of AD has been reported by demonstrating significant evidence for linkage on chromosome 3q21 [22]. In our study the presence of AD in at least 1 of the first-degree family members of the infant was the strongest risk factor for developing an allergic disease, while the biparental family history of atopy had no significant influence.

Although our study was primarily not designed to investigate the influence of a specific allergic phenotype in the family on the effect of a nutritional intervention measure, we reanalyzed the data with respect to the presence or absence of AD in the family as a hypothesis-generating exercise. After stratification for this genetic risk factor, we observed different effects of the formulas on the incidence of AD. The beneficial effect of the nutritional intervention was generally more pronounced and differently influenced in children without this genetic background. For the first time it could be demonstrated that the preventive potential of a dietary prevention measure may depend on a genetic risk factor. This result could have far-reaching implications for future approaches to allergy prevention. But since these findings resulted from an additional subgroup analysis, they should be interpreted with caution until results of follow-up data or future studies confirm or contradict the consistency of these results.

Conclusions

The findings of the GINI study AM and especially in children at 1 year of age confirm that feeding a hydrolyzed formula instead of CMF as a supplement or substitute to breast milk during the first 4 months of life reduces the risk for AD in the first year of life. However, the different hydrolysates do not offer the same degree of prevention. Neither does the effect depend on the degree of hydrolyzation or the protein source alone, but may be modified by the individual genetic background. Therefore, the effect of each hydrolyzed formula aiming for prevention of AM needs to be clinically evaluated.

References

1 Lin H, Mosmann TR, Guilbert L, et al: Synthesis of T helper 2-type cytokines at the maternal-fetal interface. J Immunol 1993;151:4562–4573.
2 Prescott SL, Macaubes C, Yabuhara A, et al: Developing patterns of T cell memory to environmental allergens in the first two years of life. Int Arch Allergy Immunol 1997;113:75–79.
3 Høst A, Koletzko B, Dreborg S, et al: Dietary products used in infants for treatment and prevention of food allergy. Joint statement of the European Society for Paediatric Allergology and Clinical Immunology (ESPACI) Committee on Hypoallergenic Formulas and the European Society for Paediatric Gastroenterology, Hepatology and Nutrition (ESPGHAN) Committee on Nutrition. Arch Dis Child 1999;81:80–84.
4 Vandenplas Y, Hauser B, van den Borre C, et al: The long-term effect of a partial whey hydrolysate formula on the prophylaxis of atopic disease. Eur J Pediatr 1995;154:488–494.
5 Chandra RK: Five-year follow-up of high-risk infants with family history of allergy who were exclusively breast-fed or fed partial whey hydrolysate, soy and conventional cow's milk formulas. J Pediatr Gastroenterol Nutr 1997;24:380–388.
6 Zeiger RS, Heller S, Mellon MH, et al: Effect of combined maternal and infant food-allergen avoidance on development of atopy in early infancy: A randomized study. J Allergy Clin Immunol 1989;84:72–78.
7 Halken S, Høst A, Hansen LG, Østerballe O: Preventive effect of feeding high-risk infants a casein hydrolysate formula or an ultrafiltrated whey hydrolysate formula. A prospective, randomized, comparative clinical study. Pediatr Allergy Immunol 1993;4:173–181.
8 Schoetzau A, Gehring U, Wichmann E: Prospective cohort studies using hydrolysed formulas for allergy prevention in atopy-prone newborns: A systematic review. Eur J Pediatr 2001;160: 323–332.
9 Halken S, Hansen KS, Jacobsen HP, et al: Comparison of a partially hydrolyzed infant formula with two extensively hydrolyzed formulas for allergy prevention: A prospective randomized study. Pediatr Allergy Immunol 2000;11:149–161.
10 Oldaeus G, Anjou K, Björksten B, et al: Extensively and partially hydrolysed infant formulas for allergy prophylaxis. Arch Dis Child 1997;77:4–10.
11 von Berg A, Koletzko S, Grübl A, et al: The effect of hydrolyzed cow's milk formula for allergy prevention in the first year of life: The German Infant Nutritional Intervention Study, a randomized double-blind trial. J Allergy Clin Immunol 2003;111:533–540.
12 Schoetzau A, Gehring U, Franke K, et al: Maternal compliance with nutritional recommendations in an allergy preventive program. Arch Dis Child 2002;86:180–184.
13 Hanifin JM, Rajka G: Diagnostic features of atopic dermatitis. Acta Derm Venerol Suppl 1980;92:44–47.
14 European Task Force on Atopic Dermatitis: Severity scoring of atopic dermatitis: The SCORAD Index. Dermatology 1993;186:23–31.
15 Sampson HA, Anderson JA: Summary and recommendations: Classification of gastrointestinal manifestations due to immunologic reactions to foods in infants and young children. J Gastroenterol Nutr 2000;30:87–94.
16 Beresteijn van ECH, Meijer RJGM, Schmidt DG: Residual antigenicity of hypoallergenic infant formulas and the occurrence of milk specific IgE antibodies in patients with clinical allergy. J Allergy Clin Immunol 1995;96:365–374.
17 Kjellman NI, Johansson SG: IgE and atopic allergy in newborns and infants with a family history of atopic disease. Acta Paediatr Scand 1976;65:601–607.
18 Ruiz RG, Kemeny DM, Price JF: Higher risk of infantile atopic dermatitis from maternal atopy than from paternal atopy. Clin Exp Allergy 1992;22:762–766.
19 Bjerke T, Hedegaard M, Henriksen TB, et al: Histamine release from cord blood basophils is influenced by plasma IgE concentration, osmolarity, gestational age at birth and atopic disposition. Pediatr Allergy Immunol 1994;5:193–201.
20 Johnson CC, Ownby DR, Peterson EL: Parental history of atopic disease and concentration of cord blood IgE. Clin Exp Allergy 1996;26:624–629.
21 Bergmann RL, Edenharter G, Bergmann KE, et al: Predictability of early atopy by cord blood-IgE and parental history. Clin Exp Allergy 1997;27:752–760.
22 Lee YA, Wahn U, Kehrt R, et al: A major susceptibility locus for atopic dermatitis maps to chromosome 3q21. Nat Genet 2000;26:470–473.

Discussion

Dr. Szajewska: I want to make a comment that is based on your article that was recently published in the *Journal of Allergy and Clinical Immunology* [1]. I think it is important to look at what your data mean to the clinicians. That is why I made some calculations from data published in the original article and I want to share them with you.

I compared the worst formula (cow's milk formula) with the best formula (extensively hydrolyzed casein formula). The calculations indicate that 13 children (95% CI 8–51) would need to be treated with extensively hydrolyzed casein formula to prevent atopic dermatitis, and 16 (95% CI 8–191) to prevent an allergic manifestations at 1 year of age. One should have this kind of information at hand during discussions with the parents. It would be even more important when the data on asthma are available.

I also looked at your data on patients with no family history of atopic dermatitis.

In this case, if you compare cow's milk formula with partially hydrolyzed whey formula, the absolute risk reduction is 7% and the number needed to treat is 16 (95% CI 8–490). But if you compare cow's milk formula with extensively hydrolyzed casein formula, the number needed to treat is 15 but with a very wide confidence interval.

Dr. Von Berg: So these subjects all have atopic dermatitis in the family.

Dr. Szajewska: Not all cases. There is no atopic dermatitis in the family history, and this is a comparison of cow's milk formula versus partially hydrolyzed whey formula, the first one, and the second one is a comparison of cow's milk formula and extensively hydrolyzed casein formula. If you look at the number needed to treat it is OK, but if you look at the confidence interval it is tremendous for this particular outcome measure in children or in families with no atopic dermatitis in the family history. This is just my comment of the results. I like your study very much and I congratulate you.

Dr. Von Berg: I think it is definitely necessary to do those calculations, and of course whatever we decide to give, we have to have several things in mind, that is for sure. But I think as the study was laid out for 3 years, one should do that by the end of 3 years.

Dr. Szajewska: I agree with you totally. One additional comment: in your study you presented the results of the analysis per protocol and I know that you have done the intention-to-treat analysis. I would much prefer having the results of the intention-to-treat analysis than the analysis per protocol.

Dr. Von Berg: The information on the intention-to-treat analysis is that the trend is absolutely the same, of course it is not as strong.

Dr. Isolauri: So do we criticize the study or the method of assessing the number needed to treat technique to analyze and inform the mothers? Statisticians have a strong criticism of using number needed to treat in this kind of approach. What do you say to the mother if you have a confidence interval of up to 20,000?

Dr. Szajewska: I think that it is a good way of presenting the data. Odds ratio does not say anything to mothers. As a matter of fact, it is sometimes difficult to interpret for the majority of the practitioners. So one has to present the results in such a way that would be easier to understand for both practitioners and parents.

Dr. Isolauri: So my question is: when we have seen the figures, what do we say about the number needed to treat to the mother? To improve our understanding some promote this method, some don't. So what have we learned from the method of showing the number needed to treat in that case?

Dr. Szajewska: I would probably recommend an extensively hydrolyzed casein formula to prevent atopic dermatitis. However, I would tell the parents not to expect very big effects. I would say that there is quite a large possibility that the child will not benefit from this particular intervention. One must also consider that an extensively hydrolyzed casein formula that is to be used in health infants is lactose free. One must take this into consideration when advising the parents.

Dr. Guesry: The differences in the efficiency of the intervention study compared to the historical studies by Chandra [2], Vandenplas et al. [3], Schmidt et al. [4] and Marini et al. [5] may be due to the fact that here all babies received breast milk for a few weeks or months.

Dr. Von Berg: 9% not.

Dr. Guesry: But 91% yes, and this period of breast-feeding tends to level off the difference between the groups because the ones who receive standard formula are probably improving slightly and the ones who receive the hydrolyzed formula are probably performing slightly less well.

Dr. Von Berg: I think that it is a good point, and coming back to the arguments of the number needed to treat, I think that if a mother asks what she should give her child, we have to talk to her and we can give her the numbers. We can say in one group we have X and in the other group we have Z, would you like to try that? There is a chance that your child profits from it, and I think one should say it positively and not negatively.

Dr. Isolauri: That was exactly my question: what would you now say to the mother with these figures at hand?

Dr. Lack: I wanted to ask you whether in your trial you had considered initially using an elemental amino acid-based formula? I don't know of any studies looking at elemental formula versus other formulas and breast-feeding.

Dr. Von Berg: When we first thought up this study in the 1980s, we had no idea about amino acid-based formulas. We used Neocate as an elimination diet in this study, and the problem was we would have liked to include other formulas as well, but then first of all the ministry said no, and we would have had to increase the number of the children included.

Dr. Exl: I would like to come back to the question that Dr. Sorensen raised in terms of feasibility and cost effectiveness. When I look at the results that you presented so nicely, I ask myself if a cost-benefit calculation was done and if feasibility was looked into. As we all know, a very bitter-tasting casein hydrolysate at extremely high cost was compared to a rather 'normal' tasting moderately hydrolyzed whey hydrolysate (pHF) at moderate costs. I guess that a cost-benefit calculation would clearly prove the advantage of the pHF. Then I must come back to Dr. Isolauri and say she is right. When there is such a huge difference between the number needed to treat and the effect and I have to recommend to a mother that she should buy this very expensive formula with a very bad taste, and the chances that her baby will not get an allergy are quite low, then the answer should be very clear. That is why, if I look at your figures, that with certainty the pHF formula would be the better choice. In addition, the last time you presented the sensitization data after 1 year so nicely and I was so fascinated with it, that I was wondering if it would be possible to share it with everybody here?

Dr. Von Berg: I can tell you that it is something which is in preparation now and it was a decision of the GINI board not to do it, sorry.

Dr. Shyur: We have done an IgE antibody study in cow's milk-allergic children in Taiwan and they show a positive cow's milk:IgE ratio and the same percentage of IgE:lactoalbumin and β-lactoglobulin:casein. In the treatment we also partially used extensive whey and extensive casein to try to improve the symptoms. We found that extensive casein hydrolysate has the highest incidence of diarrhea. We find the extensive whey causes less diarrhea than extensive casein and we still get good results. So how do you explain the difference in your study between extensive whey and extensive casein? We previously tried to use partial whey hydrolysate because of oral tolerance. In our experience extensive hydrolysates don't induce oral tolerance.

Dr. Von Berg: Did I get your comment right, you used these hydrolysates for therapy and the question is why do the two extensively hydrolyzed respond differently?

Dr. Shyur: Did you check a special IgE for casein and whey for these children, and how do you explain the difference between the whey and the casein? In our experience extensive whey is more acceptable than extensive casein.

Dr. Von Berg: The different effect of the two extensively hydrolyzed formulas was very unexpected for us and rather struggling, because we really have no idea why it is like that. There is a slight difference in molecular weight profile, there is perhaps a different processing with different enzymes used that cut at different sites in the molecule, that might be the reason but we can't actually tell you the mechanism why one is working and the other not. Maybe one of you here can tell me more about that.

Dr. R. Bergmann: As far as I know peptides of casein induce tolerance, so you don't have an elemental formula.

Dr. Von Berg: The strange thing is that in another study by Halken et al. [6], in which they used the same brand of extensively hydrolyzed casein and another brand of extensively hydrolyzed whey, both extensively hydrolyzed formulas performed absolutely the same. So at the beginning we could not believe this but it was very consistent in all the data we had.

Dr. Isolauri: I don't have any explanation of course for that. Definitely there are several extensively hydrolyzed whey formulas available even as products with more profile like the one you used for the hydrolyzed casein, which can be purer if you wish. We have measured the β-lactoglobulin concentrations in different formulas and there are huge differences, so if the issue is casein versus whey we should probably first see that we use the same level of hydrolysis and we find the difference. But definitely your outcome seems to be very much against the importance of bifidobacteria if we think that lactose is a bifidogenic, whey is a bifidogenic, so you showed us something against that and I was a little surprised.

Dr. Mantzourani: Why was recurrent wheezing not looked at?

Dr. Von Berg: Because we thought that asthma is not well defined at 1 year of age and it is mainly not allergic.

Dr. Mantzourani: Even if you had asthmatic parents?

Dr. Von Berg: We have recorded all these data and we will present them at 3 years, and of course later on we can analyze those as well, but for the outcome at 1 year we have decided not to do it, but the data are there.

Dr. Endres: The last child finished the study almost 2 years ago. When will the 3-year results will be published?

Dr. Von Berg: Very soon.

Dr. Endres: What does that mean? I am asking because it will be recorded.

Dr. Von Berg: We are going to present the data in Paris and we think that we will have the paper ready by then, not published but ready.

Dr. Lack: One of the things that puzzles me in prevention studies is that we all look at the connection between milk avoidance or manipulation of milk in the infant's diet and subsequent wheezing in childhood. I simply can't understand the connection. Is there a biological or pathophysiological basis? Why do we concentrate on the role of milk formula in relation to asthma, when we don't show sensitization to milk or milk allergy to be of any relevance in the pathogenesis of asthma? Why is this such an important part of our primary prevention in asthma and why does the manipulation of infant formulae dominate our thinking?

Dr. Von Berg: Because I think we know that in a high percentage of children with atopic dermatitis they go on having asthma, and the idea is if we can prevent atopic dermatitis maybe we can prevent asthma. From our study I don't know yet, but there is one study, I think by Chandra [2], in which he has shown that at the age of 5 years there was prevention of asthma as well.

Dr. Lack: I realize some studies have shown prevention of asthma, but other studies have not shown that. If you look at atopic dermatitis in community studies, which are lacking, what is the percentage of affected children who have a problem with cow's milk? We simply do not know. Because subgroups of children in selected studies and those at the more severe end of the spectrum seen in clinics have problems with cow's milk, I am not sure one can automatically assume that in general cow's milk allergy is a problem in eczema. If we do not know the extent of the role of cow's milk allergy in eczema, it is difficult to speculate how manipulation of infant formula may translate into subsequent allergic manifestations such as asthma.

Dr. Von Berg: I did not show the results but it is interesting: in our study hen's egg-associated atopic dermatitis, but not cow's milk-associated atopic dermatitis, was influenced by the formulas, and that is something very interesting.

Dr. Lack: The sensitization to hen's egg changes?

Dr. Von Berg: No, but the hen's egg-associated disease is reduced and there might be a link that it is not cow's milk sensitization but perhaps the association between sensitization and disease that is influenced, which I think is fascinating.

Dr. Bindslev-Jensen: I am not a pediatrician, I am a dermatologist. I see quite a lot of children and infants with atopic dermatitis. Even in our setting we have a sensitization rate of somewhere between 35 and 40%. We are publishing a prospective study in 600 newborns right now. But strangely there is no sensitization. We are not discussing whether these children with atopic dermatitis may or may not develop allergic diseases, e.g. IgE-mediated diseases, later on in their respiratory tract. If 9 of 10 patients in your study are breast-fed and then fed partial hydrolyzed or totally hydrolyzed formula, then you can get an effect with the totally hydrolyzed formula. So my question is: why is it then a question of intention to treat or number to treat when you can find something with the extensively hydrolyzed formula which you cannot find in your set up with the partial hydrolyzed formula? So you should either keep to the advice to the patients to use a cow's milk-based formula or use the extensively hydrolyzed formula because there is no difference in between, or is this something I haven't understood?

Dr. Von Berg: No, there is a difference.

Dr. Bindslev-Jensen: With the extensively?

Dr. Von Berg: Yes, and with the partially as well if you take all patients.

Dr. Bindslev-Jensen: OK, if you add everything.

Dr. Isolauri: Previous German multicenter studies [7, 8] have shown that there is some difference between exposure, sensitization and clinical disease. Was it house dust mite and cat?

Dr. Von Berg: Yes, house dust mite and cat.

Dr. Isolauri: We had the same result for our probiotic study. Antigen-specific IgE reactivity was not changed while clinical disease was changed. Though my question is: are your results along these lines here, or do you now in this study see the same effect for sensitization and clinical disease?

Dr. Von Berg: We see that the sensitization at 1 year is very similar in all groups including the breast-fed group, but the disease is modified along these lines.

Dr. Hill: I wonder if you can tell us, when you analyze your data do you just restrict your analysis to those infants who are totally bottle-fed? I think the introduction of breast-feeding is really a significant factor and you do have about 45 patients in each of those groups who seem to form a fairly homogenous groups. Have you had the opportunity to examine the outcomes in each of those groups that are just totally bottle-fed?

Dr. Von Berg: We have looked at those children, it is only 9%, that is one thing. But we have looked at the different duration of breast-feeding before introducing the study formulas.

Dr. Hill: I am sorry I thought they were a group of infants who were totally bottle-fed, and that is about 45 patients in each group, is that right? Have you had the opportunity to analyze the outcome of those patients because I see the formula-fed are a homogenous population.

Dr. Von Berg: They were homogenous, yes.

Dr. Hill: Their dietary exposure has not been confounded by breast milk?

Dr. Von Berg: What I wanted to show you is when those children are fed with study formula for longer than 12 weeks and less than 12 weeks, it is not exclusive breast-feeding, but in this analysis it was like this. There was a trend that partially hydrolyzed whey and extensively hydrolyzed casein had a lower prevalence of disease.

Dr. Hill: That was a trend?

Dr. Von Berg: That was a trend, yes.

Dr. Guesry: You have not analyzed this group of exclusively bottle-fed babies separately?

Dr. Von Berg: No.

Dr. Saavedra: Just to elaborate on the question relating to the link there might be between the use of a hydrolysate early in life and respiratory allergy later on. I think one of the organs we forget here is the gut. Atopic skin manifestations are easier to see, there is no question about that, and the respiratory symptoms clearly take time. The one thing we are not doing here, which obviously would not be ethical to do, is biopsy of the gut of these children. There is the potential that these children, and this is of course only a speculation, become sensitized from the point of view of gut allergy and develop allergic enteropathy, of which unfortunately we probably only see the tip of the iceberg. A huge number of children we discover only after endoscopy and demonstrate allergic gastritis, eosinophilic problems, and allergic enteritis and colitis. The possibility that the effect on the gut is what leads to later sensitization because of problems with permeability when these children are introduced during weaning to other proteins, and this can potentially, and I am speculating, explain why these children become sensitized to other proteins if they do not receive prophylaxis adequately early in life. And again that is not an easy study to do but it certainly allows a potential income.

Dr. Von Berg: It would be wonderful if I could do it, but I think our ethics committee would not allow it, and certainly in a study like this you can't do that.

Dr. Walker: If I understand the allergic march it is a sequential series of clinical expression of allergy once the initial sensitization has occurred and I think the question you are asking is if early introduction of allergens in the form of formula causes asthma development. As I understand it asthma also develops later on so I don't quite understand how you are going to be able to answer the question you pose by simply looking at 3 years of data. You need to go beyond that don't you?

Dr. Von Berg: Of course we do. First we got money for the first 3 years but now we started to do the 6-year examinations and questionnaires, and we do it with lung function and in some children with the bronchial responsiveness. Of course we want to follow them, but in Germany you can't get money for more than 3 years, not longitudinal money, definitely not.

Dr. Neijens: One of the concepts after the link between early manifestations like food allergy and asthma later on is that about 6% of food allergy patients seem to develop asthma, that is what we currently assess, and at a particular dose some are sensitized and have IgE-positive reactions. Most probably early sensitization, in particular not so much to milk but more to hen's egg and pollen, is a risk factor for developing allergic asthma. So the other concept is that you are able to switch off the sensitization tract by one of the measures, like food for instance, but you switch not only the sensitization to food allergens but also to the other ones. This comes from the concept of tolerance induction as has been found in immunotherapy, etc. Therefore it is important, whether this is true or not, sensitization and the development of sensitization should of course be studied, and it is very important that this aspect is documented very carefully in your study. In addition it is even better to also measure immunomodulation and then you gain insight into the effect not only of sensitization immunoregulation but also disease expression, and that is what we actually need.

Dr. Von Berg: Yes, we measure sensitization, we don't do cytokines and all that.

Dr. Neijens: When can you tell us something about the results?

Dr. Von Berg: Sensitization at 1 year is very low in our study and there is no difference between the groups. We have very little sensitization to inhalant allergens, again with no significant differences between the groups, actually a little more in the breast-fed children, and the main sensitization at 1 year is hen's egg sensitization. The disease is much more associated with hen's egg sensitization than with cow's milk sensitization.

Dr. Neijens: The best evidence we have this far is at 2 years of age from the ETAC study [9].

Dr. Von Berg: We have 3 years then again.

Dr. Neijens: So that is important, 2 and 4 years.

Dr. Von Berg: We have 1 and 3 years.

Dr. Rijntjes: I have a question about food allergy with symptoms in the gut. My first question is: when you did an elimination and afterwards a provocation, was it a blind placebo control? What is puzzling me is that the group with the cow's milk formula was the lowest one that had the positive elimination and provocation. Have you got an explanation for this?

Dr. Von Berg: It is just very small numbers and I think you can't test for anything with such small numbers. The problem is we had 12 definite cases and we had 68 parentally reported cases who thought they probably have one, but of them a very low percentage was really proven by the elimination and provocation procedure. One of the problems is that many mothers did not agree to this procedure, and therefore I think we have to look at these data with caution, on gastrointestinal manifestation.

Dr. Rijntjes: But do you think that the fact that the parents were in the study is a barrier, and is that the reason why the group is so small?

Dr. Von Berg: No, I think first of all if a mother is in the study and if a mother is interested in allergy and the development of allergy, she probably induces much more from any symptom the possibility that it might be an allergy. But we always see that, of all the children with parenterally reported food allergies, the percentage of definite cases is very low in all the studies.

Dr. Murch: These formulas are different in one important way which is the carbohydrate content and the presence of lactose. This will have at least some prebiotic effect. Did you see differences in the gut flora between the children?

Dr. Von Berg: We didn't do that.

References

1 Von Berg A, Koletzko S, Grubl A, et al: The effect of hydrolysed cow's milk formula for allergy prevention in the first year of life: The German Infant Nutritional intervention Study, a randomized double-blind trial. J Allergy Clin Immunol 2003;111:533–540.

2 Chandra RK: Five-year follow-up of high-risk infants with family history of allergy who were exclusively breast-fed or fed partial whey hydrolysate, soy, and conventional cow's milk formulas. J Pediatr Gastroenterol Nutr 1997;24:380–388.

3 Vandenplas Y, Hauser B, van den Borre C, et al: The long-term effect of a partial whey hydrolysate formula on the prophylaxis of atopic disease. Eur J Pediatr 1995;154:488–494.
4 Schmidt E, Reinhardt D, Gerke R: The use of hypoallergenic milk formulas in newborns. Kinderarzt 1987;18:1–7.
5 Marini A, Agosti M, Motta G, Mosca F: Effects of a dietary and environmental prevention program on the incidence of allergic symptoms in high atopic risk infants: Three year's follow-up. Acta Paediatr Scand 1996;85(suppl 414):1–21.
6 Halken S, Hansen KS Jacobsen HP, et al: Comparison of a partially hydrolyzed infant formula with two extensively hydrolyzed formulas for allergy prevention: A prospective randomized study. Pediatr Allergy Immunol 2000;11:149–161.
7 Lau S, Nickel R, Niggemann B, et al., MAS Group: The development of childhood asthma: Lessons from the German Multicenter Allergy Study (MAS). Paediatr Respir Rev 2002;3: 265–272.
8 Lau S, Illi S, Sommerfeld C, et al: Early exposure to house-dust mite and cat allergens and development of childhood asthma: A cohort study. Lancet 2000;356:1392–1397.
9 Warner JO, ETAC Study Group, Early Treatment of the Atopic Child: A double-blind, randomized, placebo-controlled trial of cetirizine in preventing the onset of asthma in children with atopic dermatitis: 18 months' treatment and 8 months' posttreatment follow-up. J Allergy Clin Immunol 2001;108:929–937.

Isolauri E, Walker WA (eds): Allergic Diseases and the Environment.
Nestlé Nutrition Workshop Series Pediatric Program, Vol. 53, pp. 301–313,
Nestec Ltd.; Vevey/S. Karger AG, Basel, © 2004.

Novel Approaches for the Nutritional Management of the Allergic Infant[1]

Erika Isolauri

Department of Pediatrics, University of Turku, Turku, Finland

One Child in Four Is Allergic

Allergic diseases, manifesting as atopic eczema, allergic rhinitis and asthma, are on the increase in industrialized countries, currently in fact constituting the most common chronic diseases of childhood [1]. Despite the pronounced hereditary element in allergic disease, genetic factors are unlikely to explain the increased emergence of the atopic-type immune responsiveness to environmental antigens. Rather, it would appear that environmental changes more directly shape the immune responder type of the host during a critical period of life.

Immune responses early in life are physiologically predominantly of the T-helper 2-type (Th2) due to the immunological balance prevailing in utero [2]. Interestingly, however, it has been observed that neonatal Th2 responses, including the production of interleukin (IL)-13 [3] and IL-4 [4], are actually lower in infants who develop atopic disease as compared to those who remain healthy. Healthy infants exhibit a decline in Th2 responses during the early postnatal period, whereas a converse pattern is characteristic of infants developing atopic disease [4]. Increased production of Th2 cytokines would thus appear to be the result of defective immune regulation associated with the development of atopic disease rather than a direct cause of such development. Indeed, the first allergic condition to manifest itself, atopic eczema, has been identified as a portal for the development of IgE-mediated atopic manifestations [5].

The underlying factors in allergic disease include impaired barrier functions of the skin and the gut mucosa, with altered microbiological and immunological milieu, and disturbed cytokine regulation. The environmental

[1] A Nutrition, Allergy, Mucosal Immunology and Intestinal Microbiota (NAMI) research group report.

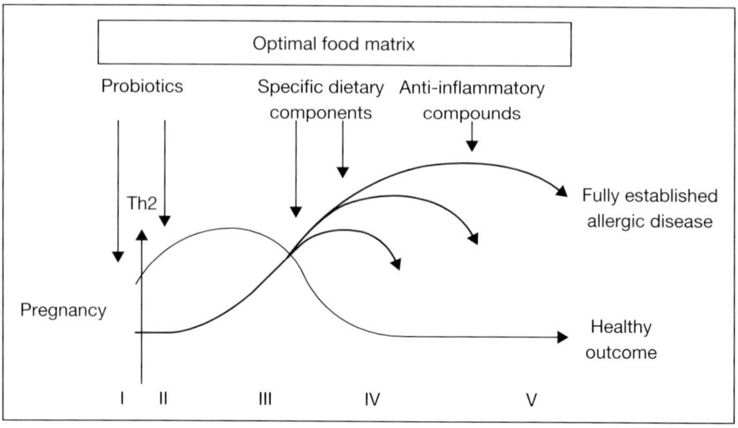

Fig. 1. Induction of allergic disease. A schematic presentation of potential targets of future research on preventive and therapeutic intervention at different stages I = Pregnancy: physiological T-helper type-2 (Th2) priming; intrauterine allergen exposure. II = Neonatal period: neonatal Th2 responses are lower in infants who develop atopic disease as compared to those who remain healthy; mode of delivery, the establishment of gut microbiota and neonatal antigen exposure. III = Critical window: healthy infants exhibit a decline in Th2 responses during the early postnatal period, whereas a converse pattern is characteristic of infants developing atopic disease; counterregulatory mechanisms. IV = Early symptoms of allergic disease: atopic eczema-food allergy; induction of tolerance, control of allergic inflammation. V = Fully established allergic disease: consolidation of the immune responder type; control of allergic inflammation.

determinants underlying the increasing incidence of allergic diseases include changes in the composition of the Western diet during the past decades. However, the specific processes which initiate the vicious circle of allergic inflammation remain unresolved. This notwithstanding, current nutrition research has improved our understanding of the heterogeneous nature of allergic disease, and has uncovered a number of targets for therapeutic and preventive applications (fig. 1).

Nutrition and Allergy – Identification of Targets for Nutritional Management and Risk Reduction

The counterregulatory processes of primary allergy prevention should exert their effects very early, as the first expression of the atopic immune responder type frequently occurs within the first months of life [6]. Furthermore, identification of these first signs and symptoms of allergic disease, in particular atopic eczema and control of allergic inflammation, constitutes the key in the allergy-prevention strategy. Several dietary factors may influence the inflammatory responses in allergic disease [7]. The nutritional theories attracting current research interest relate to identification of active compounds which reinforce an anti-inflammatory, potentially tolerogenic type of immune response to assimilate allergenic challenges.

Probiotics represent one example of immunomodulatory compounds for the allergic host. The immunomodulatory potential of the healthy gastrointestinal microbiota, the source of specific probiotic strains, is possibly associated with two structural components of bacteria, the lipopolysaccharide portion of gram-negative bacteria (endotoxin) and a specified CpG motif in bacterial DNA [8, 9]. These structures activate immunomodulatory genes via the Toll-like receptors present, e.g. on macrophages, dendritic and intestinal epithelial cells [10, 11]. The net effect on intestinal epithelial cells is immunosuppressive by way of inhibition of the transcription factor NF-κB pathway. In addition, specific strains of the gut microbiota have been shown to contribute to a Th cell population promoting oral tolerance induction [12], and to counter allergy by generation of anti-inflammatory IL-10 and transforming growth factor (TGF)-β [13–15]. The importance of the immunoregulatory potential of gut microbiota is emphasized in the recent demonstration of cross-talk between the innate and adaptive immune system; the nature of the initial immune response governs the homeostasis of the adaptive immune response.

The first condition to manifest itself is atopic eczema, and the first sensitizing antigens are frequently derived from dietary proteins [16]. Most children become tolerant to food antigens by school age, when sensitization to air-borne allergens takes over. Unlike food allergy, respiratory allergic diseases are in many cases not transient phenomena. Recent advances call in question a causal cascade of exposure to potentially allergenic proteins, sensitization and hypersensitivity [17]; the exposure to allergens sensitizing the host immune system may not necessarily induce allergic disease. Indeed, sensitization to indoor allergens such as house dust mite, as assessed by specific IgE, but not the level of exposure to these allergens, has been associated with asthma, wheeze and increased bronchial responsiveness [18]. In like manner, a modified Th2-type response, characterized as an IgG and IgG4 antibody response, without a risk of asthma upon cat allergen exposure, has been detected [19]. The same appears to hold true for dietary antigens as well. The effect of exposure to cow's milk antigen on the development of allergic symptoms was evaluated in 1,533 breast-fed neonates who randomly received dietary intervention during 3 days after birth [20]. The intervention consisted of either cow's milk-based formula or an essentially protein-free placebo formula. The children were initially followed up for 2 years, and no difference was observed between the 2 groups in the prevalence of atopic disease. The long-term effects were assessed in a subsequent study at 5 years of age [21]. One child in four was allergic; atopic disease was detected in 26.3% of the children given cow's milk-based formula neonatally and in 25.0%

of those given the placebo formula. Furthermore, prevention of food allergy by elimination diets has not resulted in prevention of asthma [22], suggesting distinct immunoregulatory processes between these allergic diseases. These data would imply that eradication of allergens from the early environment may not apply in allergy-prevention strategies, albeit that elimination of the antigen responsible, if any, constitutes the mainstay of the treatment of established allergic disease.

Recent studies on the immunomodulatory properties of fatty acids and antioxidants, including ascorbic acid, α-tocopherol, β-carotene, selenium and zinc, have shown that food not only constitutes a source of dietary antigens causing sensitization but may also contain protective factors [7]. Consequently, both macronutrients as well as micronutrients may play a role in allergic disease. Thus far, despite failure to verify any association between antigen exposure and allergic disease, the dietary approach in attempts to prevent and treat these conditions has focused on elimination diets. In future, the potential of specific dietary antigens, their processed peptides, may actually be applied in tolerance induction and thus in protection from allergic disease.

Nutritional Management of the Allergic Infant: Current Position

The current approach in the treatment of food allergy is directed towards elimination diets. The mainstay in the treatment of cow's milk allergy is thus complete avoidance of cow's milk proteins. Dietary elimination of the antigen responsible has been shown to alleviate symptoms, preserve intestinal integrity, prevent aberrant antigen absorption, and reverse the disturbance of humoral and cell-mediated immune responses [23, 24].

In infants with cow's milk allergy, it is necessary to use substitute formulas. Factors which influence the allergenicity of a protein include molecular complexity, solubility and stability, and its concentration. Heat treatment of cow's milk proteins can affect the conformational epitopes of allergens and facilitate their hydrolysis. To produce the least allergenic formulas, cow's milk proteins are modified by multiple enzymatic hydrolysis with progressive destruction of sequential epitopes. Protein hydrolysates are classified as partially hydrolyzed or extensively hydrolyzed formulas. Enzymatic hydrolysis does not necessarily render the formula nonallergenic, as the optimal extent of hydrolysis is not known and traces of the original protein are detected in the hydrolysate [25]. However, extensively hydrolyzed formulas constitute the treatment of choice for patients with cow's milk allergy. In patients with multiple food allergies not tolerating these, amino acid-derived formulas are used [26].

The advantage afforded by elimination diets seems to lie in the silencing of specific allergic inflammation induced by an offending food, not in the primary prevention of the disease. The effect is thus antigen-specific. Elimination diets may place affected infants at a constant risk of inadequate nutrition [26–28]. On this basis, these diets should be applied only in patients with proven allergy to a specific dietary protein. Conversely, in patients with documented food allergy, the completeness of the elimination diet needs to be confirmed and clinically monitored.

Future Trends in the Management of the Allergic Infants: From Elimination Diets to Active Therapeutic Compounds

The dilemma of the host immune defense is to generate an effective response to pathogens while concomitantly maintaining unresponsiveness to antigens in food and the normal host microbiota. The gastrointestinal tract provides a protective interface between the internal environment and the constant challenge from antigens in the external environment [29]. This first line of host defense is directed towards exclusion of antigens and elimination of foreign antigens penetrating the mucosa.

Apart from the barrier function, the intestinal mucosa is efficient in assimilating antigens, for which purpose there are specialized transport mechanisms in the villous epithelium [29]. Antigens are absorbed across the epithelial layer by transcytosis along two functional pathways. The main degradative pathway includes lysosomal processing of the antigen into smaller fragments, which reduces the immunogenicity of the antigen load. A minor pathway allows the transport of intact unprocessed antigens, which results in antigen-specific immune responses.

Degradation of antigens is a necessary initial step in controlling inflammatory responsiveness to dietary antigens [30, 31]. Most antigens encountered are already processed when they contact the mucosal surface. Proteases of specific strains of the intestinal microbiota contribute to the processing of food antigens in the gut and modify their immunogenicity in vitro and in vivo. This processing has been linked with the potential to generate peptides with suppressive effects on lymphocyte proliferation in healthy subjects; systemic immune responses to gut-processed antigens are preferentially directed towards suppression.

The gut not only constitutes a target of allergic inflammation but may also act as a route for tolerance induction. The major mechanism by which the gut-associated lymphoid tissue maintains homeostasis is via control of cytokine regulation. A healthy homeostasis in the gut milieu is achieved by optimizing the balance of pro- and anti-inflammatory cytokines and other mediators.

One modern approach to allergic disease might be a nutritional mode of management capable of preventing or depressing allergic inflammation. Such an approach could be based on the administration of tolerogenic gut-processed peptide fragments of the specific protein, and the use of specific dietary compounds such as fatty acids and antioxidants.

Increasing evidence suggests that dietary lipids, especially long-chain polyunsaturated fatty acids, regulate the immune function and therefore contribute to the development and severity of symptoms of allergic disease [for review see 7]. Particularly relevant to this process is arachidonic acid (20:4n-6)-derived eicosanoid prostaglandin E2 (PGE2). PGE2 induces increased IgE synthesis due to the induction of B-cell differentiation in the presence of IL-4. The effects of PGE2 may also be exerted through IgE-binding receptors. PGE2 reduces the surface expression of these receptors. Indeed, the most frequently reported abnormality in cell fatty acid composition in patients with atopic disorders has been an imbalance between series n-6 and n-3 fatty acids, which predisposes them to the adverse effects of PGE2. Despite their apparent proinflammatory role, n-6 fatty acids may also contribute to an anti-inflammatory intestinal environment in that antigen stimulation upregulates PGE2 production, which eventuates in suppression of antigen-specific T-cell proliferation in gut-associated lymphoid tissue. Enhanced synthesis of prostaglandins also contributes to an anti-inflammatory intestinal milieu through suppression of Th1-type cytokines, stimulation of anti-inflammatory IL-10 and TGF-β, and maintenance of the IgA environment.

In allergic disease, inflammatory processes result in increased endogenously generated oxidative stress. Both cellular enzyme-based antioxidants and diet-derived antioxidants may counteract this stress and may diminish the inflammatory response [7]. Although the potential role of antioxidants in the prevention of allergic disease is currently unknown, diet-derived antioxidants may be postulated to have protective effects. Low concentrations of plasma antioxidants (β-carotene, ascorbate and α-tocopherol) have been measured in patients with wheezing illness, and a low intake of antioxidants has been associated with bronchial reactivity and the risk of asthma. In addition, a higher dietary intake of vitamin E has been shown to be associated with a lower serum IgE concentration. These findings suggest that antioxidant deficiencies may be associated with symptoms of allergic disease.

The challenge for nutrition research is to identify the mechanisms of action of immunomodulatory dietary factors which may be protective in allergic disease. For example, probiotic performance has been shown to manifest itself in normalization of increased intestinal permeability and improvement of the intestine's barrier functions [17], also contributing to the capacity of specific strains to damp inflammatory responses in the gut. The effects are strain-specific; different bacteria or modifications/components thereof have defined adherence sites and immunological effects and varied effects in the healthy versus inflamed mucosal milieu.

Thus far, the experience acquired in clinical trials assessing the effects of probiotics in the prevention and treatment of atopic disease demonstrates the complexity of the challenge due to the heterogeneous nature of hypersensitivity: bifidobacteria appear to be effective in reversing the manifestation of atopy, whereas lactobacilli have proved beneficial in the prevention of atopic disease but ineffective in protection against cow's milk allergy, albeit that both bifidobacteria and lactobacilli appear to be effective in the treatment of the disorder [17].

Considering dietary lipids and antioxidants, the Nutrition, Allergy, Mucosal Immunology and Intestinal Microbiota (NAMI) research group recently demonstrated that in the diet of breast-feeding atopic mothers the intake of fat, especially saturated fatty acids, was relatively high and the intake of some antioxidants was relatively low compared to recommendations [32]. A maternal diet rich in saturated fat during breast-feeding was seen to be associated with atopy of the infant regardless of maternal atopic disease. The result corroborates recent demonstrations on a delicate balance of inflammatory and anti-inflammatory compounds in breast milk [33].The interindividual variation in fatty acid concentration, antioxidants and other immunomodulatory compounds in breast milk is considerable, and could thereby explain the inconclusive evidence on the effect of breast-feeding on allergic disease.

Importantly, recent clinical studies indicate that the potential of breast-feeding to counteract allergic disease may be promoted by dietary means [33]. When probiotic supplementation was given to the lactating mother, the amount of anti-inflammatory TGF-β in breast milk could be promoted [15], furnishing one mechanism by which the risk of infant atopic eczema could be reduced during a critical period of life (fig. 1).

In conclusion, while uncoordinated elimination diets result in a risk of general nutritional inadequacy or deficiency of essential single nutrients, a balanced diet following current dietary recommendations, specifically containing fresh fruits and vegetables (antioxidants) and fat of predominantly vegetable origin, may be associated with a lower prevalence of allergic symptoms. Rigorous scientific effort is required to elucidate the characteristics of distinct probiotic strains in different manifestations of allergic disease and the role of fatty acids and antioxidants in regulating allergic inflammatory processes. Due to interaction between nutrients; no single supplement can be expected to resolve the challenge of allergic disease. In the future, the properties of specific dietary compounds and their combinations, in an optimal food matrix, might be exploited in the development of specific prophylactic and therapeutic interventions (fig. 1).

References

1 The International Study of Asthma and Allergies in Childhood (ISAAC) Steering Committee: Worldwide variation in prevalence of symptoms of asthma, allergic rhinoconjunctivitis, and atopic eczema. Lancet 1998;351:1225–1232.

2 Piccinni MP, Beloni L, Livi C, et al: Defective production of both leukemia inhibitory factor and type 2 T-helper cytokines by decidual T cells in unexplained recurrent abortions. Nat Med 1998;4:1020–1024.
3 Williams TJ, Jones CA, Miles EA, et al: Fetal and neonatal IL-13 production during pregnancy and at birth and subsequent development of atopic symptoms. J Allergy Clin Immunol 2000;105:951–959.
4 Prescott SL, Macaubas C, Smallacombe T, et al: Development of allergen-specific T-cell memory in atopic and normal children. Lancet 1999;353:196–200.
5 Hanifin JM: Atopiform dermatitis: Do we need another confusing name for atopic dermatitis? Br J Dermatol 2002;147:430–432.
6 Kilpi T, Kero J, Jokinen J, et al: Common respiratory infections early in life may reduce the risk of atopic dermatitis. Clin Infect Dis 2002;34:620–626.
7 Laiho K, Hoppu U, Ouwehand A, et al: Probiotics: On-going research on atopic individuals. B J Nutr 2002;88:19–27.
8 Hartmann G, Weiner GJ, Krieg AM: CpG DNA: A potent signal for growth, activation, and maturation of human dendritic cells. Proc Natl Acad Sci USA 1999;96:9305–9319.
9 Kranzer K, Bauer M, Lipford GB, et al: CpG-oligodeoxynucleotides enhance T-cell receptor-triggered interferon-gamma production and up-regulation of CD69 via induction of antigen-presenting cell-derived interferon type I and interleukin-12. Immunology 2000;99:170–178.
10 Cario E, Rosenberg IM, Brandwein SL, et al: Lipopolysaccharide activates distinct signaling pathways in intestinal epithelial cell lines expressing Toll-like receptors. J Immunol 2000; 164:966–972.
11 Hemmi H, Takeuchi O, Kawai T, et al: A toll-like receptor recognizes bacterial DNA. Nature 2000;408:740–745.
12 Sudo N, Sawamura S, Tanaka K, et al: The requirement of intestinal bacterial flora for the development of an IgE production system fully susceptible to oral tolerance induction. J Immunol 1997;159:1739–1745.
13 Pessi T, Sütas Y, Hurme M, et al: Interleukin-10 generation in atopic children following oral *Lactobacillus rhamnosus* GG. Clin Exp Allergy 2000;30:1804–1808.
14 von der Weid T, Bulliard C, Schiffrin EJ: Induction by a lactic acid bacterium of a population of CD4+ T cells with low proliferative capacity that produce transforming growth factor beta and interleukin-10. Clin Diagn Lab Immunol 2001;8:695–701.
15 Rautava S, Kalliomaki M, Isolauri E: Probiotics during pregnancy and breast-feeding might confer immunomodulatory protection against atopic disease in the infant. J Allergy Clin Immunol 2002;109:119–121.
16 Isolauri E, Turjanmaa K: Combined skin prick and patch testing enhances identification of food allergy in infants with atopic dermatitis. J Allergy Clin Immunol 1995;97:9–15.
17 Isolauri E, Rautava S, Kalliomäki M, et al: Role of probiotics in food hypersensitivity. Curr Opin Immunol Clin Allergol 2002;2:263–271.
18 Lau S, Illi S, Sommerfeld C, et al: Early exposure to house-dust mite and cat allergens and development of childhood asthma: A cohort study. Lancet 2000;356:1392–1397.
19 Platts-Mills T, Vaughan J, Squillace S, et al: Sensitisation, asthma, and a modified Th2 response in children exposed to cat allergen: A population-based cross-sectional study. Lancet 2001;357:752–756.
20 de Jong MH, Scharp-van der Linden VETM, Aalberse RC, et al: Randomised controlled trial of brief neonatal exposure to cows' milk on the development of atopy. Arch Dis Child 1998;79:126–130.
21 de Jong MH, Scharp-van der Linden VETM, Aalberse RC, et al: The effect of brief neonatal exposure to cows' milk on atopic symptoms up to age 5. Arch Dis Child 2002;86:365–369.
22 Zeiger RS, Heller S: The development and prediction of atopy in high-risk children: Follow-up at age seven years in a prospective randomized study combined maternal and infanty food allergen avoidance. J Allergy Clin Immunol 1995;95:1179–1190.
23 Agata H, Kondo N, Fukutomi O, et al: Effect of elimination diets on food-specific IgE antibodies and lymphocyte proliferative responses to food antigens in atopic dermatitis patients exhibiting sensitivity to food allergens. J Allergy Clin Immunol 1993;91:668–679
24 Isolauri E, Suomalainen H, Kaila M, et al: Local immune response in patients with cow milk allergy- follow-up of patients retaining allergy or becoming tolerant. J Pediatr 1992;120: 9–15.

25 Mäkinen-Kiljunen S, Sorva R: Bovine β-lactoglobulin levels in hydrolysed protein formulas for infant feeding. Clin Exp Allergy 1993;23:287–291.
26 Isolauri E, Sütas Y, Mäkinen-Kiljunen S, et al: Efficacy and safety of hydrolysed cow milk and amino acid-derived formulas in infants with cow milk allergy. J Pediatr 1995;127:550–557.
27 Isolauri E, Sütas Y, Salo MK, et al: Elimination diet in cow milk allergy: risk for impaired growth in young children. J Pediatr 1998;132:1004–1010.
28 Eggesbo M, Botten G, Stigum H: Restricted diets in children with reactions to milk and egg perceived by their parents. J Pediatr 2001;139:583–587.
29 Sanderson IR, Walker WA: Uptake and transport of macromolecules by the intestine: possible role in clinical disorders (an update). Gastroenterology 1993;104:622–639.
30 Strober W, Kelsall B, Marth T: Oral tolerance. J Clin Immunol 1998;18:1–30.
31 Barone KS, Reilly MR, Flanagan MP, Michael JG: Abrogation of oral tolerance by feeding encapsulated antigen. Cellular Immunology 2000;199:65–72.
32 Hoppu U, Kalliomäki M, Isolauri E: Maternal diet rich in saturated fat during breastfeeding is associated with atopic sensitisation of the infant. Eur J Clin Nutr 2000;54:702–705.
33 Hoppu U, Kalliomäki M, Laiho K, Isolauri E: Breast milk – Immunomodulatory signals against allergic diseases. Allergy 2001;56:23–26.

Discussion

Dr. Rijntjes: In practice we always have the problem, especially in atopic dermatitis, that we have sensitization for a lot of allergens, but this doesn't mean that it is causing the symptoms. When a patient is sensitized to a lot of allergens what do you suggest: elimination or just a normal diet?

Dr. Isolauri: My first slide showed that it is part of the intention pattern in sensitization but there is multiple sensitization, and first of all probably the best advise is not to test those oral sensitizations. So if you have a patient with this clinical problem try to make a diagnosis. I think diagnosis is very easy in a baby. When I see a 3-month-old infant with atopic eczema the question is very simple: is it allergy to milk or is it allergy to wheat or something else. Of course when the baby is being breast-fed we ask the mother to think about taking a diet. It is the experience of several groups in Europe that this is a marker of disease like asthma. It means that I have to take care and look very carefully for the specific diagnosis. We perform food challenges in infants to make a diagnosis of specific food allergies if we need an elimination diet; if this isn't needed we do not modulate the clinical practice.

Dr. Rijntjes: A lot of pediatricians are advising the elimination of all kinds of food.

Dr. Isolauri: That is good to hear because, as I mentioned, that is done in Finland even before the infant has atopic eczema, 60%.

Dr. Rijntjes: So when your elimination and provocation tests are negative you advise giving cow's milk, for instance. Can you speculate then on the reason why there are symptoms as the cause is not cow's milk according to your elimination and provocation tests?

Dr. Isolauri: I don't understand the elimination and provocation thing. If I have an exclusively breast-fed baby who has atopic eczema of course I do not challenge the baby until the mother is planning to stop breast-feeding, because I am definitely not the first one to introduce the baby to a cow's milk formula. So when the time comes I ask the mother to see me again before starting a standard infant formula. Unless the infant has a specific food allergy, elimination is not the answer.

Dr. Szajewska: I am very much interested in your studies on the use of probiotics in the treatment of atopic dermatitis. Could you please comment because as I understand you have 2 studies with rather small numbers of patients, 27 in one study and probably the same number in the second study. My question is: do you have any other ongoing trials on a larger sample size in which the result is still the same?

Dr. Isolauri: We started with probiotic intervention studies 12 years ago. The first clinical study in allergic infants was published in 1997 [1]. Dr. Holt told me that their ethical committee does not allow a trial with probiotics in pregnant mothers. So 12 years ago we could not think of going to 2,000 babies and supplementing them during breastfeeding with probiotics. The only way to do that is to make a very well-controlled pilot study with a sufficient number of patients needed for the outcome you are interested in. We were allowed to do that and had money for it. Nobody was funding us because the allergologist community was denying our approach because they thought it was dangerous. But anyway I don't have large numbers, but I have provided the back up data for prevention studies and that is what we were aiming for. We were interested in prevention with probiotics, not treating with probiotics. I know that other groups have done that and for functional food claims we need these studies to be done in different centers. Michaelson et al. had the same findings for atopic eczema, and I know there are ongoing studies in Holland.

Dr. Szajewska: But with different probiotic strains.

Dr. Isolauri: Yes, but the effect was the same, as the same effect could be shown with two different probiotic strains. The studies were done and we went on to prevention studies. At this time we are doing a prevention study with 150 infants. The second part of the study will be published next month, and we will then follow up the patients at 7 years with a asthma provocation test. We have 3 other ongoing studies with different probiotic preparations in combination. So we have something like 1,000 infants treated so far.

Dr. Shyur: In our country we have some infant formulas enriched with bifidobacteria. Do you suggest that only high-risk atopic newborns should be fed a formula enriched with probiotics?

Dr. Isolauri: I refer to what Dr. Bergmann has shown: the frequency of infants with atopic outcomes. A number of them are from no-risk families. So I see that as an advance in infant feeding; I see that as a definitely better choice than standard infant formula.

Dr. Shyur: In our country we now promote yogurt as a healthy food. Would you suggest yogurt for a newborn baby?

Dr. Isolauri: No, pediatricians advise not to use any other milk products than infant formula for infants because we have achieved the situation of the 1970s when we had unadapted formulas. So formulas are for infants until they 1.5 years, and yogurts and such are for adults or from a certain age. In our country most of the population uses the product and mothers are consuming large amounts of probiotic preparations themselves while they are lactating. I cannot advise them otherwise even though I would be interested to do research on that.

Dr. Shyur: You showed that BB12 seems better than LGG. Do you have any studies on these two probiotics.

Dr. Isolauri: That study was not aimed at looking at the clinical outcome, it was aimed to look at certain inflammatory markers. The message from that study was that there were different immunomodulatory effects. So if the clinical outcome is similar with 2 probiotic preparations, probably 3 preparations, we can most likely find 5 successful probiotic preparations which achieve the same clinical effect. But the clinical outcome is not very sensitive. It would be interesting to find out if they have different immunomodulatory effects, so I am aiming at specific interventions. Once we know what the reason for atopic eczema is, what the target is there, and once we learn what the mechanisms of several probiotic strains are, we could hit that target, but we are not that far.

Dr. Ham Pong: One of your earlier slides showed that secondary prevention of food allergy is antigen-specific.

Dr. Isolauri: No, treatment of food allergy is antigen-specific.

Dr. Ham Pong: Two examples I can provide tend to suggest that this may not be so. For example, the frequent coexistence of cow's milk protein and soy protein allergy in infants has been attributed to the leaky gut following an allergic reaction which enhances the absorption of macromolecules and facilitates the development of a soy allergy. The second example is in regard to respiratory allergies. We recently studied infants who were mono-sensitized to mites and received mite immunotherapy after a year, they had lower rates of sensitization to other allergens, suggesting a nonspecific effect.

Dr. Isolauri: I fully agree with that. Soy formulas are not used very much in our country because many infants who have cow's milk allergy are also sensitized to soy. That is a very well-known association in our country as well, so therefore we need to make the diagnosis and have the treatment and that treatment is antigen-specific. Elimination is harmful, since many of these food components may provide immunoregulatory functions in breast milk.

Dr. Aylott: I just wanted to make a comment about elimination diets. There has been a maternal egg avoidance study in Southampton in the UK looking at pregnant women trying to avoid egg in their diet. This was an FSA-funded study and has not yet been published. One of the main observations from that study was that it is very difficult to avoid a food in pregnancy, and I think it was found that only 16% of the women were completely egg free in that diet.

Dr. Isolauri: I would say that half of this audience doesn't know where egg is hidden in our diet. It is not only on your breakfast table; you eliminate what looks like an egg, but you have to know how you prepare cakes and so on, and it is not easy.

Dr. Aylott: I think it is very important to remember that when we try to give public health advice to women.

Dr. Hill: I would like to pick on an important point that some of us are trying to come to terms with. We have had some very elegant results from a GINI study and your own work showing that interventions are effective. But the question we are often asked by the government, by health administrators, is what is the cost effectiveness of that, what are the numbers you need to treat to show a benefit? I think that is a move from this sort of conference that in fact we now get to start looking at those issues and really address the issue for a severely atopic eczema child. What is the place of probiotic treatment?

Dr. Isolauri: The number needed to treat is a very friendly figure for allergic diseases because it is not only the statistical effect but the incidence and the prevalence of that disease in our community that affects the number. So for probiotics the number needed to treat is 4 something, so the 5th child benefits from that.

Dr. Hill: But the point is what for the average atopy eczema child is the benefit of that? How adaptable are the data to a general atopy eczema population out there.

Dr. Isolauri: Our results, which will come out in a month, show that the effect is not transient. We see the effect continue until the age of 4, and next year we are going to look at asthma. I am not very optimistic for asthma because there are different allergens in respiratory allergies, but we have managed to prevent half the cases with atopic eczema and we will definitely continue to follow up this cohort. So far this is considered effective and the costs are very low. We did not use any special diets, only the supplementation.

Dr. Schiffrin: I don't know if I understood well. The milk quality of mothers who are breast-feeding and consuming probiotics changes with regard to the quantity of TGF-β. Do you know if other immunomodulatory molecules change at the same time? How long does it last during lactation?

Dr. Isolauri: We have data published in *Pediatric Research* [2] showing differences in eicosanoid levels in nonallergic mothers. So there are many immunomodulatory compounds that we can look at, and I think that one complete product that we would like to see would be the anti-allergenic probiotics there. There are beneficial fatty acids that have been proven anti-allergic for that population. For other patients, like Crohn's disease, we might think of something else, and the product supplemented with TGF-β that Dr. Murch mentioned sounds very nice. So I think once we have a very good product, we will learn from such studies, but I cannot say how long that effect continues. The breast-feeding continued for 3 months, that is all I know.

Dr. Walker: I just wanted to comment on something said earlier on. I don't think you can consider yogurt as a probiotic. I think by definition it doesn't contain enough organisms to constitute the criteria necessary to function as a probiotic.

Dr. Isolauri: We have probiotic yogurts on the market, yogurts supplemented with probiotics.

Dr. Von Berg: We know that hydrolysates have a preventive effect, as do microbes. Do you see any additional effect of the combination of both?

Dr. Isolauri: Think about your level. You actually used extensively hydrolyzed and partially hydrolyzed formulas similar to the level in breast-feeding, as I understood. The level of breast-feeding is a given in our population, but we could go lower than that. Before such a trial is initiated, we must learn about the healthy gut microbes of the healthy at-risk infant who remains healthy: how does it differ from the flora of the infant who develops allergy? Then that strain must be used in the product. The probiotics we are currently using might be the best ones.

Dr. Saavedra: I just wanted to follow up on a comment that has to do with what is then the best way to adapt whatever we do know so far, particularly from the point of view of prevention, and it also has to do with the issues of cost and benefit. One of things we were talking about here is the conceptual change from the point of view of diet in terms of the modifications we talked about, protein and particularly something radically different which is adding bacteria to the diet. If we are going to look for cost effectiveness as well as a conceptual change, we must give infant formulas to those children who unfortunately just don't have the benefit of breast-feeding. The concept must be changed in terms of how nutrition needs to modify this old idea that we need to chemically copy breast milk or we need to copy the functionality of breast milk.

Dr. Isolauri: We need to copy the breast-fed baby.

Dr. Saavedra: Exactly, our gold standard should be the child, not the liquid, not the milk. If that is what we need to accomplish, it should be accomplished with infant nutrition. The defense and protection that breast-feeding provides for those children is when these concepts begin emerging. What we have done with other interventions, such as iron, calcium, iodine, is to incorporate those changes into the diet rather than into these capsules or therapies or treatment, so that we modify the approach that we have to nutrition to get the costs and benefits that we can in the long-term, which will also reduce cost dramatically.

Dr. Isolauri: That is very important, I agree with both of your points. One recent study in our lactating mothers where we tried to modulate the diet with supplements was unsuccessful. The problem is that the mothers think that they don't need to eat properly, just take the vitamin, and it was unsuccessful.

Dr. Lack: I wonder if you could comment on the discrepancy in your findings between prevention on reduction in eczema as opposed to specific IgE sensitization I believe primarily to foods. If this approach is going to be successful in halting the allergic march, it is going to actually prevent the expression of IgE-mediated allergies. The fact that you didn't see differences in sensitization doesn't actually mean that you haven't prevented the expression of allergic disease. I think Dr. van den Biggelaar spoke the other day about how in certain parasitic infections you might not change Th2 responses or IgE responses but you might change their expression through regulatory mechanisms. So the question is, do these children have a different expression of IgE-mediated allergic disease on challenges or subsequently? I think that is information that is going to be key in having an idea to whether the subsequent atopic march is prevented.

Dr. Isolauri: I did not show the data on sensitization here today. I tried to avoid that as we discussed earlier that there is a clear discrepancy between exposure to antigen sensitization and the development of disease, and we don't understand why. It has been in all the clinical studies so far. So I don't know a prospective prevention study showing that you first prevent sensitization and thereby you prevent disease. Do you see sensitization and clinical disease go in the same line? We don't see that. So TGF-β could be one mechanism and probably other regulatory cells. If we think about the data I showed from Prescott et al. [3], healthy outcome starts with a strong Th2-type immunity. It decreases with age, while allergic infants have the opposite, an increase: first it starts lower and then it increases and increases. What is the appropriate age to test that, and since up to the age of 6 months we know that there is a huge overlap in skin prick test reactivity between patients who have and don't have atopic disease. Probably the optimal age to achieve an answer to your question is the age of 7.

Dr. Lack: Perhaps not so much for IgE-mediated food allergy if one wants to find out about reactivity to egg, where early testing in the first 2 years of life is reliable.

Dr. Isolauri: I was not referring to food allergy. Food allergy frequency in our country has not increased and cow's milk allergy is something we can manage. We should think about other sensitizations as you said, hen's egg sensitization, a marker, something coming out, we need to learn more about that.

References

1 Majamaa H, Isolauri E: Probiotics: A novel approach in the management of food allergy. J Allergy Clin Immunol 1997;99:179–186.
2 Laiho K, Lampi AM, Hämäläinen M, et al: Breast milk fatty acids, eicosanoids and cytokines in mother with and without allergic disease. Pediatr Res 2003;53:642–647.
3 Prescott SL, Macaubas C, Smallacombe T, et al: Development of allergen-specific T-cell memory in atopic and normal children. Lancet 1999;353:196–200.

Isolauri E, Walker WA (eds): Allergic Diseases and the Environment.
Nestlé Nutrition Workshop Series Pediatric Program, Vol. 53, pp. 315–318,
Nestec Ltd.; Vevey/S. Karger AG, Basel, © 2004.

Concluding Remarks

There are number of ingredients to a successful conference which, I hope you will agree with me, existed over the last 3 days, so that a number of concepts have been clarified. We need to thank the organizers, particularly *Philippe Steenhout* and *Wolf Endres*, for putting on a very good conference, particularly under the extremely stressful conditions of having to change the venue within the last 2 weeks. I would also like to thank our speakers for providing very provocative presentations and the participants for very stimulating discussion. The format of providing a short overview followed by extensive discussions is the best way to address the complex topics we considered in this week's conference. *Erika Isolauri* summarized what was discussed today and, if you allow me, I just want to make a couple of observations about the sessions we held on Monday and Tuesday.

In our first session on clinical aspects and definitions, we heard about the changing and increasing incidence of food allergy and I heard a term which I had not heard before, 'the allergic march', which is, I understand, a progression of symptoms over a period of the child's early life after an initial sensitization. From the allergy perspective, we have also learned the complexity of defining allergy and atopy, and that symptoms of allergy, such as dermatitis and asthma, may not necessarily be caused by an IgE-mediated effect, it could be non-IgE-mediated as perhaps it is not even immunologically based, so this is still an area of confusion. We had a particularly insightful presentation by *David Hill* on the prevalence and clinical profile of food allergy and some of his concepts were extremely remarkable. Others suggested that there has been an increase in allergy over the last decade, but he stressed that symptoms need to be carefully documented and defined as allergic in nature, particularly those that are related to the gastrointestinal tract. Of interest and very important, was his showing that eosinophilia and pH probes overlap and may not necessarily prove disease. The other point that *Dr. Hill* made is that it is very important to carefully document disease in your own clinical setting and treat objectively based on the patients seen, in his case in Australia. You can't necessarily generalize to other areas. This concept is very important.

In the second session on environmental factors we had an excellent description of the 'hygiene hypothesis' and its refinement by one of the originators of the hypothesis. He emphasized the importance of a balance between Th1 and Th2 responses, and that early balance seems to be an important component to a healthy lifestyle as opposed to an allergic lifestyle. There was a very enthusiastic discussion of allergy as an IgE-mediated Th2 response which may be balanced by factors that affect Th1 responsiveness. Finally in this environmental factor session we heard that worm infestation, which is a typical Th2 stimulus, may also protect against allergy. Thus we need to think in terms of other ways that allergy, at least symptomatic responses, can be prevented through counter-regulatory mechanisms with cytokines released, such as IL-10.

In session 3 on oral tolerance, we had a review of the mechanisms of non-responsiveness and some of the experimental observations regarding the counter-regulatory cytokine IL-10 and its effect on IL-13 blocking the actual production of specific IgE instead of symptoms, again in a worm-infested model. We also heard of the importance of innate immunity, not only in producing an appropriate immune response but also oral tolerance. We then had a discussion on gut maturation where regulatory cytokines, such as IL-10 and TGF-β, were very important in modulating the development of appropriate host defense. The fact of establishing oral tolerance in infancy as a developmentally regulated process requires stimulation by actual colonization and an important component of this is how the antigen-presenting cell functions. A very salient point was made that the timing of exposure to antigens may be a very important means of preventing the so-called 'allergic march'.

Finally, in the session on microbial–gut interaction it was emphasized that there is a need for early appropriate colonization for normal development of host defense, and that with inappropriate colonization under conditions of an immature gut it may result in an adverse effect which leads to disease. Then, as a substitute for the original speaker, we had a lecture emphasizing that the means by which we measure intestinal flora as a reflection of the microbiota that colonize the gut appears to cover only a fraction of what actually exists within the gut. Stool cultures really don't tell you the whole story of colonization, so we need to find new ways of quantifying bacteria. We need also to utilize some of the new molecular techniques in identifying bacteria to get a better sense of where we stand. This was addressed in the context of colonizing bacteria which may be different in atopic compared to nonatopic patients, and that colonizing bacteria differ less than they used to with regard to formula versus breast-feeding. A very interesting observation that hydrolysate seems to produce colonization that is more similar to breast milk was made. However, the bottom line is we need more research.

Again I would like to thank everyone for participating. This has been a very fruitful and well-discussed conference and hopefully we now have some 'food for thought' for additional studies. Thank you.

Allan Walker

It is a great pleasure to see you here at the closure of this conference and, although I was not able to attend last week, it is clear that this has been a successful conference because most of you are still awake and sitting straight, which are usually good signs. I thank your for your flexibility in the change of venue from such a nice location in Malaysia to Switzerland, and I hope you have not been too disappointed by the weather and the surroundings here. I am sure you have not been disappointed here at the laboratory.

I have worked here myself for a year and half, and every day I walk into the building with a smile on my face because without a doubt it is the most beautiful laboratory in the world. In addition, as you have noticed this is a very nice room and the kitchen staff is also one of the best in Switzerland. So I take this opportunity to give you two messages to convince you of the fact that, scientifically speaking, we are perhaps not the best but among the best in the world and certainly the most complete laboratory when it comes to nutrition.

The first message I have to give you is that we are not alone. This is the R of the Nestlé R&D system. So research takes place here and, as you can see, the map contains many dots which stand for our polytechnology centers, the research centers that are individually devoted to a product category: there is one for water in Vittel for instance, one for dairy in Konolfingen here, coffee in Orbe, and so on all around the world. The second set of dots are R&D centers where we adapt our products to the local conditions of a country or the local conditions of a whole part of the world. We also do the opposite: we try to obtain local knowledge, local experts who we use all over the world. So the dot here is our laboratory in Singapore for instance, and this one our laboratory in Shanghai which is growing very rapidly.

Here in Vevey there are about 570 people, and I should say we are not here alone. We also have active collaborations outside with the scientific community at various universities and institutions all over the world, and to be able to do that we also have to provide very good science. Last year with these 300 scientists, we had more than 200 scientific publications, and this is a level that we keep up regularly in addition to all the work that we don't publish and keep secret.

The second message is what do we do here. All 570 of us work on various aspects of nutrition. We have a very large department of food science in which we work on things like texture, structure, how the ingredients behave, how we can keep them stable. Food safety of course is a very important aspect and we have about 100 people working on this with special emphasis on new solutions. When we eat food, when food meets the consumer, the consumer can be a human, can be a pet, but the food has to be tasteful and the consumer must take pleasure from eating it. So we have a large group of people looking into flavor in terms of molecules, receptors for tasting, and how these signals reach the brain. The same group of people then look at the responses from the consumer. Another topic is satiety: how can we stop people from eating too much, and how can we increase their appetite if they don't eat enough.

And then of course, human nutrition itself. I will take very big steps to where we see our targets in the future. Firstly we look at bioavailability, indisposition, and it is amazing how many common nutrients, ingredients there are. We don't know how well they are absorbed and where indisposition takes place. Secondly if we think about Nestlé as a food company, ingredients are usually preparatory to the point at which they reach the alimentary canal. When they cross the gastrointestinal barrier they are anybody's ingredients. Up to this point they can be ours, and bioavailability is one way of providing some preparatoriness to our products. Thirdly, of course, health effects and their biomarkers are very important, and here we have the newest techniques available today, we work with genomics.

The last point, one that I very much believe in, is individual variation in the future. We are all different as we sit here and of course we all have different needs for certain ingredients. So although it may seem far away to talk about a passport for everybody to show how much they need to eat, this can sometimes be very dangerous by providing different frozen meals for women or for men. So this is where we see the future developing.

I should thank several people in particular for bringing you here: in the first place *Pierre Guesry* who you already met, *Barbara Marchesini*, and *Sylvie Helfer* and her people. So thank you all once again and have a nice dinner and then a good trip home. Thank you very much.

Peter Van Bladeren

Subject Index